EMERGENCY PLASTIC SURGERY

EMERGENCY PLASTIC SURGERY

Edited by

RICHARD J. GRECO

Instructor in Plastic Surgery, University of Pittsburgh School of Medicine; Attending Physician, Plastic and Reconstructive Surgery, Presbyterian-University Hospital, Pittsburgh

Little, Brown and Company
Boston/Toronto/London

To those physicians and residents called upon to provide acute care to the injured patient in the early hours of the morning.

And to my wife Robin and my children, Richard, Blake, Apryl, and Dean, who have sacrificed so that I could complete this task.

CONTENTS

CONTRIBUTING AUTHORS

Pat L. Aulicino, M.D.
Associate Professor of Orthopedic Surgery, Eastern Virginia
Medical School, Norfolk

Haven J. Barlow, Jr., M.D.
Fellow, Hand and Microsurgery, University of Pittsburgh School of
Medicine, Pittsburgh

Robert A. Chase, M.D.
Emily Homan Professor of Surgery, Stanford University School of
Medicine, Stanford

Holly W. Davis, M.D.
Associate Professor of Pediatrics, University of Pittsburgh School of
Medicine; Medical Director, Emergency Department, Children's
Hospital of Pittsburgh, Pittsburgh

Howard D. Edington, M.D.
Assistant Professor, Division of Plastic Surgery, University of Pittsburgh School of Medicine; Attending Physician, Plastic and Reconstructive Surgery, Presbyterian-University Hospital, Pittsburgh

Paul D. Fischer, M.D.
Attending Surgeon, Division of Plastic Surgery, Hospital of St.
Raphael's, New Haven

I. William Goldfarb, M.D.
Clinical Assistant Professor of Surgery, University of Pittsburgh
School of Medicine, Pittsburgh; Associate Director, Burn Trauma
Center, The Chicago Medical School, Chicago

Mark S. Granick, M.D.
Clinical Assistant Professor of Plastic Surgery, Hahnemann
University School of Medicine; Associate Professor of Plastic Sur-
gery, Medical College of Pennsylvania, Philadelphia

Richard J. Greco, M.D.
Instructor in Plastic Surgery, University of Pittsburgh School of
Medicine; Attending Physician, Plastic and Reconstructive Surgery,
Presbyterian-University Hospital, Pittsburgh

Frederick R. Heckler, M.D.
Clinical Associate Professor of Plastic Surgery, University of
Pittsburgh School of Medicine; Head, Division of Plastic Surgery,
Allegheny General Hospital, Allegheny

James H. Herndon, M.D.
David Silver Professor and Chairman, Department of Orthopedic Surgery, University of Pittsburgh School of Medicine; Chief, Department of Orthopedics and Rehabilitation, Presbyterian-University Hospital, Pittsburgh

James Hunter, M.D.
Professor, Orthopaedic Surgery, Jefferson Medical College of Thomas Jefferson University; Chief, Hand Surgery Service, Department of Orthopaedics, Thomas Jefferson University Hospital, Philadelphia

Dennis J. Hurwitz, M.D.
Clinical Associate Professor of Plastic Surgery, University of Pittsburgh School of Medicine; Attending Surgeon, Montefiore Hospital, Pittsburgh

Joseph E. Imbriglia, M.D.
Associate Professor, Orthopedic Surgery, Medical College of Pennsylvania, Philadelphia; Director, Division of Hand Surgery, Allegheny General Hospital, Allegheny

Timothy R. Jones, M.D.
Fellow, Plastic and Reconstructive Surgery, University of Pittsburgh School of Medicine; Presbyterian-University Hospital, Pittsburgh

Neil Ford Jones, M.D.
Associate Professor of Plastic and Reconstructive Surgery, University of Pittsburgh School of Medicine; Attending Surgeon and Chief, Division of Hand Surgery, Presbyterian-University Hospital, Pittsburgh

Scott E. Kasden, M.D.
Chief Surgical Resident, The Western Pennsylvania Hospital, Pittsburgh

Harold E. Kleinert, M.D.
Clinical Professor of Surgery, University of Louisville School of Medicine, Louisville; Clinical Professor of Surgery, Indiana University School of Medicine, Indianapolis

Marc D. Liang, M.D.
Assistant Professor of Plastic Surgery, University of Pittsburgh School of Medicine; Head, Division of Plastic Surgery, Montefiore Hospital, Pittsburgh

H. Wolfgang Losken, M.B.Ch.B.
Associate Professor of Plastic Surgery, University of Pittsburgh School of Medicine; Director, Pediatric Plastic Surgery, Children's Hospital of Pittsburgh, Pittsburgh

Mary H. McGrath, M.D.
Professor of Surgery and Chief of Plastic Surgery, George Washington University School of Medicine and Health Sciences;

Attending Surgeon, George Washington University Medical Center and Children's Hospital National Medical Center, Washington, D.C.

John H. Moore, Jr., M.D.
Assistant Professor of Plastic Surgery, Jefferson Medical College of Thomas Jefferson University; Attending Surgeon, Thomas Jefferson University Hospital and Jefferson Park Hospital, Philadelphia

Ross Musgrave, M.D.
Clinical Professor of Plastic Surgery, University of Pittsburgh School of Medicine; Attending Physician, Presbyterian-University Hospital, Pittsburgh

Krishna Narayanan, M.D.
Fellow, Department of Surgery, University of Pittsburgh School of Medicine; Attending Physician, Montefiore Hospital, Pittsburgh

E. Douglas Newton, M.D.
Plastic Surgeon, Division of Surgery, Western Pennsylvania Hospital, Pittsburgh

Gary Patterson, D.M.D.
Assistant Professor of Surgery, University of Pittsburgh School of Medicine; Associate Director, Oral-Maxillofacial Surgery, Presbyterian-University Hospital, Pittsburgh

Sai S. Ramasastry, M.D.
Associate Professor of Plastic Surgery, University of Pittsburgh School of Medicine, Pittsburgh

Bruce W. Rosenthal, M.D.
Assistant Professor of Pediatrics, University of Pittsburgh School of Medicine; Attending Physician, Emergency Department, Children's Hospital of Pittsburgh, Pittsburgh

James M. Russavage, M.D., D.M.D.
Oral and Maxillofacial Surgeon, University of Pittsburgh School of Medicine; Chief Resident, Oral Surgery, Presbyterian-University Hospital, Pittsburgh

Robert C. Russell, M.D.
Professor of Surgery, Southern Illinois University School of Medicine; Attending Surgeon, Division of Plastic Surgery, Memorial Medical Center and St. John's Hospital, Springfield

Roger E. Salisbury, M.D.
Professor of Surgery and Chief, Plastic and Reconstructive Surgery, New York Medical College; Director, Burn Center, Westchester County Medical Center, Valhalla

Lawrence H. Schneider, M.D.
Clinical Professor of Orthopaedic Surgery, Jefferson Medical College of Thomas Jefferson University; Attending

Orthopaedic Surgeon, Thomas Jefferson University Hospital, Philadelphia

Kenneth C. Shestak, M.D.
Assistant Professor of Plastic Surgery, University of Pittsburgh School of Medicine; Chief of Plastic Surgery, Magee-Women's Hospital, Pittsburgh

Harvey Slater, M.D., F.A.C.S.
Clinical Assistant Professor of Surgery, University of Pittsburgh School of Medicine; Director, Burn Trauma Center, Jefferson Medical College, Philadelphia

James K. Smith, M.D.
Clinical Associate Professor of Surgery, University of Pittsburgh School of Medicine; Attending Surgeon, Division of Plastic and Reconstructive Surgery, Western Pennsylvania Hospital, Pittsburgh

George C. Sotereanos, D.M.D.
Associate Professor, Department of Oral-Maxillofacial Surgery, University of Pittsburgh School of Medicine; Director, Graduate Training in Oral and Maxillofacial Surgery, Presbyterian-University Hospital, Pittsburgh

William M. Swartz, M.D.
Professor and Chief of Plastic Surgery, Tulane University Medical School; Chief of Plastic Surgery, Tulane University Medical Center, New Orleans

Angela M. Tangredi, M.D.
Fellow, Pediatric Emergency Medicine, University of Pittsburgh School of Medicine; Attending Physician, Emergency Department, Children's Hospital of Pittsburgh, Pittsburgh

Jeanine M. Walenga, Ph.D.
Assistant Professor of Thoracic and Cardiovascular Surgery and Pathology, Loyola University of Chicago Stritch School of Medicine, Maywood

Michael J. White, M.D.
Attending Physician, Plastic and Reconstructive Surgery, University of Pittsburgh School of Medicine, Pittsburgh; Allegheny General Hospital, Allegheny

PREFACE

"Did I ever tell you about my first day in the emergency room? I was called to see a patient with a severely traumatized face, and I didn't really know where to start." This feeling is all too common for emergency room, general surgery, and plastic surgery residents. The goal of this book is to offer a concise, practical approach to the major plastic surgical injuries seen in the emergency room and how to provide the first 24 hours of care.

The first portion of each chapter is aimed at the primary caretaker and discusses structurally important anatomic details, basic concepts in evaluation of the injury, and how to deal with the injury.

The second portion of each chapter is aimed at giving the operating resident enough technical information to have an accepted approach to the injury. This operation need not be performed in the first 24 hours, but is part of the treatment path decided on at that time. References are given so that a more thorough review can be done in the hospital library if necessary before the operation.

The commentary at the end of each chapter is provided to offer some perspective from a "voice of experience" and should stimulate discussion with attending staff during the repair.

A special thanks to all of the contributors of this book. Their efforts and revisions allowed us to provide a practical and readable approach to the topics of *Emergency Plastic Surgery.*

Appreciation is due to Susan Pioli, Executive Editor at Little, Brown and Company, for her guidance and assistance throughout the development and completion of this project.

The book would not have been possible without the efforts of all the contributors' secretaries, the Medical Media Department of the Pittsburgh V.A. — in particular, Saul Weis — and the illustrations created by Dean Robinson and Robin Greco.

The continued support and guidance of my mentors, J. William Futrell, Neil Jones, Victor F. Greco, Wolfgang Losken, Ross Musgrave, and others, made this book possible. Special appreciation is due to Neil Jones and Wolfgang Losken for their assistance in editing the hand and craniofacial chapters.

And a special thanks goes to my family — Robin, Richard, Blake, Apryl, and Dean — for their sacrifices, support, and understanding. Also, thanks to all my fellow residents — we have learned from each other, so that we can teach others.

R.J.G.

I SKIN AND SOFT TISSUE

NOTICE

The indications and dosages of all drugs in this book have been recommended in the medical literature and conform to the practices of the general medical community. The medications described do not necessarily have specific approval by the Food and Drug Administration for use in the diseases and dosages for which they are recommended. The package insert for each drug should be consulted for use and dosage as approved by the FDA. Because standards for usage change, it is advisable to keep abreast of revised recommendations, particularly those concerning new drugs.

1 BASIC CONCEPTS AND ACUTE WOUND CARE

Howard D. Edington

Perhaps paramount to the acute management of the injured patient are the history and the physical examination. The process must be succinct, goal-directed, and based on an understanding of the regional anatomy of the injured part and the pathophysiology of the injury. Problems arise because the emergency room visit is obviously unscheduled, the physician may be rushed, and the patient is often uncooperative or intoxicated. The appropriate evaluation, moreover, may require a concerted effort. The additional care and effort, however, are well invested. The patient who has been treated for facial or hand injuries particularly is reminded daily of treatment either well done or poorly executed.

INITIAL EVALUATION

The most important goal of the initial evaluation is to identify all injuries and, in particular, to anticipate and actively rule out associated occult injuries that may be life threatening or potentially outweigh the importance of the injury that prompted the initial consultation. For example, the spectacular nature of severe facial trauma frequently focuses attention away from the less obvious, or completely unrecognized, cervical spine or airway injury — with catastrophic consequences. The consultant must share the responsibility for the patient's safety.

The history should identify the time and mechanism of injury, pertinent past or current medical problems, tetanus immunization status, and the presence of any drug allergies. During the physical examination the injury is defined, occult injuries are ruled out, and treatment is planned. The examination is guided by the history and knowledge of the regional anatomy. Appropriate radiographs and wound exploration augment the physical examination. Often the most pressing initial decision is whether the patient must be taken to the operating room for treatment. Such a decision is somewhat subjective and depends on the nature of the injuries, the age and cooperation of the patient, and the availability of facilities. Tetanus prophylaxis should be performed according to U.S. Public Health Service recommendations (Table 1-1).

Table 1-1. Guidelines for tetanus prophylaxis

Tetanus toxoid immunization	Wound type[a]	Tetanus toxoid	Tetanus immune globulin
Three or more, the last within 5 years	Clean, minor	No	No
Three or more, the last within 5 years	Significant	No	No
Three or more, the last within 10 years	Clean, minor	No	No
Three or more, the last within 10 years	Significant	Yes	No
Three or more, the last > 10 years	Clean, minor	Yes	No
Three or more, the last > 10 years	Significant	Yes	No
Unknown or < three	Clean, minor	Yes	No
Unknown or < three	Significant	Yes	Yes

[a] Clean, minor = clean, superficial wounds. Significant = contaminated wounds, punctures, burns, frostbite, crush injuries, suturable lacerations.
Source: D. D. Zukin and R. R. Simon, *Emergency Wound Care—Principles and Practice.* Rockville, MD: Aspen, 1987. With permission.

WOUND HEALING

There are few if any "rules" regarding the emergency management of wounds. Therapy must be guided by a basic knowledge of wound healing balanced by an understanding of the potential risks versus benefits of the elected therapy. A basic synopsis of normal wound healing is presented: Wound healing is classically divided into three phases that differ with respect to the biochemistry and cellular anatomy and physiology of the wound's microenvironment.

Inflammatory Phase

The initial response to injury, whether mechanical, immunologic or chemical, is a nonspecific inflammatory response. Immediately following an injury there is a period of vasoconstriction, lasting 5 to 10 minutes. Activation of platelets and the coagulation cascade effects hemostasis. A period of vasodilatation, probably mediated by histamine, occurs. There is margination and diapedesis of leukocytes through "leaky" vascular endothelium in the zone of injury. The predominant initial cell type is the polymorphonuclear leukocyte, whose primary function is presumed to be débridement. By day 3, the predominant cell type in the wound is the macrophage, which continues phagocytic activities. It probably also regulates activities of

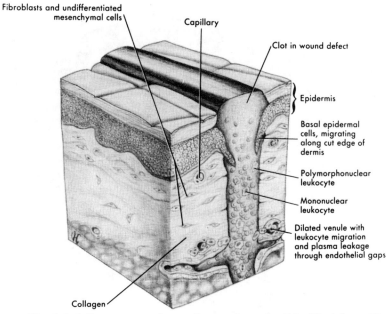

Fig. 1-1. Inflammatory phase of wound repair. (Modified from W. M. Bryant. *Clinical Symposium (Ciba)* 29(3):1, 1977.)

fibroblasts, myofibroblasts, and their precursors, as well as wound angiogenesis (Fig. 1-1).

Phase of Fibroplasia   Activities of the fibroblast and its congeners dominate the fibroplasia phase, which lasts from day 4 to 3 weeks. Elaboration of glycosaminoglycan ground substance and, later, collagen are biochemical events characterizing this phase. Although collagen deposition can be detected at 3 days, collagen elevation and wound tensile strength do not occur until day 4 or 5. Wound collagen contents increase dramatically for about 3 weeks (Fig. 1-2).

Maturation Phase   During the maturation phase, which lasts about 3 weeks, collagen synthesis and degradation rates are increased, so the net collagen content remains the same. This phase is characterized by maturation and remodeling. The type 3 collagen, initially laid down, is replaced by the more mature type 1 collagen. The duration of this phase is variable but may be 1 year or more. Along with internal scar remodeling, the external appearance of the scar changes, with normal flattening and decreased erythema pruritus. Pragmatically, patients should be advised that scar changes occur for at least 1 year, so cosmetic scar revision generally is not advised until at least 1 year has passed since the time of injury (Fig 1-3).

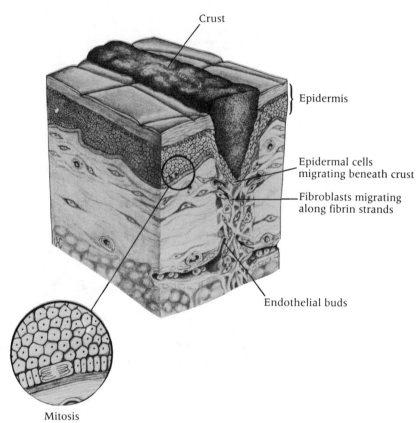

Crust

Epidermis

Epidermal cells
migrating beneath crust

Fibroblasts migrating
along fibrin strands

Endothelial buds

Mitosis

Fig. 1-2. Early proliferative phase of wound repair. (Modified from W. M. Bryant. *Clinical Symposium (Ciba)* 29(3):1, 1977.)

**Clinical Wound
Healing**

The basic wound healing process appears to be the same, regardless of how the wound is managed. Clinically, wound healing may be separated into primary, secondary, and delayed primary intention.

Primary-intention healing follows acute closure of wounds, which results in the quickest healing with minimal scarring. However, the risk of clinically significant infection is greater than with healing by second or third intention.

Second-intention healing occurs when the wound does not close but heals by contraction granulation and reepithelialization. This approach is most appropriate for heavily contaminated or infected wounds, as well as for some fingertip injuries (see Chapter 5).

Third-intention healing, or delayed primary closure, occurs when a wound that has been treated open is closed by opposing edges of granulation tissue 4 to 6 days after injury.

The management of any wound must be individualized, particularly open soft-tissue injuries, all of which are contaminated. To adhere rigidly to the classic "6-hour golden period" makes little biologic clinical sense. Most wounds can be cleaned by appropriate

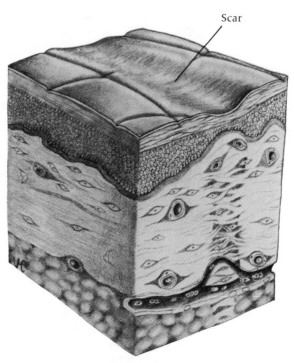

Fig. 1-3. Early maturation phase of wound repair. (Modified from W. M. Bryant. *Clinical Symposium (Ciba)* 29(3):1, 1977.)

irrigation/débridement and, in some instances, excision. The decision to close a wound or to treat it open must be made within the context of the situation. How old is the wound? How heavily and with what is it contaminated? What would be the morbidity in this particular patient if an infection should develop? Generally, when possible, human bites, blast injuries, and wounds heavily contaminated with fecal debris are managed in an open manner. When a delay in definitive wound management is anticipated (i.e., a patient with additional severe injuries), the wound should be irrigated thoroughly with saline, the skin edges approximated loosely, and the wound dressed with saline-moistened gauze. Injured extremities should be splinted.

Wound Management

Once the decision has been made to treat the wound outside the operating room, basic wound management consists of four parts: planning, wound preparation, wound closure, and wound dressing.

Planning

Most wounds are contaminated. Débridement is a necessary, and perhaps the most important, part of treatment. Sharp débridement or wound excision may be used to change the direction of the wound so it is more aesthetically pleasing or functional. Whenever possible, wounds should be excised to coincide with Langer's lines or lines of

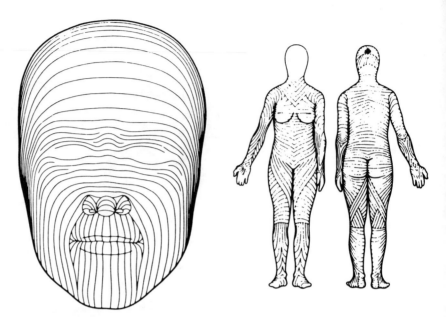

Fig. 1-4. Basic pattern of the body's skin tension lines. There is, of course, a fair amount of variation from person to person. (From R. R. Simons and B. E. Brennan. *Procedures and Techniques in Emergency Medicine.* Baltimore: Williams & Wilkins, 1982. With permission.)

skin tension (Fig. 1-4). A scar that lies parallel to these lines is aesthetically more pleasing than those at 90 degrees to lines of skin tension (LST). Incisions for débridement should also be planned with functional considerations in mind. For example, periorbital tissue avulsions, if closed incorrectly, may lead to ectropion.

Wound Preparation

Skin Antiseptics and Wound Cleansing. The most commonly used antiseptics are quaternary ammonium salts, hexachlorophene (pHisoHex), and complexed iodine compounds (Betadine). Most antiseptics should not be used on the wounds themselves, as they are generally toxic to cells (Table 1-2). Wounds should be irrigated with saline. For removal of particulate matter, studies have shown irrigation with at least 200 ml of saline through a 35-ml syringe and 19-gauge needle (pressure exerted at more than 8 psi) is more effective than bulb syringe irrigation alone.

Anesthesia. Local anesthesia techniques are discussed in greater detail elsewhere (see Chapter 20). Lidocaine (Xylocaine) 0.5 to 2.0% is generally used. Lidocaine with epinephrine is useful for prolonging the anesthetic effect and decreasing blood loss but should not be used in the digit, earlobe, nasal tip, or penis, as tissue loss may occur. Total dosage (without epinephrine) should not exceed 4.5 mg per kilogram. *Note:* 1% solution contains 10 mg/ml. One millimeter of 10%

Table 1-2. Toxicity of topical agents[a]

Agent	Relative toxicity
Saline	0
Pluronic F-68	0
Betadine prep solution (povidone-iodine solution)	1+
Hexachlorophene solution	2+
Quaternary ammonia solution	3+
Hydrogen peroxide	6+
Betadine surgical scrub (povidone-iodine and detergent)	8+
pHisoHex (hexachlorophene and detergent)	8+
Isopropyl alcohol	10+

[a] Saline (0) is the standard. The higher the number, the more caustic the agent.
Source: D. D. Zukin, and R. R. Simon. Toxicity of topical agents. In: *Emergency Wound Care — Principles and Practice.* Rockville, MD: Aspen, 1987.

sodium bicarbonate can be added to 10 ml of lidocaine prior to injection. The bicarbonate increases the pH of the anesthetic and results in less pain on infiltration. Topical anesthetics include ethylene glycol spray, lidocaine spray, and a topical solution of tetracaine (0.5%) + epinephrine (1:2000) + cocaine (11.8%) (TAC) and are discussed in depth in Chapter 20.

Sharp Débridement. Sharp débridement aims to convert a dirty wound to a clean wound, reorient lacerations or avulsions, and remove devitalized tissue. Most wounds associated with an impact have a zone of surrounding damaged skin, which should be removed for optimal cosmetic results. Excisions must be planned with both cosmetic and functional considerations in mind. Wound edges are generally trimmed perpendicular to the skin, except in hair-bearing regions, where edges should be beveled in the direction of the hair follicles (Fig. 1-5). Heavily contaminated wounds that are to heal by second or third intention should be thoroughly irrigated and débrided, and then packed or dressed with packing or gauze soaked in saline or antibiotic solution (Table 1-2). Abrasions should be managed by meticulous cleansing, using either a sponge or a toothbrush. All embedded dirt must be removed, or a traumatic tattoo will result. Children with extensive abrasions may require a general anesthetic for adequate cleansing. Abrasions may then be treated with serial saline-soaked gauze dressings or antibiotic ointment. Wounds are then allowed to "scab over" and reepithelialize. An excellent cosmetic result is the rule for abrasions that are correctly managed. Lacerations within abrasions should be closed with absorbable sutures, as their removal is made difficult if not impossible by the surrounding coagulum, particularly in small children.

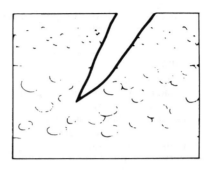

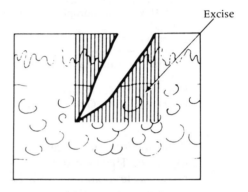

Excise

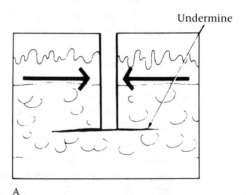

Undermine

A

Fig. 1-5. A. Excision of edges of the wound perpendicular to the skin surface and subsequent undermining for a tension-free repair.

Wound Closure

Prior to closing any wound one must choose the appropriate therapy from a hierarchy of choices, starting with the least complicated. The simplest solution is often to clean and dress the wound and then allow healing by contraction and secondary intention. This treatment often produces the most cosmetically acceptable result and must be considered prior to ascending the ladder of complexity. Simple, superficial lacerations may be appropriately managed with an adhesive strip (Steri-Strip) closure, assuming adequate wound edge alignment can be obtained. For deeper, more complex injuries, a layered tension-free closure is required.

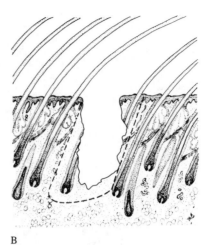

B

Fig. 1-5 (continued) B. Excision of wounds in hair-bearing area (eyebrow, scalp) should be tangential, in the direction of the hair shafts. (From D. D. Zukin and R. R. Simon. *Emergency Wound Care — Principles and Practice.* Rockville, MD: Aspen, 1987. With permission.)

Undermining may be required to facilitate tension-free skin closure and should be performed at either the subdermal or the facial layer. Apices of elliptical wounds must also be undermined. A layered closure is required in all but the most superficial wounds, particularly when early skin suture removal is anticipated (especially in facial wounds). Deadspace should be eliminated using the least amount of suture material possible and preferably the least reactive.

Buried dermal sutures of absorbable suture can align skin edges and permit accurate, tension-free skin edge approximation. Skin sutures may then be removed early without fear of wound dehiscence or scar widening.

Suture Techniques. Skin sutures should achieve skin-edge alignment with deadspace obliteration and slight wound eversion (Fig. 1-6). Eversion is obtained by passing the needle through the skin at 90 degrees (or more) and tying the knot next to the wound. An inverting suture is achieved by entering the skin at an acute angle (Fig. 1-6). Inverting sutures are occasionally appropriate (i.e., at the junction of the nasal ala with the face). Generally, interrupted simple or mattress-type sutures are most appropriate for skin closure.

Suture and Needle Selection. Most sutures used in the emergency room are the swaged type. The needle and suture material form a continuous unit, cause less trauma, and are more convenient than either closed or split (French) eye needles. A variety of needle shapes and point designs are available for specific applications, however (Fig. 1-7). The ⅜ circle conventional cutting needle is most frequently used. The half-circle is more difficult to use but results in more reliable wound eversion.

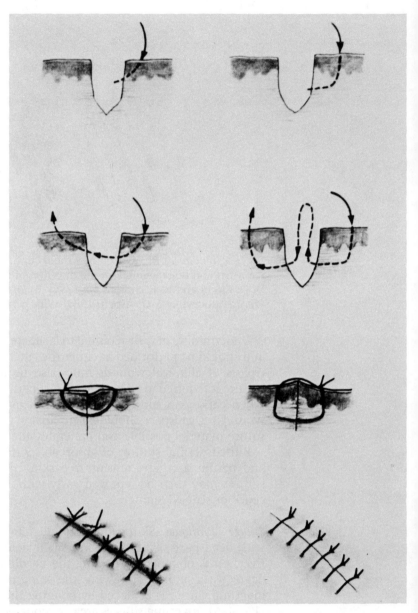

Fig. 1-6. Improper (*left*) and proper (*right*) paths of simple percutaneous suture.

A variety of suture materials, both absorbable and nonabsorbable, is available. Sutures differ with respect to their tensile strength, absorption rate, and tissue reaction, as well as their manageability (Table 1-3). Generally, absorbable sutures are used to close deep layers of the wound, and monofilament nonabsorbable sutures are used for the skin: size 6.0 on the face, 4.0 on the scalp, and 4.0 or 5.0 elsewhere.

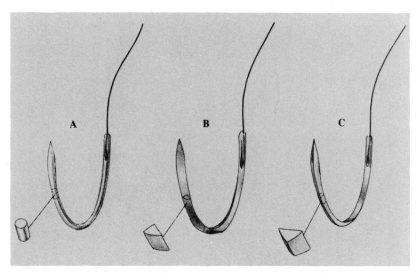

Fig. 1-7. Three types of needle tip (points). *A.* Round. *B.* Cutting. *C.* Reverse cutting. (From D. D. Zukin and R. R. Simon. *Emergency Wound Care — Principles and Practice.* Rockville, MD: Aspen, 1987. With permission.)

Dressings

Acute care dressings are discussed thoroughly in Chapter 18. Generally, a dry gauze dressing suffices. In the pediatric group, where small fingers are likely to explore it (unless put on deviously), the dressing usually lasts only for the trip home. Dressings therefore may need to be protected by fiber glass or plaster casts. Facial wounds may be dressed with simple Steri-Strips or kept covered with a layer of antibiotic ointment (particularly wounds around the mouth, eyes, lips, or hairline, where bulky dressings are not feasible). Alternatively, membrane dressings such as Op-site may be applied.

The efficacy of prophylactic antibiotics remains to be proved, although when properly used they appear to decrease infection rates. The antibiotics should be administered as soon as possible after the injury (i.e., in the emergency room) and should be effective against the microbe(s) most likely to cause a clinical infection (Table 1-4).

SPECIAL WOUNDS
Complex Wounds

Stellate Wounds

Stellate wound edges should be trimmed and débrided. The edges should be perpendicular to the skin surface and approximated with a half-buried mattress suture (Fig. 1-8).

Table 1-3. Suture materials commonly used for surgery

Suture	Types	Color of material	Raw material	Tensile strength retention in vivo	Absorption rate	Tissue reaction	Contra-indications	Warnings	Frequent uses
Surgical gut	Plain	Yellowish-tan Blue dyed	Collagen derived from healthy mammals	Lost within 7–10 days. Individual patient characteristics can affect rate of tensile strength loss	Digested by body enzymes within 70 days	Moderate	Should not be used in tissues that heal slowly and require support	Absorbs relatively quickly	Ligate superficial vessels; suture subcutaneous and other tissues that heal rapidly; sometimes used in presence of infection, in contrast to a braided nonabsorbable suture Ophthalmology
Surgical gut	Chromic	Brown Blue dyed	Collagen derived from healthy mammals. Treated to resist digestion by body tissues	Lost within 21–28 days. Individual patient characteristics can affect rate of tensile strength loss	Digested by body enzymes within 90 days	Moderate, but less than plain surgical gut	Being absorbable, should not be used where prolonged approximation of tissues under stress is required	Protein-based absorbable, sutures have a tendency to fray when tied	One of the most versatile of all materials; may be used in presence of infection; used in tissues that heal slowly but intended for use as absorbable suture or ligature Ophthalmology
Coated Vicryl (polyglactin 910)[a]	Braided	Violet Undyed (natural)	Copolymer of lactide and glycolide coated with polyglactin 370 and calcium stearate	Approximately 60% remains at 2 weeks. Approximately 30% remains at 3 weeks	Minimal until about 40th day. Essentially complete at 60–90 days. Absorbed by slow hydrolysis	Mild	Being absorbable, should not be used where prolonged approximation of tissues under stress is required	Safety and effectiveness in neural and cardiovascular tissue have not been established	Ligate or suture tissues where an absorbable suture is desirable except where approximation under stress is required

PDS (polydioxanone)[a]	Monofilament	Violet Clear	Polyester polymer	Approximately 70% remains at 2 weeks. Approximately 50% remains at 4 weeks. Approximately 25% remains at 6 weeks	Minimal until about 90th day. Essentially complete within 210 days. Absorbed by slow hydrolysis	Slight	Being absorbable, should not be used where prolonged approximation of tissues under stress is required	Safety and effectiveness in neural and cardiovascular tissue have not been established	Abdominal and thoracic closure, subcutaneous tissue, colon and rectal surgery; can use in presence of infection Orthopedic, plastic
Surgical silk	Braided	Black White	Natural protein fiber of raw silk spun by silkworm	Loses most or all in about 1 year	Usually cannot be found after 2 years	Moderate	Should not be used for placement of vascular prostheses and artificial heart valves	Slowly absorbs	Most body tissues for ligating and suturing. General surgery, ophthalmology, and plastic surgery
Ethilon (nylon)	Monofilament	Black Green Clear	Polyamide polymer	Loses 15–20% per year	Degrades at a rate of about 15–20% per year	Extremely low	None	None	Skin closure; retention; plastic surgery, ophthalmology, and microsurgery
Nurolon (nylon)	Braided	Black White	Polyamide polymer	Loses 15–20% per year	Degrades at a rate of about 15–20% per year	Extremely low	None	None	Most body tissues for ligating and suturing. General closure; neurosurgery
Ethibond (polyester fiber)[a]	Braided	Green White	Polyester polyethylene terephthalate coated with polybutylate	Indefinite	Nonabsorbable: remains encapsulated in body tissues	Minimal	None	Has not been evaluated for ophthalmic surgery	General surgery, cardiovascular and plastic surgery; retention

Table 1-3. (*continued*)

Suture	Types	Color of material	Raw material	Tensile strength retention in vivo	Absorption rate	Tissue reaction	Contra-indications	Warnings	Frequent uses
Prolene (polypropylene)[a]	Monofilament	Clear Blue	Polymer of propylene	Indefinite	Nonabsorbable: remains encapsulated in body tissues	Minimal transient acute inflammatory reaction	None	None	General, plastic, cardiovascular surgery and skin closure; ophthalmology

[a] See package insert for complete product information.
Source: *Ethicon Wound Closure Manual.* Sommerville, N.J.: Johnson and Johnson.

Table 1-4. Choice of antimicrobials for prevention of infection in specific wounds[a]

Type of wound	Antimicrobial of choice	Adult dose (g)[b]
Human bite seen within 1–2 days	Penicillin or ampicillin (alternative: erythromycin)	0.5–1.0
		0.5
Human bite older than 2 days	Dicloxacillin (alternative: erythromycin)	0.5
		0.5
Animal bites	Ampicillin (penicillin for cat bites) (alternative: tetracycline)	0.5
		0.5
Other wounds	Dicloxacillin (alternative: erythromycin)	0.5
		0.5
		0.5

[a] These recommendations apply only to wounds *without* evidence of infection at the time of examination.
[b] Four times daily orally for 3 to 5 days.
Source: J. Mills et al. Choice of an antimicrobial for prevention of infection in specific types of wounds. In: *Current Emergency Diagnosis and Treatment.* Los Altos, CA: Lange, 1985.

Circular Wounds
Most circular wounds are best managed by their conversion to an ellipse (Fig. 1-9). Elliptical wounds are closed as described below. Alternatively, circular wounds may be closed with a rotation flap or skin graft (see below).

Irregular Wounds
Not all wounds need to be closed in a straight line. Appropriate débridement allows acceptable zigzag closure (Fig. 1-10).

Elliptical Wounds
Wounds of various shapes (e.g., circular, triangular, square, irregular) may be converted to an ellipse and closed in a straight line. Wound edge undermining may be required. Generally, the total width of undermining should equal the short diameter of the wound. When the long diameter is less than four times the length of the short diameter, a straight line closure may result in "dog ears" (Fig. 1-11). This problem may be corrected by an additional elliptical incision or by Burow's triangle techniques (Fig. 1-12).

Large Defects
When a soft-tissue defect is too large to be closed primarily, or when primary closure will result in unwanted tension, producing distortion (e.g., eyelid, eyebrow, mouth), either a local flap or a skin graft (see

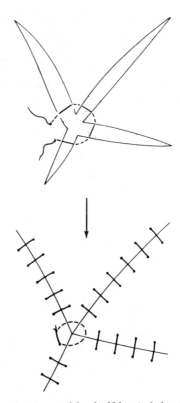

Fig. 1-8. Stellate laceration treated by half-buried, horizontal mattress sutures. (From D. D. Zukin and R. R. Simon. *Emergency Wound Care — Principles and Practice.* Rockville, MD: Aspen, 1987. With permission.)

below) may be used. These techniques are particularly valuable when cartilage, nerve, blood vessels, or tendons are exposed in the base of the wound. Care must be taken to not use flaps or grafts indiscriminately, as wound complications result in a defect that is larger than the one originally present.

Skin Grafts. Some wounds cannot be closed completely primarily because of loss of tissue, and they may require skin grafts. Donor site considerations involve donor scar, color match, and the size and thickness of skin required. Obviously, hair-bearing skin should not be used to graft a non-hair-bearing region. Appropriate donor sites for optimum color match for facial grafts include pre- and postauricular skin as well as skin from the supraclavicular region. Buttocks, upper inner arm, and thigh are commonly used donor sites for grafts below the head and neck. Split-thickness skin grafts are harvested at a thickness of 0.012 to 0.018 inch using either a dermatome or, rarely, freehand techniques with special skin grafting knives (Humby, Weck, or Goulian). A freehand technique requires more

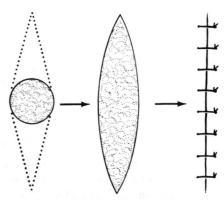

Fig. 1-9. Conversion of a circle to an ellipse. This technique allows closure of the circle without the formation of buckles in neighboring skin. The dotted lines on the left indicate the pattern of excision. The drawing on the right shows the finished repair. (From D. D. Zukin and R. R. Simon. *Emergency Wound Care — Principles and Practice.* Rockville, MD: Aspen, 1987. With permission.)

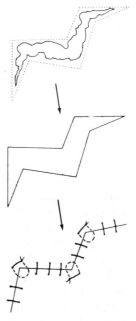

Fig. 1-10. Repair of an irregular wound. Note that the corners are repaired using half-buried horizontal mattress sutures. (From D. D. Zukin and R. R. Simon. *Emergency Wound Care — Principles and Practice.* Rockville, MD: Aspen, 1987. With permission.)

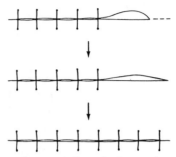

Fig. 1-11. Dog ear repair by extending the laceration. This method is especially useful for small tissue buckles. (From D. D. Zukin and R. R. Simon. *Emergency Wound Care — Principles and Practice.* Rockville, MD: Aspen, 1987. With permission.)

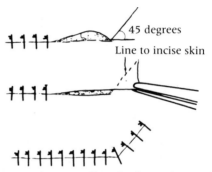

Fig. 1-12. Dog ear repair by extending the laceration at 45 degrees to the injury and removing an adequate Burow's triangle of tissue. (From D. D. Zukin and R. R. Simon. *Emergency Wound Care — Principles and Practice.* Rockville, MD: Aspen, 1987. With permission.)

skill and practice than the dermatome method. Donor sites may be covered with impregnated gauze (e.g., Xeroform, scarlet red) and allowed to dry as a scab. The gauze then drops off within 1 to 2 weeks as the wound epithelializes underneath. Alternatively, polyethylene film (Op-site) may be applied.

Full-thickness grafts (epidermis and dermis) are usually harvested as an ellipse to facilitate primary closure of the donor site. All adherent subcutaneous fat must be removed from the graft before it is transferred to the recipient site.

Grafts are avascular and survive for 48 hours by imbibition or absorption from the graft bed. Any factor that disrupts this process results in graft loss or poor take. In particular, hematoma, edema, or shearing forces must be avoided. The grafts should be sutured and placed with enough tension to ensure contact with the graft bed. Sutures are left long. Xeroform or Adaptic gauze is placed over the graft, and long suture ends are then used to secure a tie-over bolster dressing, usually of cotton or gauze (Fig. 1-13). After 4

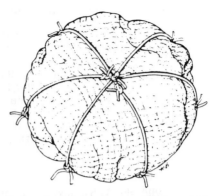

Fig. 1-13. Skin graft dressing. A buttress consisting of Xeroform wrapped around cotton is secured with the free ends of the sutures used to stitch the graft to the skin. (From D. D. Zukin and R. R. Simon. *Emergency Wound Care — Principles and Practice.* Rockville, MD: Aspen, 1987. With permission.)

to 5 days the bolster is removed and the graft inspected. The graft is then treated with a lubricating antibiotic ointment for 1 to 2 weeks.

Bite Wounds

All bites should be thoroughly débrided and irrigated or excised when possible. If the bite is acute, lacerations may be closed after suitable débridement. Small puncture wounds should always be left open. Bites of the hand, especially human bites, are infection-prone and probably should be treated open or by delayed primary closure (see Chapter 12 for further details). All bites should be considered tetanus-prone and appropriate tetanus prophylaxis administered according to guidelines established by the U.S. Public Health Service (Table 1-1).

Rabies
In the United States carnivores and scavengers are the animals most likely to transmit rabies. Rodents, rabbits, and squirrels are rare transmitters. (U.S. Public Health Service recommendations for post-exposure prophylaxis are listed in Table 1-5.) The decision to give antirabies prophylaxis is based on the animal and the circumstances of the bite. Because the prevalence of rabies is geographically variable, management decisions should be tempered by recommendations of regional and national public health officials, and consultations should be obtained when indicated. Prophylaxis is obtained using both active and passive immunization. Passive immunization consists in rabies immune globulin (RIG; 20 IU per kilogram), one-half of the dose being given in and around the wound. Active immunization is preferably done with human diploid cell rabies vaccine (HDCV), or if HDCV is not available duck embryo vaccine (DEV) may be used (Table 1-6).

Table 1-5. Rabies postexposure prophylaxis guide[a]

Animal species	Condition of animal at time of attack	Treatment of exposed person[b]
Domestic: dog and cat	Healthy and available for 10 days of observation	None, unless animal develops rabies[c]
	Rabid or suspected rabid	RIG[d] and HDCV[e]
	Unknown (escaped)	Consult public health officials. If treatment is indicated, give RIG[d] and HDCV.[e]
Wild: skunk, bat, fox, coyote, raccoon, bobcat, and other carnivores	Regard as rabid unless proved negative by laboratory tests[f]	RIG[d] and HDCV[e]
Other: livestock, rodents, and lagomorphs (rabbits and hares)	Consider individually. Local and state public health officials should be consulted on questions about the need for rabies prophylaxis. Bites of squirrels, hamsters, guinea pigs, gerbils, chipmunks, rats, mice, other rodents, rabbits, and hares almost never call for antirabies prophylaxis.	

[a] These recommendations are only a guide. When applying them, take into account the species involved, the circumstances of the bite or other exposure, the vaccination status of the animal, and the presence of rabies in the region. Local or state public health officials should be consulted if questions arise about the need for rabies prophylaxis.

[b] All bites and wounds should immediately be thoroughly cleansed with soap and water. If antirabies treatment is indicated, both rabies immune globulin (RIG) and human diploid cell rabies vaccine (HDCV) should be given as soon as possible, regardless of the interval from exposure.

[c] During the usual holding period of 10 days, begin treatment with RIG and vaccine (preferably with HDCV) at first sign of rabies in a dog or cat that has bitten someone. The symptomatic animal should be killed immediately and tested.

[d] If RIG is not available, use antirabies serum, equine (ARS). Do not use more than the recommended dosage.

[e] If HDCV is not available, use duck embryo vaccine (DEV) or other rabies vaccine. Local reactions to vaccines are common and do not contraindicate continuing treatment. Discontinue vaccine if fluorescent antibody tests of the animal are negative.

[f] The animal should be killed and tested as soon as possible. Holding for observation is not recommended.

Source: J. Mills et al. Rabies post exposure prophylaxis. In: *Current Emergency Diagnosis and Treatment.* Los Altos, CA: Lange, 1985.

Table 1-6. Rabies immunization regimens

Rabies vaccine	No. of 1-ml doses	Route of administration	Intervals between doses	If no antibody response to primary series[b]
HDCV	3	Intramuscular	1 Week between first and second; 2–3 weeks between second and third[c]	1 Booster dose[c]
DEV	3 or 4	Subcutaneous	1 Month between first and second; 6–7 months between second and third[c] *or* 1 Week between first, second, and third; 3 months between third and fourth[c]	2 Booster doses[c] 1 week apart
Postexposure[d] HDCV	5[e]	Intramuscular	Doses to be given on days 0, 3, 7, 14, and 28	Additional booster dose[f]
DEV	23	Subcutaneous	21 Daily doses followed by a booster on day 31 and another on day 41[c] *or* 2 Daily doses in the first 7 days, followed by 7 daily doses; then 1 booster on day 24 and another on day 34[c]	3 Doses of HDCV at weekly intervals[c]

[a] Preexposure rabies prophylaxis for persons with special risks of exposure to rabies (e.g., animal care and control personnel and selected laboratory workers) consists in immunization with either human diploid cell rabies vaccine (HDCV) or duck embryo vaccine (DEV), according to the following schedule, followed by a booster dose every 2 years.

[b] If no antibody response is documented after the recommended additional booster dose(s), consult the state health department or CDC.

[c] Serum for rabies antibody testing should be collected 2–3 weeks after the last dose only in immunocompromised patients.

[d] Postexposure rabies prophylaxis for persons exposed to rabies consists of the immediate, thorough cleansing of all wounds with soap and water, administration of rabies immune globulin (RIG) or (if RIG is not available) antirabies serum, equine (ARS), and the initiation of either HDCV or DEV, according to schedule outlined.

[e] The World Health Organization recommends a sixth dose 90 days after the first dose.

[f] An additional booster dose should be given only to immunocompromised patients.

Infected Wounds

Infected wounds and particularly bite wounds should be opened, cultured, and drained. Antibiotic therapy may be initiated according to Table 1-4 and then guided by culture results. Antibiotic therapy is indicated by local erythema and evidence of systemic or local toxicity. Patients with systemic toxicity or infected bites of the hand should be admitted for parenteral antibiotic therapy. After débridement and drainage, the hand is splinted in the position of function and elevated. Evidence of tenosynovitis mandates operative management (see Chapter 12).

FOLLOW-UP MANAGEMENT

Early conscientious follow-up is mandatory not only to identify and treat early complications or "problem wounds" but also to reassess the patient for any additional injuries or difficulties that were missed during the initial encounter. One can learn much from close critical evaluation of results obtained from surgical repair of a wound.Photographs of the injury, repair, and result allow one to change an operative technique and ultimately help obtain improved results.

SUGGESTED READING

Mills, J., et al. *Current Emergency Diagnosis and Treatment.* Los Altos, CA: Lange, 1985.

Zukin, D. D., and Simon, R. R. *Emergency Wound Care — Principles and Practice.* Rockville, MD: Aspen, 1987.

Commentary on Chapter 1

Richard J. Greco

I am in agreement with the basic tenets of Dr. Edington's basic concepts of acute wound care. Specifically, it is important for the examining physician to remember the basic ABCs and to rule out all significant internal and intracranial injuries prior to dealing with the soft-tissue injuries.

As a plastic surgeon, one is called upon to deal with various types of wounds; from a small laceration on a child's face to devastating blast and degloving injuries of the upper extremity. It is important to remember an old adage taught to me by Dr. J. William Futrell, when discussing the operative repair of a child with a cleft lip deformity he would say this day is the most important day of this child's life because the quality of the surgical repair will make a significant difference in the way both he and his peers perceive him in his social environment. This adage applies to a child with a facial laceration, and therefore, after appropriate evaluation of the patient, one should demand of the emergency room staff adequate lighting and appropriate instruments and suture material to perform the best repair that one can for this patient. Small children should be sedated as necessary because it is very difficult to perform a meticulous repair on a child who is screaming and moving about.

My own personal preference is to excise the margin of wounds caused by crushing or tearing mechanisms and to irrigate the wound with at least 250 ml of saline using a 20 ml syringe and an 18 gauge needle. I then attempt to perform a layered closure using deep layers of either vicryl or PDS suture. The skin is then closed using fine, interrupted sutures of 6-0 nylon suture on the face. These sutures are removed within five days. An appropriate dressing should be placed over the injured site, and I have found mastiosol and layered application of steri-strips to help stabilize the wound. After the sutures are removed I typically will use steri-strips for an additional 5–7 days, at which time the complete dressing is removed.

In areas with large, abrased surfaces I suture the wounds with chromic suture, do not use steri-strips, and use bacitracin ointment as the dressing three times a day. Although many of the lacerations of the face and body can be dealt with by emergency room physicians, if there is any doubt in the physician's mind as to his ability to achieve an acceptable result, it is appropriate to consider consulting a plastic surgeon or another physician who feels comfortable with the treatment of the particular wound.

2 MANAGEMENT OF PHYSICAL AND CHEMICAL INJURIES

James K. Smith

Industrialization of society has meant an increased exposure to new chemical agents and solvents, many of which cause significant injury to the human skin and respiratory systems. The description of each agent and its chemical properties, clinical presentation, pathophysiology of injury, and treatment provide the treating physician with the basic database to initiate logical therapy. Common considerations to all of these injuries include (1) the location and amount of surface area exposed to the agent, (2) the chemical composition and concentration of the agent, (3) the physical state of the agent, (4) the duration of exposure, (5) the amount of time before initiation of appropriate therapy, and (6) the general condition of the patient prior to exposure and any concomitant injuries they have suffered.

ACIDS

Hydrochloric and *sulfuric acids* are common industrial agents and are frequently used in low-concentration, liquid states. Their mechanisms of injury are similar and are caused by the exothermic reaction of the hydrogen ion.

The exposed skin presents with a varying clinical appearance depending on the concentration and duration of exposure. Mild exposures present with erythema and tenderness, and heavy exposures lead to full-thickness coagulation necrosis. Regardless of the acid or site of injury, immediate therapy includes removing the exposure and saturated clothing and applying copious lavage with water and antibacterial burn dressings. Extensive exposure requires fluid resuscitation as for equivalent thermal insults.

Hydrofluoric acid (HF) is used as a solvent and catalyst in the petrochemical, ceramic, semiconductor, and glass etching industries. It causes injury not only by desiccation and exothermic reaction, as with other mineral acids, but also by release of free fluoride ions. The fluoride ion's affinity for calcium destroys cell walls and renders mitochondria dysfunctional until the fluoride ion is bound and neutralized. Instability of the neuron's cell membrane leads to a release of potassium and subsequent excruciating pain associated

Table 2-1. Correlation of hydrofluoric acid strength with degree of injury

Acid strength (%)	Degree of injury
<20	No symptoms for 24 hours
20–50	Pain and erythema noticeable within 8 hours
>50	Immediate pain and obvious tissue destruction

with HF burns. The U.S. Public Health Service has proposed three categories of injury severity, primarily depending on the concentration of acid to which the patient was exposed (Table 2-1).

Current treatment recommendations include immediate removal of any and all clothing that may be contaminated, washing with copious amounts of water or sodium bicarbonate solutions, and application of iced benzethonium chloride (Hyamine 1622, 2 g per liter of ice water) or benzalkonium chloride (1.3 g per liter of ice water) for 15 minutes to 6 hours until symptomatic relief, and then application of 2.5% calcium gluconate gel. Calcium gluconate solution (10%) should be subcutaneously injected without hesitation if symptomatic relief is not obtained or there has been an exposure to more than 20% HF. Reinjection is indicated if the pain returns.

Hydrofluoric acid penetrates nails and nail beds, readily causing intense pain and destruction of the subungal areas. Removal of the nails under digital block and treatment of the nail beds is indicated. Patients with more than 1 percent total body surface area (BSA) exposure to high concentration HF, more than 5% BSA exposure to low concentration HF, or inhalation of more than 60% HF fumes should be monitored for hypocalcemia with cardiac monitoring and serial serum calcium levels. Treatment with intravenous calcium should be early and aggressive (1 g $CaCl_2$ every 15 to 30 minutes) until the calcium level is normalized. The victim's airways can develop severe mucosal swelling and may require intubation or tracheostomy [1–3].

White phosphorus, an ingredient of gunpowder, produces burns seen in munitions accidents. This substance often becomes embedded in the soft tissues and, if incompletely spent, oxidizes spontaneously with air, causing further thermal destruction. Initial therapy includes removal of contaminated clothing, copious lavage with water, and wet saline soaks to prevent further oxidation injury. The Wood's lamp is useful for identifying retained phosphoric materials, all of which should be removed. After the complete removal of this compound, immediate or early dermabrasion of traumatic tattooing is recommended. Electrocardiographic abnormalities and ventricular arrhythmia secondary to abrupt shifts of calcium/phosphate ratios can occur with systemic absorption of phosphate compounds [2,4].

Chromic acids are used for chrome plating, textile printing, dyeing, and the manufacturing of wallpaper and rubber goods. Hexavalent chromium is more physiologically mobile and thus more systemically toxic than trivalent chromium. Clinical manifestations of its toxicity include diarrhea, gastrointestinal bleeding, hemolysis, hepatic necrosis, and acute renal failure. Emergency excision of the exposed skin has been advocated as a first line treatment to reduce the systemic absorption and toxicity. EDTA creams and baths as well as topical dimercaprol have also been recommended for less intense burns [5].

Nitric acid injuries are treated with water lavage and local wound care. Systemic absorption of substantial quantities of nitrates can occur through the burn wound and lead to methemoglobinemia and hypoxia, which require treatment with intravenous methylene blue and high flow oxygen [4].

Formic acid, like other agents in this class, causes local coagulation necrosis, and can lead to significant systemic absorption, leading to metabolic acidosis, hemolysis, and hemoglobinuria. The hemolysis is secondary to the direct toxic effect on the erythrocytes. One should treat the cutaneous injury with ice water lavage and intravenous bicarbonate, mannitol, exchange transfusion, and hemodialysis as indicated.

Phenol (carbonic acid), a highly lipid-soluble substance, is used in the medical and industrial fields. Coagulation necrosis occurs rapidly because of its solubility, and treatment consists in removal of all contaminated clothing, immediate lavage with 50% polyethylene glycol solution in water, or a high flow shower followed by treatment according to guidelines for local thermal injuries. Individual supportive measures may be necessary for the systemic toxic effects of phenol: myocardial depression, vasomotor collapse, clinical pneumonitis, hemolysis, and renal failure.

ALKALIS

Sodium hydroxide is by far the most common and widely publicized caustic agent. Most cutaneous injuries are caused by direct contact with plumbing solutions or crystals. Rapid protein precipitation and continued coagulative necrosis occurs because of the strength of this base. Immediate copious lavage with water and local wound care for thermal injury are in order.

Cement is a hydroscopic alkaline substance made up of primarily calcium oxide (about 63 percent). The addition of gypsum to cement controls the amount of excessive exothermic reaction and subsequent local thermal injury. The addition of water leads to the formation of calcium hydroxide and a pH of almost 12.9. This substance causes protein denaturation when in contact with the skin and can produce third degree burns after 2 hours of contact. Treatment is similar to that for sodium hydroxide exposure [6,7].

PSORALENS

Topical and oral psoralens, as pigment-inducing medications, can cause a serious photosensitivity reaction. Specifically, this phototoxicity is manifested as an increased sensitization to ultraviolet A radiation. Intraepidermal edema and necrosis occurs with sparing of the underlying dermis. The strongest oral photosensitizer is 8-methoxypsoralen, and the strongest topical agent is trimethylpsoralen. Treatment is similar to that for a second degree burn because the basal layer and skin appendages are frequently spared with the dermis [8].

HYDROCARBON/ PETROLEUM DISTILLATES

The depth of injury associated with hydrocarbons is directly related to the duration of exposure to the agent. This group is highly lipid-soluble and causes cellular dehydration and systemic absorption. Fortunately, most of these injuries are halted at the partial-thickness injury level. Treatment consists of removing solvent-containing clothing, lavage or soaking in water, and local wound care for second degree burns.

Complications of systemic absorption include vascular endothelial damage of the cardiovascular, neurologic, renal, and hepatic systems. If continued systemic absorption is occurring, full-thickness débridement is indicated. One must be cognizant that *methylene chloride,* an additive in many hydrocarbon solvents, is metabolized to carbon monoxide, and such ancillary poisoning may require supportive hyperbaric oxygen support [9].

INFUSION/ EXTRAVASATION INJURIES

There are two basic types of infusion/extravasation injury: (1) hospital-acquired extravasation of medications and intravenous fluids; and (2) less sterile injection of narcotics and impure pharmaceuticals by the parenteral drug abuser. The treatments for these injuries are similar, but frequently the sequela are much different.

The minor extravasation of intravenous fluids, common antibiotics, and nonantineoplastic pharmaceuticals rarely cause permanent sequela, provided a hydrostatic vascular compromise has not been created. Immobilization and elevation of the affected extremity with frequent Doppler and clinical examinations are required.

If the hydrostatic pressure in the fascial compartment is in excess of approximately 40 mm Hg, a compartment syndrome is created. The clinical examination and findings of pain, paresthesias, paralysis, and pulselessness are helpful guides. If there is any doubt, serial compartment pressures can be obtained. Decompression is warranted in symptomatic patients or those with elevated pressures.

Hypertonic and highly ionic media can cause overlying skin necrosis by direct cellular injury, leading to increased edema and swelling. Unless the agent has vasoconstricting properties, the areas are treated topically and then débrided and grafted when demarcation is complete.

Antineoplastic agents are by nature directly cytotoxic. The significance of the extravasation injury is potentially magnified by the patient population in which it has occurred. Oncologic patients often metabolize these agents more slowly and frequently have poor wound healing. The ultimate wound is a function of the drug's mode of action and is directly proportional to the total amount of drug extravasated and the time elapsed prior to initiating therapy. Although few of these agents have specific antidotes, immediate direct cooling of the exposed area limits the rate of cellular drug uptake and is followed immediately by subcutaneous clysis with 20 ml or more of hyaluronidase and saline solution (150 U/1000 ml). Clysis is currently thought to limit ulceration by diluting the local concentration of the drug and therefore its cytotoxic effects.

Extravasation of agents with vasoconstrictive properties (e.g., epinephrine, narcotics) may cause significant ischemic injury to the surrounding skin and tissues. Local infiltration with α-blockers (e.g., phentolamine) help prevent or limit the amount of tissue at risk. Fasciotomies are required frequently, and acute vascular reconstruction may be necessary if vasodilatory and thrombolytic agents are ineffective.

In all instances, the area of injection must be promptly explored, irrigated with saline solution, and débrided of all foreign substances and necrotic tissues. The tendon sheath must often be sacrificed, and pulleys are salvaged whenever possible. Frequent wet dressing changes to the open wound with splinting and elevation of the involved extremity are utilized. Secondary delayed closure is then performed [10,11].

BLAST INJURIES

Blast injuries present as a spectrum of injuries because there are many types of explosive. The injury depends on: (1) the total energy released by the explosion; (2) the rate of energy released; (3) the proximity of the victim to the blast; (4) the size, velocity, and composition of blast debris that strikes the victim (including shotgun pellets); and (5) associated heat, steam, or fire caused by or contributing to the blast, which includes the composition of the blast materials.

No matter what the source of the explosion, these injuries do have many similarities. It is almost impossible to predict the extent of deep tissue injury or what the likely aesthetic or functional result will be. The energy force can splinter underlying bones and irreversibly damage vascular intima, causing thrombosis and tissue infarction (Table 2-2). Doppler evaluation of local vessels and radiographic studies should be done in addition to visual inspection of the injured areas.

If vascular integrity is compromised because of direct tissue loss or thrombosis, the skin and fascia are decompressed, followed by immediate reconstruction using autogenous or synthetic conduits. Anastomoses must be performed proximal and distal to the zone of injury. If this step is not possible, operative failure is likely.

Table 2-2. Spectrum of tissue destruction with blast injuries

Cutaneous laceration, abrasion, avulsion, or burn
Bone and cartilage fractures (open, closed, comminuted)
Tendon laceration or avulsion
Nervous lacerations, contusion, or avulsion
Vascular thrombosis, laceration, or avulsion
Truncal visceral organ involvement

HIGH PRESSURE INJECTION INJURIES

The three most common devices involved in high pressure injection injuries are (1) grease guns, (2) spray guns, and (3) diesel fuel injectors. A wide variety of products with inherent noxious physical and chemical properties is propelled through these systems, including substances such as water, sand, paint, and petroleum products.

The most common site of injury is in the nondominant "steady" hand and in particular the distal index or middle finger. Despite the innocuous appearance of the small entry wound, it is a surgical emergency. The site of injection is frequently painless, but the affected area is or becomes progressively more swollen owing to the volume of injected material and the local tissue reaction. If the area is restricted by overlying skin or fascia, vascular compromise ensues.

The clinical course depends on the volume and composition of the injected material, the anatomic site injected, the time lapse between incident and treatment, and the local tissue reaction. The acute phase is characterized by progressive tissue necrosis and is due to pressure, chemical irritation, and secondary infection.

The chronic phase involves slow tissue reaction of the retained petroleum products and is characterized by chronic inflammation with foreign body reactions. Oleomas, oil-containing tumors, and recurrent abscesses form if the wound is not adequately treated.

Frequently, one can only débride embedded missiles and devitalized tissue. Treatment then consists in intravenous antibiotics, immobilization and elevation of the affected part, and a planned second look 48 hours later. Closure is delayed until the tissue edema subsides and demarcation is complete [12] (Table 2-3).

Predictions of the degree of joint stiffness, tendon excursion, or neurologic return after blast are uncertain. Hyperbaric oxygen has been promoted for decreased swelling and increased tissue salvage in blast injuries.

VENOMS
Insects

Hymenoptera (bees, wasps, hornets, yellow jackets, ants) constitute the vanguard in nature's army of venomous pests. Local reactions rarely require the attention of plastic surgeons; however, occasionally the reaction is extensive and leads to massive edema with compromised vascular integrity. Fasciotomies may be required.

The patient often experiences throbbing pain and immobility

Table 2-3. Immediate treatment protocol for severe blast injuries

1. Reestablish vascular integrity.
2. Implement skeletal fixation.
3. Irrigate aggressively, and débride conservatively.
4. Fasciotomy as required.
5. Apply biologic dressing.
6. Elevate the affected extremities.
7. Mandatory second look and delayed closure.

secondary to the edema, and the area is diffusely tender. The site of envenomation must be examined for signs of secondary infection and drained as necessary. Vascular integrity is evaluated with Doppler examination of the hand and careful neurologic assessment.

If any question exists, compartmental pressures can be measured and decompressive fasciotomies performed as necessary. Commonly the vessels are patent, and decompression and elevation are all that is needed. Rarely, thrombectomy or surgical revascularization is required.

Spider Bites

In the United States there are three spiders capable of envenomation: black widow, brown recluse, and scorpion. Black widow (*Latrodectus mactans*) poisoning results in latrodectism, a specific syndrome that incudes sharp pain at the site of attack, which is marked by two red fang marks close together. Within 15 minutes the neurotoxin causes pain and cramps in the bite region, progressing to involve all striated muscle, generally resulting in a telltale rigid abdomen, vomiting, tremor, increased salivation, and possible shock.

Envenomation can lead to either acute severe or delayed hypersensitivity reactions with acute paralysis, hemolysis, renal failure, intense puritus, and coma. Treatment includes 10 ml of 10% calcium gluconate over 15 minutes, muscle relaxants, Lyovac antivenin in severe cases, and general supportive measures.

The brown recluse (*Loxosceles reclusa*) bite results in a chronologic reaction: minor irritation, local erythema with central blistering, a halo of pallor, and a delayed severe necrotic arachnidism with hemolysis and disseminated intravascular coagulation. Relatively few of these bites ultimately lead to a significant local wound or systemic reactions. A predictive test of which wounds are likely to progress can be performed if the wound is less than 48 hours old. One gives the patient intravenous fluorescein and examines the wound with a Wood's lamp. If an area of more than 1 cm^2 illuminates, this area is likely to necrose and the wound should be directly excised.

Dapsone (50 or 100 mg PO b.i.d.) has emerged as an effective agent for aborting the cutaneous sequela of these bites by its effect on polymorphonuclear leukocytes (PMNs). The PMNs are thought to mediate not only the local cutaneous effects but systemic loxoscelism as well [13].

Table 2-4. Grades of snake bite severity

Grade	Sign
0	No sign of bite
1	Minimal swelling
2	Progressive swelling and discoloration
3	Marked local tissue necrosis and systemic illness

SNAKE BITES

Most snake bites are by nonpoisonous snakes, and those caused by poisonous snakes involve little or no envenomation. Fortunately, most patients seek medical attention promptly. A careful history and thorough examination of the involved area may alleviate many of the patient's fears. Information important to obtain includes the type and size of the snake, the anatomic site of the bite, the time elapsed since the bite, the interval between injury and signs or symptoms, and the local and systemic signs and symptoms.

Local manifestations of pit viper envenomation (the most common) include fang marks, edema, erythema, pain, bluish discoloration, blistering, ecchymosis, persistent bleeding, and local tissue necrosis, depending on the severity. Systemic manifestations progress through perioral tingling, metallic taste, muscle fasciculation, vomiting, hypotension, generalized ecchymosis, coagulopathy, respiratory distress, and renal failure. Copperhead snake bites rarely progress to the advanced state seen with other poisonous snake bites.

Patients may present in a state of circulatory collapse, and treatment of shock must be immediate, including the administration of three to five vials of intravenous antivenin over 1 hour in a glucose or saline drip. Patients may require up to 20 vials for severe reactions; most patients develop serum sickness if more than five vials are administered because of the equine source of the antiserum.

The grading system of snake bites and their degree of envenomation is determined by the degree of local tissue reaction and systemic toxicity (Table 2-4). All patients with suspected poisoning require close observation, elevation of the involved extremity, and local wound care. Observation for compartment syndromes is necessary, and decompression is performed as necessary. The use of local wound exploration and antivenin in patients without systemic toxicity is controversial. Only grade 3 bites — with systemic symptoms — definitely require antivenin and exploration.

Coral snake bites are rare, usually resulting from direct handling of the species. They require antivenin. Fortunately, most of these bites are superficial, and envenomation rarely occurs unless the digits are involved [13,14].

REFERENCES

1. Flood, S. Hydrofluoric acid burns. *Am. Fam. Physician* 37:175, 1988.
2. Connel, S. J., and Defranzo, A. J. Principles and management of injuries from physical and chemical agents. In N. G. Georgaide (ed.),

Essentials of Plastic, Maxillofacial, and Reconstructive Surgery. Baltimore: Williams & Wilkins, 1987.

3. Greco, R. J., et al. Hydrofluoric acid induced hypocalcemia. *J. Trauma* 28:1593, 1988.
4. Mozingo, D. W., et al. Chemical burns. *J. Trauma* 28:642, 1988.
5. Laitung, J. K. G., and Earley, M. The role of surgery in chromic acid burns: our experience with two patients. *Burns* 10:378, 1984.
6. Peters, W. J. Alkali burns from wet cement. *Can. Med. Assoc. J.* 130:7, 1984.
7. Early, S. H., and Simpson, R. L. Caustic burns from contact with wet cement. *J.A.M.A.* 254:528, 1985.
8. Berakha, G. J., and Lefkovits, G. Psoralen phototherapy and phototoxicity. *Ann. Plast. Surg.* 14:458, 1985.
9. Hansbrough, J. F., et al. Hydrocarbon contact injuries. *J. Trauma* 25:250, 1985.
10. Harter, B. T., and Harter, K. C. High pressure injection injuries. *Hand Clin.* 2:547, 1986.
11. Smith, T. E., Canady, J. W., and Jones, C. D. Cervicofacial high-pressure injection injuries. *Arch. Otolaryngol.* 108:452, 1982.
12. Parsons, R. W. The management of traumatic tattoos. *Clin. Plast. Surg.* 2:517, 1975.
13. Pennell, T. C., Babu, S. S., and Meredith, J. W. The management of snake bites in the southeastern United States. *Am. Surg.* 53:198, 1987.
14. *Emergency Department Management of Poisonous Snake Bites.* Philadelphia: American College of Surgeon's Committee on Trauma, 1981.

Commentary on Chapter 2

Roger E. Salisbury

One must congratulate the author for presenting a great deal of information in an abbreviated but rational fashion in this chapter. The chapter is valuable more for the problems it raises than for any didactic solutions. The wide variety of possible injuries due to acids and alkalis defies simple memorization. Yet the systemic complications of contact with some of these agents can be catastrophic. Each emergency room should have a chart readily available that lists the offending agent with its possible complications and treatments. Physicians on call should have a pocket copy of this same chart. Many patients are referred from great distances, and rapid treatment response is imperative. Although most physicians appreciate that local care should consist in removal of clothing and dilutional lavage with water, many have never seen a hydrofluoric acid burn and are not aware of the hypocalcemia and cardiac complications that may result. Few realize that acute renal failure may complicate chromic acid or formic acid injury. Thus it is also advisable, in anticipation of systemic problems, to have early consultation with the medicine department when managing these patients.

The authors rightly emphasize that tissue necrosis following high pressure injury may be due to chemical irritation as well as pressure. The most common treatment error with these injuries is delay of exploration. The wound should be explored when edema begins, not after vascular compromise occurs. One should not employ simplistic thinking and believe it is possible to remove mechanically all the injected materials, e.g., oil or paint. Multiple débridements of necrotic tissue may be necessary, and often the surgeon is unable to close the wound because of edema and friable tissue. Such wounds close gradually over several weeks by contraction or may even require skin grafting.

For blast injuries this reviewer emphasizes even more strongly than the author that the plastic surgeon be in a *consulting* capacity to the general surgeon rather than managing the patient himself or herself. Blast injuries are notorious for their variability and occult tissue damage. Severe retroperitoneal injury, dead bowel, or lethal pulmonary dysfunction may not be immediately obvious. Although a dramatic regional problem (e.g., subtotal amputation of the extremity) may have caused the patient to be referred to the subspecialist, the general surgeon-traumatologist should be in charge of the case to ensure that the priorities of the injury are addressed properly.

The author's management of snake bites may seem aggressive but is a sound, conservative approach. Most often the snake does not linger and invite identification. Thus the treating physician is often working "blind." Admission of the patient and following the guidelines suggested prevents undertreatment. Although extremity bites are discussed, one should also mention management of truncal injuries. Toddlers playing in the grass are frequently bitten in the chest or abdomen (unlike adults who are usually struck in the lower extremity). Thus the general or pediatric surgeon should be consulted to consider early exploration and débridement of the wound.

3 ACUTE CARE BURN MANAGEMENT

Scott E. Kasden

Burns are among the most devastating injuries seen in the emergency department. They range in severity from sunburn to lethal injury. Excluding motor vehicle injuries, they are the most common cause of accidental death in the United States, with more than two million burns per year resulting in over 100,000 burn hospitalizations per year. The most severe burns occur in dwelling fires [1,2].

Thermal injuries result from transfer of heat to body tissues. The depth of burn depends on the duration of exposure and the intensity of the thermal gradient. Conduction damage rarely occurs at temperatures of less than 45° to 50°C. The most common cause of thermal injury is direct exposure to an open flame, with scalds and burns due to direct contact also presenting frequently. Chemical and electrical injuries are relatively rare.

Burns seen in the emergency department vary according to age distribution. Children less than 3 years of age are most frequently scalded as a result of kitchen accidents, bathroom accidents, and abuse or neglect. Children between the ages of 3 and 14 years are burned most frequently by clothing catching fire. Girls are more frequently and more severely burned than boys because girls wear more clothing that is highly flammable. The second leading cause of burns in this age group is the dwelling fire. Burn patients between 15 and 60 years of age are most frequently burned in work-related accidents, usually industrial. Although relatively rare, chemical and electrical burns are most commonly seen in this category of patients. Burn patients 65 years and older present primarily with injuries secondary to fire. This age group usually has contributing factors of co-morbidity (e.g., decreased mobility, decreased level of consciousness, seizure disorders, and alcohol and drug abuse [1,3].

ANATOMY AND HISTOLOGY OF SKIN

Skin is the largest organ of the body, comprising 16 percent of the total body weight. It functions as the first line of defense in immunity. Skin also functions as a diffusion and exchange barrier, as a thermal regulator, in sensory reception, in metabolism, in emotional expression, and in coloration [4–7].

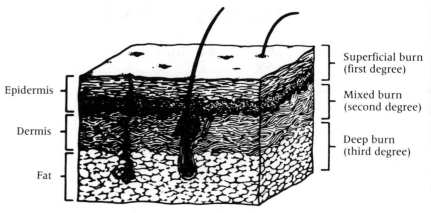

Fig. 3-1. Three depths of burn. (From W. B. Conolly. *Color Atlas of Hand Conditions*. London: Wolfe Publishing, 1980. With permission.)

Skin has a total thickness of 1.5 to 4.0 mm and is composed histologically of the epidermis and dermis. The most superficial layer is the epidermis and the deeper layer the dermis [4–7]. The stratified composition of skin is demonstrated in Figures 3-1 and 3-2.

Burn Trauma Physical Examination

After the trauma workup has been completed and the burn trauma history obtained, the burn trauma physical examination is undertaken. The most logical approach is a systematic and thorough examination starting at the head and proceeding to the toes.

Burns on the head pose special hazards. Burns of the ears must be documented and treated early and aggressively to avoid the grave complication of chondritis. Eye burns must also be carefully evaluated. If there is any question of injury, a fluorescein investigation under Wood's light must be performed. Any injury to the eye must be followed up with an ophthalmologic consultation within 24 hours.

The airway is at risk with a burn injury not only because of heat and smoke but also inhaled toxins. An initially asymptomatic patient may develop airway obstruction secondary to edema within 48 to 72 hours after exposure. Usually the injury is to the larynx and supraglottic airway. Suggestive findings on physical examination include facial burns, singed nasal and facial hairs, inflammation of the oronasopharynx, hoarseness, and carbonaceous sputum [8,9].

When the signs and symptoms of inhalation injury are present with the appropriate history, bronchoscopy is the diagnostic tool of choice. Bronchoscopy is safe, is relatively easy, and can be performed through an endotracheal tube. Moreover, it can be used to assist in difficult endotracheal or nasotracheal intubations.

Inhalation injury is diagnosed and is classified according to anatomic location.

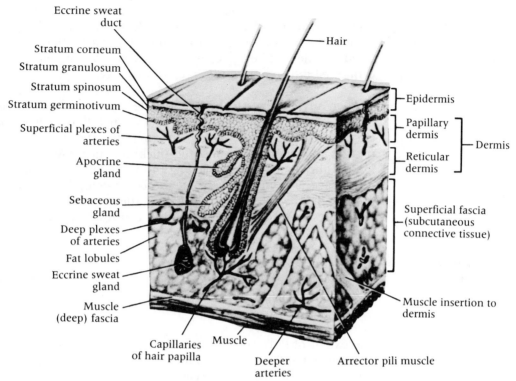

Fig. 3-2. Cross section of histology of skin and skin appendages. (From R. J. Bennett. *Fundamentals of Cutaneous Surgery.* St. Louis: Mosby, 1988. With permission.)

1. *Supraglottic inhalation injury.* Supraglottic inhalation injury is a direct result of heat transferred to the upper airway. Patients who sustain this injury generally present with marked oral and lip edema. Lip edema is generally a good indicator of vocal cord edema and, when severe, indicates the need for transient endotracheal intubation. Airway edema is usually present within 6 to 24 hours after the burn and generally resolves in 3 to 5 days. Because the oro- and nasopharynx are efficient heat exchangers, it is uncommon to see a heat injury below the vocal cords.

2. *Tracheobronchial injury.* Tracheobronchial injury is due to inhalation of incomplete products of combustion, causing injury to the tracheobronchial mucosa. Agents commonly associated with this injury are nitrates, polyvinyls, sulfa radicals, and polyurethane gases. In addition to chemically "burning" the mucosa of the tracheobronchial tree, these agents injure the mucociliary escalator. Ultimately, mucosal sloughing and associated tracheobronchitis occur, leading to a pneumonic process.

3. *Alveolar inhalation injury.* Some patients present with alveolar inhalation injury, which is manifested by hypoxia immediately

following extrication from the fire. This inhalation injury is generally due to severe alveolar damage, which leads to an adult respiratory distress-type syndrome. The usual clinical course for these patients is rapid decline despite aggressive intervention. Approximately 5 percent of all inhalation injuries present this way.

After airway assessment is complete, the examination should proceed in an orderly caudad fashion. Special note is made of circumferential burns involving the extremities and chest wall. These injuries are important because full-thickness burns lose their elasticity and these areas are unyielding to the underlying swelling. The eschar acts as a tourniquet and the circumferential burns, when present on the chest, can result in respiratory insufficiency; and when present on the extremities, they can result in vascular insufficiency.

Classification and Extent of Burns

Burns are classified as first degree, partial thickness (superficial or deep — second degree), full thickness (third degree), and fourth degree. Characteristics of these burns are demonstrated in Figure 3-3.

Extent of Burn Injury
The extent of burn injury can be simply and accurately estimated using the Lund Browder diagram. An accurate estimate can be made using the "rule of nines" (Fig. 3-4). The rule-of-nines method divides the adult body into surface areas of 9 percent, or fractions or multiples of 9 percent; burn severity and extent are then estimated. A crude estimate of burn size can be made utilizing the size of the patient's hand, which is approximately 1.5 percent total body surface area (BSA). All burns are expressed as percent BSA.

In the pediatric patient the head and neck constitute a large proportion of the BSA and the lower extremities a smaller proportion compared to the adult patient. It is the proportion of partial-thickness and full-thickness burns that determine resuscitation requirements and the need for admission (Tables 3-1 and 3-2).

RESUSCITATION

Adequate resuscitation of the acute burn patient is essential to prevent "burn shock." Burn shock is due to rapid fluid shifts and fluid losses, creating a state of intravascular hypovolemia that leads to cardiovascular collapse and end-organ hypoperfusion. The fluid shift phenomenon is due to a temporary increase in capillary permeability. This derangement in permeability is not usually observed in patients sustaining BSA burns of less than about 25 percent.

Burns larger than approximately 25 percent BSA produce a rather stereotypical derangement in physiology and homeostasis in general. The derangement evolves over time, generally following an orderly progression, although the time spent in any one phase may vary somewhat.

Depth of Burn	Signs & Symptoms	Severity
Second Degree Second-degree burns are of greater depth than first-degree burns and involve partial thickness. They result from a very deep sunburn, contact with hot liquids, or flash burns from gasolines flames. They are usually more painful than deeper burns that destroy nerve endings in the skin. 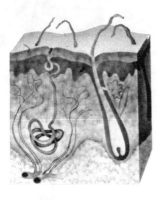	Red or mottled appearance Blisters and broken epidermis Considerable swelling Weeping, wet surface Painful Sensitive to cold air	**Critical:** Burns complicated by respiratory tract injury and fractures. Burns involving more than 30% of body surface. **Moderate:** Burns involving 15% to 30% of body surface. **Minor:** Burns of less than 15% of body surface.
Third Degree Third-degree burns cause damage to all layers of the skin and involve subcutaneous tissue. They can be caused by fire, prolonged exposure to hot liquids, contact with hot objects, or electricity. 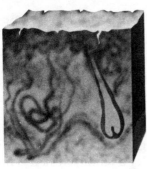	Pale white or charred appearance, leathery (At first, may resemble second-degree burn) Broken skin with fat exposed Dry surface Painless, insensitive to pinprick Edema	**Critical:** Burns complicated by respiratory tract injury and fractures. Burns involving the critical areas of the face, hands, and feet. Burns involving more than 10% of body surface. **Moderate:** Burns of 2% to 10% of body surface and not involving face, hands, or feet. **Minor:** Burns of less than 2% of body surface.

Fig. 3-3. Second and third degree burn classification. (From *Advanced Trauma Life Support Course for Physicians Manual.* Philadelphia: American College of Surgeons, Committee on Trauma, 1983. With permission.)

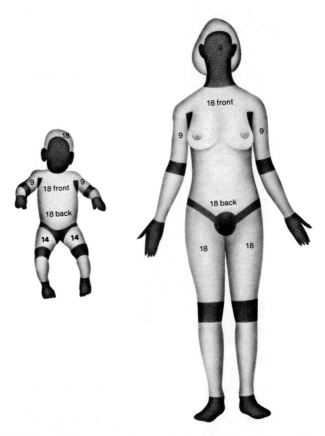

Fig. 3-4. Body surface area estimates: "rule of nines." (From *Advanced Trauma Life Support Course for Physicians Manual.* Philadelphia: American College of Surgeons, Committee on Trauma, 1983. With permission.)

Phase 1: acute phase (first 24 hours). The acute phase is marked by increased capillary leakiness causing intravascular hypovolemia, which, if uncorrected, leads to cardiovascular collapse and burn shock.

Phase 2: subacute phase (day 2 to day 4). This period is marked by a hyperdynamic state (cardiac output reaching 2.0 to 2.5 times normal) if resuscitation efforts have been adequate.

Phase 3: diuretic phase (day 5 to day 7). If the patient has been adequately resuscitated during the first two phases, diuresis occurs on about the fifth to seventh day after the burn. It is not uncommon during this period for the urinary output to exceed 100 ml per hour in the adult. During this phase, the patient's fluid status must be carefully monitored, and it is important not to increase intravenous fluids to compensate for the increased urinary output. During this phase only maintenance fluids are required.

Table 3-1. Indications for hospitalization and referral to a burn center

Hospitalization
Full-thickness burns covering > 2% BSA
Partial-thickness burns exceeding 10% BSA
Any serious burns of the face, hands, or feet
Burns of the perianal or genital areas
Burns that cross flexion creases or are circumferential
Referral to a burn center
Burns that involve > 25% BSA (20% if < 10 or > 40 years old)
Full-thickness burns involving > 10% BSA
All burns of the face, eyes, ears, hands, feet, or perineum
Burns associated with multisystem trauma
High-voltage electrical burns
Suspected inhalation injuries
Lesser burns in patients with significant, preexisting disease

BSA = body surface area.

Many "formulas" for fluid resuscitation of the acutely burned patient have been developed [10–13]. These formulas are not absolute laws but, rather, guidelines from which to *estimate* fluid requirements. These formulas generally base fluid resuscitation requirements on various intravenous solutions, body weight in kilograms, and percent total body surface burn comprising partial-thickness and full-thickness burns. The most commonly used acute burn resuscitation formulas are shown in Table 3-3.

It is beyond the scope of this chapter to elaborate on the pros and cons of each formula. Regardless of the formula utilized, however, it is important to monitor the fluid status constantly. The most accurate indicator of the adequacy of resuscitation is hourly urinary output. In the adult a urinary output of 0.5 ml/kg/hr is ideal; and in the pediatric age group a urinary output of 1 ml/kg/hr is recommended. For more severely burned individuals, the elderly, and patients who do not respond to resuscitative efforts as expected, central venous and possibly Swan-Ganz monitoring are indicated. Escharotomies are indicated in patients with circumferential, deep burns to avoid respiratory or neurovascular compromise (Figure 3-5).

ROUTINE LABORATORY STUDIES

Routine laboratory studies on admission should include a complete blood count with differential, complete chemical profile, and arterial blood gases. These studies often identify electrolyte and metabolic abnormalities induced by the injury or that are present owing to preexisting illnesses or medications. Additionally, a toxicology screen may be helpful for evaluating patients with altered mental status. Chest radiographs should be obtained on admission. Although the lung fields are usually clear at this time, they serve as a good baseline. Routine urinalysis should be performed for every patient to identify possible renal injuries or the myoglobinuria that is commonly seen with electrical and crush injuries.

Table 3-2. Criteria of burn injury severity (American Burn Assocation)

| Severity | Degree and % of BSA | |
	Adults	Children
Minor	Second (< 15)	Second + third (< 10)
	Third (< 2)	
Moderate	Second (15–25)	Second (10–20)
	Third (< 10)	Third (< 10)
Major	Second (> 25)	Second (> 20)
	Third (> 10)	Third (> 10)

Table 3-3. Burn resuscitation formulas

Formula	First 24 hours	Second 24 hours
Brooke	Ringer's lactate	Colloid
	2 ml/% burn/kg	0.3–0.5 ml/% burn/kg
	½ in first 8 hr	
	½ each of next 8 hr	
Parkland	Ringer's lactate	Colloid
	4 ml/% burn/kg	0.3–0.5 cc/% burn/kg
	½ in first 8 hr	
	¼ in each next 8 hr	
Hypertonic solution	300 mEq Na, 200 mEq lactate, 100 mEq Cl; Infused at a rate sufficient to maintain urine output 30 ml/hr	Same combination as for first 24 hours ⅓ to ½ of first 24 hr volume

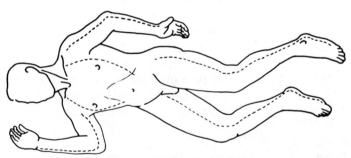

Fig. 3-5. Sites for escharotomy. Escharotomies should be placed so that scar contracture bands are not produced and so that they relieve the constrictive effect of the circumferential burn. (From J. W. Golfarb. The initial management of burn injuries. In: *Masters of Surgery Series.* Research Triangle Park, NC: Galaxo Drug Company, 1985. With permission.)

ELECTRICAL INJURIES

Unlike thermal injuries, where damage at the surface is extensive and internal injuries usually minor, electrical injuries usually present with minimal surface damage and extensive internal injury. The internal injuries resulting from electrical trauma are caused by falls, tonic-clonic contractions, and passage of electrical current along lines of least resistance (blood vessels, nerves, and muscles). In patients with electrical injuries, one must rule out associated injuries of the pneumothorax, perforated viscus, myonecrosis with myoglobinuria, and compartment syndromes.

The diagnosis of myoglobinuria should be entertained upon visualizing port wine or mahogany-colored urine in the high risk patient. The diagnosis may be confirmed in the laboratory. In the event that myoglobinuria occurs, it is best treated by early hydration, alkalinization of the urine with intravenous bicarbonate boluses, and use of mannitol to maintain a urinary output of more than 100 ml per hour. Inadequately treated myoglobinuria may lead to renal failure and anuria.

Electrocardiographic monitoring during the first 24 hours often reveals myocardial infarction or electrically induced malignant dysrhythmias.

FROSTBITE

Frostbite rarely occurs in areas other than the extremities, chin, cheeks, nose, and ears. Injuries similar to frostbite include trench foot and immersion foot. Frostbite, which appears after exposure to temperatures near freezing (10°C), occurs less frequently in acclimatized individuals and less frequently in whites than in blacks. The environmental factors important in determining severity of frostbite include humidity, wind, and immobility of the patient.

Frostbite occurs as freezing between cells begins, causing cellular osmotic dehydration. Eventually this process progresses to intracellular ice crystal formation, arterial constriction, thrombosis, and edema. The severity of the frostbite is proportional to the length of exposure and the temperature gradient. Interestingly, the patient is often unaware of the severity of the injury.

Frostbite injuries, like thermal injuries, are classified according to severity. First degree frostbite presents with edema and erythema without tissue necrosis. Second degree frostbite is manifested by blister formation, which usually occurs within 24 to 36 hours of injury. Third degree frostbite is present with skin necrosis. Fourth degree frostbite presents as gangrene, which requires amputation.

A more clinically useful classification is based on the depth of the cold injury. "Superficial frostbite" is characterized by a white, firm, exterior surface of exposed tissue, with soft underlying tissue. When the affected area is rewarmed, the skin becomes mottled and a burning sensation is experienced. The skin may go on to form blisters.

The more severe form of frostbite is termed "deep frostbite." The superficial tissues are hard to solid, and the deeper tissues cannot be indented by gentle to moderate pressure. Tissue destruction may be complete and involve bone. On rewarming, the tissue is blue to gray, and throbbing pain is experienced. Blisters usually form on days 3 to 7 after exposure, and necrotic tissue generally demarcates after 2 to 3 weeks. Infection increases tissue loss.

The best treatment for frostbite is prevention. It is easily prevented by wearing appropriately insulated, loosely fitting dry clothes and avoiding prolonged immobility in cold environments. If frostbite occurs, the most effective treatment is rapid rewarming by placing the affected part in warm water (40°–44°C). Rewarming is usually complete in about 20 minutes. Care must be taken to avoid higher rewarming temperatures or exposure of the affected limb to open fire or dry heat, as these conditions tend to damage viable tissue.

Once rewarming is complete, the affected part should be elevated to minimize edema and hyperemia. The injury must be protected by a soft, sterile dressing; and antibiotics should be started. Tetanus vaccinations must be updated.

In addition to these measures, sympathectomy performed within the first few days of injury has been found to be of some benefit in reducing tissue loss and late complications of hyperhidrosis, coldness, paresthesias, and vasospasticity. The optimal time for sympathectomy is 36 to 72 hours after exposure; earlier treatment increases edema, and later treatment is ineffective. Although vascular injury with vasospasm and thrombosis is the etiology of tissue loss, the theoretical advantages of heparin and dextran therapy have not been realized in practice.

Viability of affected limbs *cannot* be immediately assessed: it often takes several weeks for demarcation of gangrenous areas to be fully manifested. Moreover, tissue initially thought nonviable may prove viable with time.

Frostbite often presents with hypothermia. The normal body temperature ranges between 36.4° and 37.5°C. Temperatures less than 35°C are defined as hypothermic. The extent of hypothermia can be evaluated only with a low-reading *rectal* thermometer.

The clinical presentation of hypothermia varies with severity. Severe shivering and peripheral cutaneous vasoconstriction manifest at core body temperatures below 35°C. In such cases the patient is alert and oriented, and hypothermia is easily reversed. Severe hypothermia occurs when core body temperature falls below 32°C. The level of consciousness here decreases to obtundation and full stupor. Although blood pressure may not be detectable, strong femoral or carotid pulses are usually present. As the temperature decreases, the pulse slows and respiration becomes irregular and shallow. Profound hypothermia occurs when the core temperature falls below 27°C. Deep coma and muscular rigidity are seen, and pulmonary edema and ventricular dysrhythmia may develop.

Hypothermia must be treated when first recognized. The patient is removed from the cold exposure, all wet garments are removed, and warm blankets are placed until the patient can get to the hospital. Patients with severe, profound hypothermia should have their core temperatures raised. *Note:* Immersion or surface warming causes vasodilatation with return of cool blood to the core, which exacerbates hypothermia.

The most effective way to warm the core body temperatures is through peritoneal dialysis or lavage. It is performed with a peritoneal dialysis catheter, infusing normal sterile saline that has been heated in a blood warmer to 35° to 37°C. Two liters are exchanged every 20 to 30 minutes until the rectal temperature is greater than 30°C. Once this temperature is more than 30°C, a hypothermia blanket can be used. During the rewarming process, intravenous fluid support is necessary to maintain blood pressure, and endotracheal intubation is required to protect against aspiration.

OUTPATIENT CARE

Small burns comprise up to 95 percent of all treated burns in the United States. Most are less than 10 percent of the total body surface area, heal regardless of treatment, and are amenable to outpatient care. Minor burns (based on American Burn Association guidelines) are best treated by outpatient management. Careful patient selection, accurate assessment of the depth and extent of injury, initiation of appropriate simplified therapy, education of the patient, and careful follow-up are the essential elements of effective outpatient burn management.

Patient Selection

Many "nonmedical" factors must be considered prior to considering the patient a candidate for outpatient care. Such factors include the competence level of the patient, the ability of the patient to obtain outpatient supplies, his or her ability to safely and reliably return for follow-up visits, the dedication of the patient to self-treat, and various social factors such as alcohol/drug abuse and family support systems. The nonmedical factors must be evaluated thoroughly, and it is here that social service consultation can be helpful.

Assessment of Burn Extent

Ideally, only patients with partial-thickness burns are considered candidates for outpatient management. Burns should not involve the face, hands, feet, or perineum [14]. Wounds covering up to approximately 10 percent of the total body surface area in the healthy adult or toddler, who has undergone proper patient selection, may be safely managed on an outpatient basis.

Treatment

Treatment begins in the office. The patient is made comfortable with mild analgesics, when indicated, and reassured. The wound is débrided using clean but not necessarily sterile instruments. Small blisters or bullae are left intact, and large bullae are unroofed using scissors; any coagulum under the blisters is gently rinsed away with warm tap water. Nonviable tissue may be débrided by gentle scrubbing with gauze or surgical instruments. The burn is then washed with a gentle hand soap and tap water, gently blotted dry, and a topical agent such as silver sulfadiazine cream applied (Table 3-4). For patients allergic to silver sulfadiazine, another topical agent such as a polysporin may be used. Polysporin or neomycin is preferred for facial burns. Following such topical application, the

Table 3-4. Commonly used topical antimicrobial burn wound agents

Sulfamylon (mafenide acetate cream)
    Advantage: penetrates eschar; wound is readily visible; no gram-resistance identified, compatible with other therapies and joint motion
    Disadvantages: Painful for 20–30 minutes after application to second degree burns; delays spontaneous eschar separation; 7% hypersensitivity reactions
Silvadene (silver sulfadiazine cream)
    Advantage: painless application; wound is readily visible; compatible with other therapies and joint motion
    Disadvantage: poor penetration of eschar; gram-resistance occurs, bone marrow suppression with neutropenia, hypersensitivity reported

wound is dressed with a nonsterile gauze dressing that is secured in place by either a circular gauze wrap or gauze netting.

Instruction on dressing changes is given to the patient or the patient's home caregiver, one of whom must show competence with dressing changes prior to the patient's discharge. On discharge, the patient is instructed to carry out the dressing changes twice a day. Additionally, procedures that complicate the dressing change are eliminated in order to ensure optimal patient cooperation.

Antibiotic prophylaxis is not indicated, but tetanus prophylaxis is updated. Analgesia with codeine is occasionally prescribed where indicated. On discharge, a step-by-step instruction sheet should be provided to the patient.

Education

Once the patient has demonstrated proficiency and competence with dressing changes, he or she is further educated on trouble signs. The patient is instructed to call immediately if the wound becomes red, hot, or tender, or if it develops a discharge. The patient is further instructed to call immediately should a fever or chills develop. These instructions should also be included on the dressing change information sheet.

Follow-up

Because of the dynamic nature of the burn injury, adequate and frequent follow-up is perhaps the most essential consideration of outpatient burn management. Patients initially seen in the emergency department or office are instructed to return the next day, regardless of weekends or holidays, to confirm the diagnosis of partial-thickness injury. The immediate follow-up is also an excellent means of testing patient cooperation. After this initial visit, the next one is scheduled based on the patient's ability to comply with the treatment protocol, the level of anxiety, and the appearance of the wound. On average, wound healing is accomplished within 8 or 9 days and requires an average of three office visits. Only about 2 percent of the patient population requires admission to hospital, usually for cellulitis [15]. The patient should be seen in the office frequently until wound closure is evident and less frequently until wound healing is complete. The need for pressure garments to prevent hypertrophic scar formation is assessed during these outpatient visits.

Comment

Using these criteria, almost all small burns can be managed on an outpatient basis. The cornerstone of management is use of a simplified dressing technique and adequate and reliable follow-up. Proper patient selection is of paramount importance to ensure compliance with the recommended procedures. Thus identification of patients who are candidates for outpatient management coupled with implementation of an effective dressing technique and reliable follow-up can eliminate the unnecessary expense of hospitalization for a large number of burn patients.

AREAS OF SPECIAL CONSIDERATION

Face

Superficial burns on the face may be treated with lanolin or aloe cream. Lips may be treated with petroleum ointment or bacitracin cream to prevent cracking.

Eyes

Fluorescein evaluation of the eyes is necessary to rule out corneal injury. If injury is present or any ophthalmologic abnormalities are noted, a consultation with an ophthalmologic surgeon must be obtained within 24 hours.

Ears

The ears must be protected from the dread complication of chondritis. Protection is best accomplished with mafenide acetate cream applied generously. For ears with totally denuded cartilage, early soft tissue coverage with local temporo-parietal or subgaleal fascial flaps is necessary.

Extremities

Elevation of the extremity for the first 48 to 72 hours is necessary to minimize edema. Bulky hand dressings and splinting in the position of function are necessary. Careful observation for compartment syndrome is essential. Circumferential burns should be closely evaluated; and if the burns are deeper than partial thickness, the patient should be hospitalized for observation. A pressure garment (e.g., Jobst garment) appropriately fitted and applied after the edema subsides assists in ambulation and minimizes hypertrophic scar formation.

REFERENCES

1. May, H. L. (ed.), *Emergency Medicine.* New York: Wiley, 1984.
2. Curreri, P. W., and Luterman, A. In S. I. Schwartz et al. (eds.), *Principles of Surgery,* 5th ed. New York: McGraw-Hill, 1989. Pp. 285–305.
3. Boswick, J. A. Clinical symposium on burns. *Surg. Clin. North Am.* 58:6, 1978.
4. Bloom, W., and Fawcett, D. W. *A Textbook of Histology.* Philadelphia: Saunders, 1975.

5. Wheater, P. R., Burkitt, H. G., and Daniels, V. G. *Functional Histology: A Text and Color Atlas*. Edinburgh: Churchill Livingstone, 1979. Pp. 116–127.

6. Leeson, R. C., and Leeson, T. S. *Histology*, 3rd ed. Philadelphia: Saunders, 1976. Pp. 93–106.

7. Sauer, G. C. *Manual of Skin Diseases*, 4th ed. Philadelphia: Lippincott, 1980. Pp. 1–5.

8. McIntyre, K. M., and Lewis, A. J. (eds.), *Textbook of Advanced Cardiac Life Support*. New York: American Heart Association, 1981.

9. Gaisford, J. C., Slater, H., and Goldfarb, I. W. *The Management of Burn Trauma. A Unified Approach*. Pittsburgh: Synapse Publications, 1983.

10. Evans, E. I. The early management of the severely burned patient. *Surg. Gynecol. Obstet.* 94:274, 1952.

11. Evans, E. I., et al. Fluid and electrolytes requirements in severe burns. *Ann. Surg.* 134:804, 1951.

12. Artz, C. P., Moncrief, J. A., and Pruitt, B. A., Jr. (eds.), *Burns — A Team Approach*. Philadelphia: Saunders, 1979.

13. Monafo, W. W., Chuntrasakul, C., and Ayvazianvh, V. H. Hypertonic sodium solutions in the treatment of burn shock. *Am. J. Surg.* 126:778, 1973.

14. Archauer, B. M. *Management of the Burned Patient*, Vol. 1. Norwalk, CT: Appleton & Lange, 1987. Pp. 15–16.

15. Kauric, B. M., Goldfarb, I. W., and Slater, H. S. *Outpatient Mangement of Small Total Body Surface Burns*. Pittsburgh: Synapse Publications, 1988.

Commentary on Chapter 3

Harvey Slater
I. William Goldfarb

Advances in the management of patients with burns have presented new opportunities and new challenges to the physician caring for these patients. Our experience in managing more than 3500 burn patients has led us to a more aggressive approach for patients with full-thickness burns and a simplified approach for outpatient management.

The resuscitation of patients with moderate and even extensive burn injuries is usually straightforward and successful. Various formulas that predict the quantity of intravenous fluids likely to be required during the first 24 hours are helpful guides to resuscitation. The treating physician must understand that the formulas are estimates and do not predict absolute quantities of the intravenous fluids to be delivered regardless of the patient's response.

We have had equal success using the Parkland (Baxter) formula and various modifications of the Brooke formula. The important concept is that the initial intravenous infusion rate may be calculated from these formulas.

The subsequent rate of infusion should be varied on an hourly basis using urine output as a guide to adequacy of resuscitation. Unfortunately, a subgroup of burn patients continues to be a major problem in regard to early resuscitation. Patients with extensive and deep full-thickness burns often require massive infusions of fluid, which are followed by severe edema and weight gain. Weight gain following resuscitation is often a reliable predictor of mortality: the greater the weight gain the greater the chance of the patient dying during the early phase of treatment.

Smoke inhalation complicating extensive burns dramatically increases the fluid requirements for resuscitation. The use of isotonic crystalloid solution in such patients is often unsuccessful and may be undesirable. We and others have had some success with the use of hypertonic crystalloid solutions, and we have been impressed with the use of fresh frozen plasma to augment resuscitation in patients with massive burns.

The role of various solutions in such patients is still to be determined. In patients with extensive and deep burns complicated by smoke inhalation, the Swan-Ganz catheter may be a valuable adjunct to resuscitation. This technique provides information that allows the treating physician to deliver with confidence what appear to be unreasonably large amounts of intravenous fluid.

We have found that early excision with wound closure decreases the length of hospitalization and decreases joint immobility, and we believe that it decreases mortality following burns. After excision of eschar, the wounds should be covered with a split-thickness skin graft. It is our practice to make excision of nonviable tissue a priority, with considerations for wound coverage a secondary issue. When it is not practical to apply an autograft immediately, the wound may be safely treated with various synthetic covers, cadaver skin, or composite dressings (that will soon be available). A permanent replacement for the patient's own skin will be a great advance in the management of burn patients, but unfortunately such material is not available at this time.

Nutritional support for critically injured patients is a well established treatment modality. High calorie–high protein tube feedings may be started within 24 hours of hospital admission in many burn patients. This method is a safe and economical alternative to intravenous nutrition. The establishment of intral nutrition early in the patient's course preserves the integrity of the gut mucosa, provides adequate calories and protein, and may diminish the incidence and severity of sepsis. All critical care modalities, e.g., monitoring cardiac and respiratory function, sophisticated monitoring of renal function, and pharmacologic support for blood pressure and cardiac output, should be used when indicated.

Careful attention must be paid to intraoperative blood and blood component replacement. Burn patients undergoing extensive excisions can become dangerously hypothermic. Careful monitoring of the patient's body temperature and the provision of a warmed operating environment are important to prevent this problem.

Successful management of burn patients is greatly enhanced by close collaboration with an anesthesia department whose staff members are both skilled and interested in the management of such patients. An anesthesiologist can be of great assistance by providing various pain control techniques for patients undergoing burn treatment.

We have simplified our approach to the outpatient management of burns over the years and thereby obtained increased patient cooperation and decreased morbidity and disability. The selection of patients who are able to follow instructions and participate in their own care is more important than the specific choice of agents used to treat their injuries.

We believe that health care professionals should demonstrate wound care to the patient by mimicking as closely as possible the conditions under which the patients must work in their homes. The unnecessary use of surgical instruments and the use of the elaborate and often unnecessary drapes and gowns have often frightened our patients and have resulted in resistance to outpatient management. We believe that the use of soap and water is the fundamental key to successful outpatient management. We prefer the use of silver sulfadiazene cream and gauze dressings to the use of occlusive adherent dressings. This simplified approach involves the patients in their own care from the beginning, and they may be monitored with intermittent office visits as the wound heals. We do not use whirlpool treatments or other physical therapy techniques early in management. Our experience has been that such treatment increases patient dependency and delays their return to function.

A rational approach to the management of burn patients should result in optimum restoration of both form and function. Follow-up should be sufficiently long that hypertrophy and contracture of scarred areas do not occur. When this potential is recognized, the use of pressure garments and special splints may be indicated.

The physician caring for burn patients must understand the dynamics of wound healing so that treatment is both rational and effective.

II HAND AND UPPER EXTREMITY

4 BASIC EVALUATION OF UPPER EXTREMITY INJURY

Richard J. Greco

When evaluating an upper extremity injury it is well to remember a quote from Sterling Bunnel, "Next to the brain, the hand is the greatest asset to man, and to it is due the development of Man's handiwork."

The most important factors in the prognosis of a serious injury of the upper extremity include the initial evaluation and the acute management of these injuries. Although hand injuries are obvious and often disfiguring, rarely are they fatal. It is imperative that the patient be completely assessed by a physician adequately trained in traumatology and that management of the injuries be carried out with the appropriate priorities in mind.

ANATOMY

A broad overview of the anatomy is offered here, but the reader is referred to subsequent chapters for more detailed descriptions of each functional system of the hand.

Skin

Characteristics specific to the hand include a dorsal skin that is thin, pliable, and elastic and that allows wrist and digit flexion and extension as well as tendon gliding. The volar skin is much thicker, irregular, and hairless and is adherent to the underlying palmar fascia, providing traction for pinch and grasp and wearability to the palmar skin.

Vascular Supply

The vascular supply to the upper extremity is based on the axillary artery and its continuation in the arm, the branchial artery. The branchial artery courses along the medial intermuscular septum between the biceps and triceps muscles to enter the antecubital fossa medial to the bicipital aponeurosis. The major branches of the branchial artery include the profunda branchi, superior and inferior ulnar collateral, and biceps myocutaneous arteries, as well as direct cutaneous perforators (Fig. 4-1). The artery ends by dividing into the radial and ulnar arteries 1 cm distal to the elbow joint (Fig. 4-2).

The radial artery courses laterally over the tendon of the biceps muscle, the body of the supinator and pronator teres muscles, and

59

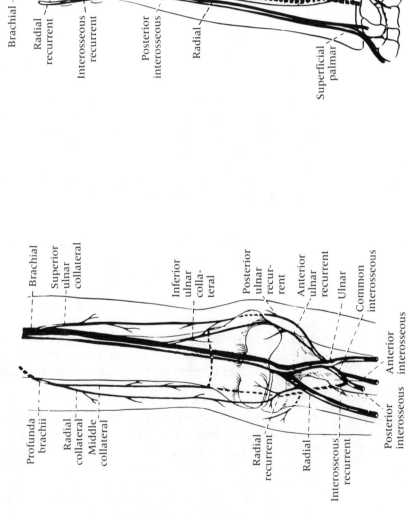

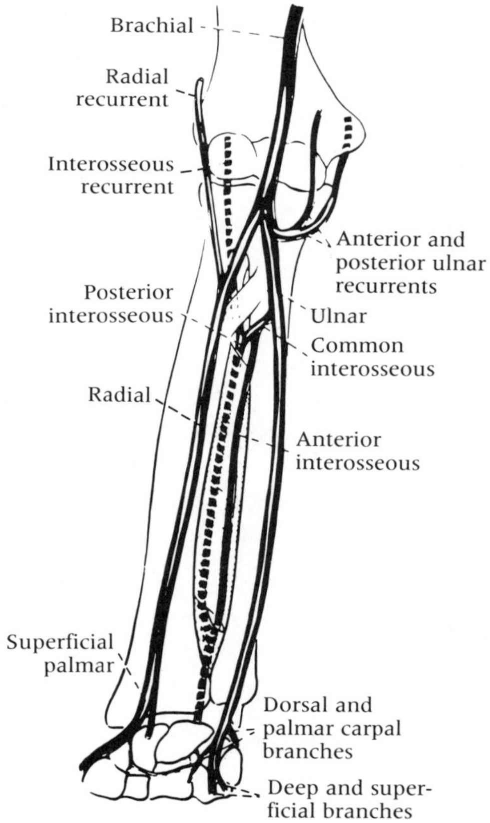

Fig. 4-2. Division of branchial artery in the forearm. (From W. H. Hollinshead et al. *Textbook of Anatomy*, 4th ed. Philadelphia: Lippincott, 1985. With permission.)

Fig. 4-1. Major branches of the branchial artery. (From W. H. Hollinshead et al. *Textbook of Anatomy*, 4th ed. Philadelphia: Lippincott, 1985. With permission.)

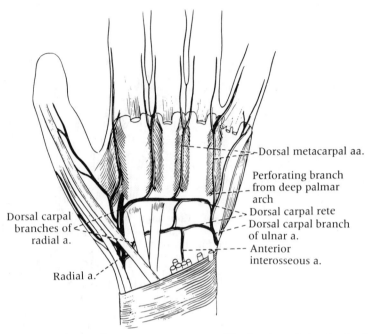

Fig. 4-3. Dorsal carpal rete. (From W. H. Hollinshead et al. *Textbook of Anatomy*, 4th ed. Philadelphia: Lippincott, 1985. With permission.)

over the fascia of the flexor digitorum superficiales muscles. The artery courses down the forearm between the flexor carpi radialis and branchioradialis to the level of the wrist. At the wrist it turns radially and dorsally underneath the abductor pollicis longus and extensor pollicis brevis. After traversing the "anatomic snuffbox," the radial artery courses underneath the extensor pollicis longus onto the dorsum of the hand. The dorsal carpal branches of the radial artery unite with a similar contribution from the ulnar artery and branches from the interosseous arteries to form a dorsal carpal rete, which supplies the dorsal skin and dorsal metacarpal arteries (Fig. 4-3).

The radial artery also gives off a large deep branch that travels volarly between the two heads of the first dorsal interossei and divides into the princeps pollicis and the deep palmar arch (Fig. 4-4).

The ulnar artery is the larger branch of the branchial artery and courses medially underneath the median nerve and the two heads of the flexor digitorum superficialis. The main artery then travels between the flexor digitorum profundus and the flexor carpi ulnaris until the level of the wrist. Near the wrist the ulnar artery appears central to the flexor carpi ulnaris, and it traverses the transverse carpal ligament with the ulnar nerve. At the base of the hypothenar musculature, the vessel divides into a deep and a superficial arch of the hand.

The ulnar recurrent artery branches from the ulnar artery at the level of the flexor digitorum superficialis origin (Fig. 4-2), and the

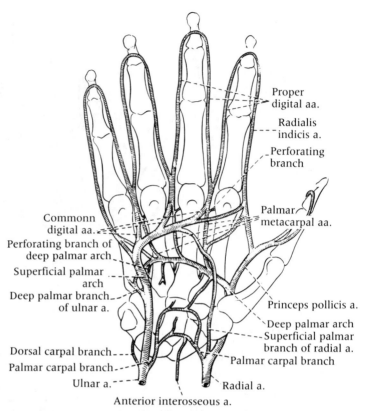

Proper
digital aa.

Radialis
indicis a.

Perforating
branch

Palmar
metacarpal aa.

Commonn
digital aa.

Perforating branch of
deep palmar arch

Superficial palmar
arch

Deep palmar branch
of ulnar a.

Princeps pollicis a.

Deep palmar arch
Superficial palmar
branch of radial a.

Palmar carpal branch

Dorsal carpal branch

Palmar carpal branch

Ulnar a.

Radial a.

Anterior interosseous a.

Fig. 4-4. Arterial anatomy of the palm. (From W. H. Hollinshead et al. *Textbook of Anatomy,* 4th ed. Philadelphia: Lippincott, 1985. With permission.)

common interosseous artery arises deep to the pronator teres and divides into the anterior and posterior interosseous arteries. The posterior interosseous artery traverses the interosseous membrane to supply the dorsal extensor compartment.

The superficial palmar arch is the continuation of the ulnar artery that crossed the transverse carpal ligament and is completed by the superficial branch of the radial artery (Fig. 4-4). It crosses the palm above the flexor tendons and common digital nerves but underneath the palmar fascia. This arch provides a palmar digital branch to the ulnar side of the ring finger, three common digital arteries, and a branch to the thumb web space. The common digital arteries divide into proper digital arteries for adjacent digits and travel volar and then dorsal to the digital nerves.

Nerves

Branchial Plexus
The branchial plexus arises from the rootlets of C5 to C8 and T1 with occasional contributions from C4 and T2 (Fig. 4-5). The upper, middle, and lower nerve trunks arise from the roots of the spinal cord and travel in close association with the subclavian vessels. At a

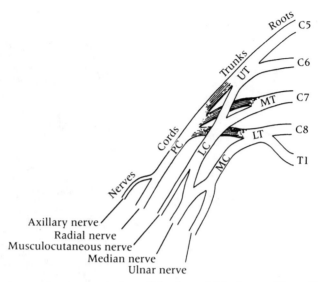

Fig. 4-5. Anatomic representation of the branchial plexus. (From W. W. Shaw and D. A. Hidalgo. *Microsurgery in Trauma.* Mount Kisco, NY: Futura, 1987. With permission.)

point just distal to the clavicle, the trunks intermingle to form the posterior, lateral, and medial cords; and subsequently these structures divide into the major peripheral nerves of the upper extremity.

The posterior cord gives rise to the axillary and radial nerves. The lateral cord gives rise to the musculocutaneous nerve and contributes to the median nerve. The medial cord contributes to the median nerve and forms the ulnar nerve. Thus the median, ulnar, and musculocutaneous nerves are susceptible in a penetrating injury because of their superficial position; the axillary and radial nerves are commonly injured during shoulder dislocation.

The axillary nerve provides motor innervation to the deltoid muscle and sensation to the posterior aspect of the shoulder. The musculocutaneous nerve innervates the coracobranchialis, biceps branchi, and branchialis muscles and supplies sensation to the proximal, radial portion of the forearm.

Median Nerve
The median nerve is the principal motor and sensory unit of the upper extremity. It originates from the lateral and medial cords of the branchial plexus and is paired with the branchial artery in the upper arm. There are no motor or sensory branches in the arm, and the median nerve enters the forearm between the two heads of the pronator teres muscle (Fig. 4-6).

The median nerve courses on the inferior surface of the flexor digitorum superficialis muscle belly and gives off direct motor

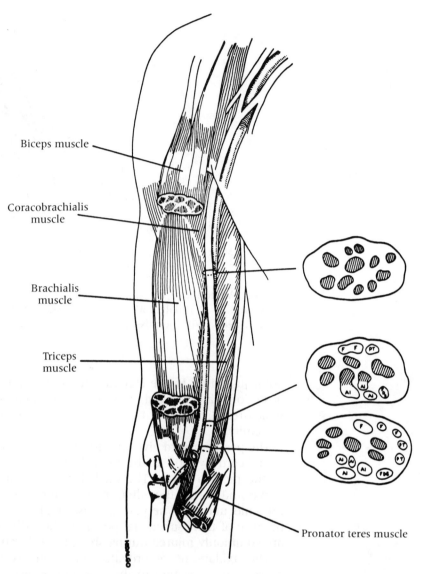

Biceps muscle

Coracobrachialis
muscle

Brachialis
muscle

Triceps
muscle

Pronator teres muscle

Fig. 4-6. Median nerve, upper arm. (From W. W. Shaw and D. A. Hidalgo. *Microsurgery in Trauma.* Mount Kisco, NY: Futura, 1987. With permission.)

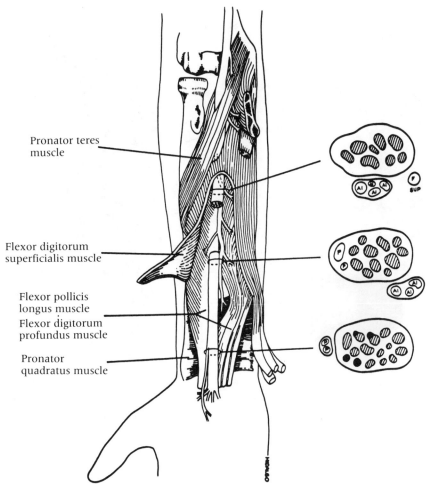

Pronator teres
muscle

Flexor digitorum
superficialis muscle

Flexor pollicis
longus muscle

Flexor digitorum
profundus muscle

Pronator
quadratus muscle

Fig. 4-7. Median nerve; forearm. (From W. W. Shaw and D. A. Hidalgo.
Microsurgery in Trauma. Mount Kisco, NY: Futura, 1987. With
permission.)

branches to the pronator teres, flexor carpi radialis, flexor digitorum
superficialis, and palmaris longus. The anterior interosseous branch
forms at the level of the elbow and runs on the volar surface of the
interosseus membrane. It innervates the flexor digitorum profundus
to the index and long fingers, the flexor pollicus longus, and
pronator quadratus (Fig. 4-7).

In the distal forearm, the median nerve travels under the tendon of
the palmaris longus and the transverse carpal ligament. In the hand,
the nerve provides motor innervation to the muscles of the thenar
eminence and the first and second lumbricales. The palmar cutaneous sensory branch begins in the distal forearm and supplies
sensation to the palmar and thenar eminence (Fig. 4-7).

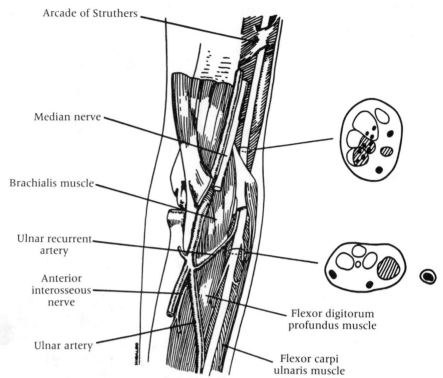

Fig. 4-8. Ulnar nerve, elbow. (From W. W. Shaw and D. A. Hidalgo. *Microsurgery in Trauma.* Mount Kisco, NY: Futura, 1987. With permission.)

Ulnar Nerve

The ulnar nerve originates from the medial cord of the branchial plexus and travels along the medial aspect of the arm. The medial antebranchial cutaneous nerve arises at the mid-arm level and supplies sensation to the medial arm and forearm. The ulnar nerve enters the forearm between the two heads of the flexor carpi ulnaris (FCU) and gives off its first motor branches, which supply the FCU (Fig. 4-8).

The ulnar nerve continues through the forearm in a plane between the FCU and the flexor digitorum profundus (FDP) muscle units. Motor branches are supplied to the FCU and the FDP muscles of the ring and little fingers en route to the hand.

At the wrist, a dorsal ulnar sensory branch arises before the ulnar nerve traverses Guyon's canal (Fig. 4-9). The nerve then separates into superficial sensory digital nerves and a deep motor branch to the hypothenar muscles, third and fourth lumbricales, all palmar and dorsal interossei, adductor pollicis, and the deep head of the flexor pollicis brevis.

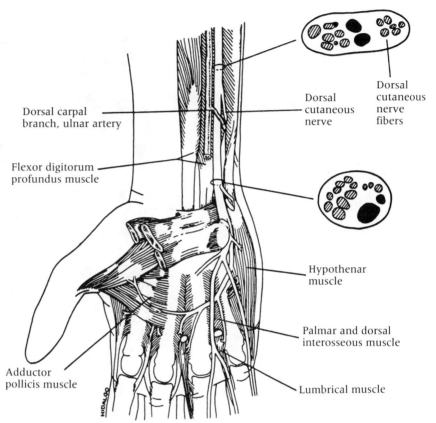

Dorsal carpal
branch, ulnar artery

Flexor digitorum
profundus muscle

Dorsal
cutaneous
nerve

Dorsal
cutaneous
nerve
fibers

Hypothenar
muscle

Palmar and dorsal
interosseous muscle

Adductor
pollicis muscle

Lumbrical muscle

Fig. 4-9. Ulnar nerve at the wrist. (From W. W. Shaw and D. A. Hidalgo. *Microsurgery in Trauma.* Mount Kisco, NY: Futura, 1987. With permission.)

Radial Nerve

The radial nerve originates from the posterior cord of the branchial plexus. It begins medial to the triceps and travels posteriorly through the muscle and behind the shaft of the humerus. The nerve then courses anteromedially between the branchialis and branchioradialis over the lateral epicondyle (Fig. 4-10). In the arm it innervates the teres major, deltoid, triceps, brachioradialis, aconeus, and extensor carpi radialis longus (ECRL).

Just distal to the lateral epicondyle, the main nerve divides into two branches. The superficial branch innervates the ECRL and the extensor carpi radialis brevis (ECRB) and provides radial sensation to the hand. The deep branch, the posterior interossei nerve, runs through the two heads of the supinator underneath the arcade of Forshe and innervates the supinator, extensor digitorum, extensor digiti minimi, extensor carpi ulnaris, extensor pollicis longus, abductor pollicis longus, extensor pollicis brevis, and extensor indicis.

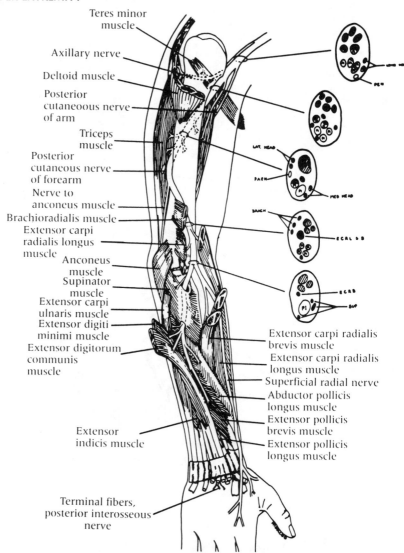

Teres minor
muscle

Axillary nerve

Deltoid muscle

Posterior
cutaneoous nerve
of arm

Triceps
muscle

Posterior
cutaneous nerve
of forearm

Nerve to
anconeus muscle

Brachioradialis muscle

Extensor carpi
radialis longus
muscle

Anconeus
muscle

Supinator
muscle

Extensor carpi
ulnaris muscle

Extensor digiti
minimi muscle

Extensor digitorum
communis
muscle

Extensor
indicis muscle

Extensor carpi radialis
brevis muscle

Extensor carpi radialis
longus muscle

Superficial radial nerve

Abductor pollicis
longus muscle

Extensor pollicis
brevis muscle

Extensor pollicis
longus muscle

Terminal fibers,
posterior interosseous
nerve

Fig. 4-10. Radial nerve, overview. (From W. W. Shaw and D. A. Hidalgo.
Microsurgery in Trauma. Mount Kisco, NY: Futura, 1987. With
permission.)

Digital Nerves

The common digital nerves, purely sensory, arise from the median
and ulnar nerves (Fig. 4-11). They course underneath the palmar
fascia and give rise to the individual digital nerves of the fingers.

The median nerve gives rise to four branches that supply innervation to the thumb, index and middle fingers, and the radial aspect
of the ring finger. The ulnar nerve gives rise to two branches that
supply innervation to the little finger and the ulnar aspect of the ring
finger.

Digital nerves lie in the palmar aspect of the hand (Fig 4-12). In
the digit, the nerve is intimately associated with the digital artery and
is bordered by Cleland's ligament and the digital artery dorsally and

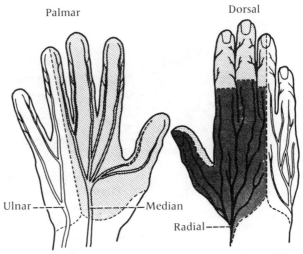

Fig. 4-11. Distribution of major nerve sensory innervation of the hand. (From American Society of the Hand. *The Hand: Examination and Diagnosis,* 2nd ed. New York: Churchill Livingstone, 1983. With permission.)

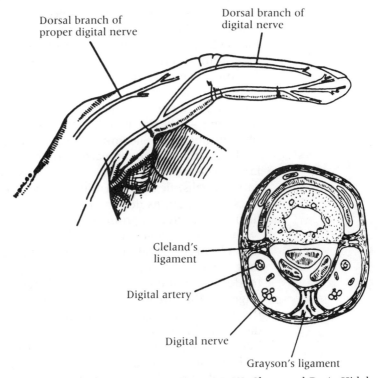

Fig. 4-12. Digital nerve anatomy. (From W. W. Shaw and D. A. Hidalgo. *Microsurgery in Trauma.* Mount Kisco, NY: Futura, 1987. With permission.)

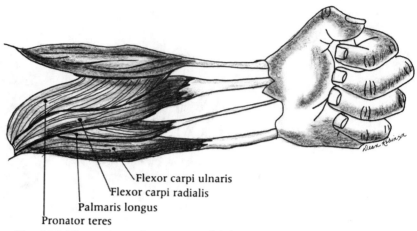

Flexor carpi ulnaris
Flexor carpi radialis
Palmaris longus
Pronator teres

Fig. 4-13. Flexor musculature, superficial group.

Grayson's ligament volarly. At the level of the distal interphalangeal (DIP) joint, the digital nerve terminates into three branches: nail bed, tip, and pulp.

Muscles

Volar Compartment

The flexor system comprises muscle bellies originating in the proximal two-thirds of the volar compartment of the forearm and tendinous extensions that insert into the wrist or digits. There are two tendons for each finger and one for the thumb. In the fingers, the flexor digitorum superficialis inserts into the middle phalanx and creates flexion at the proximal interphalangeal (PIP) joint. The flexor digitorum profundus inserts into the distal phalanx and flexes the DIP joint of the respective finger. There is only one long flexor tendon to the thumb — the flexor pollicis longus — and it inserts into the distal phalanx and causes flexion of the interphalangeal joint of the thumb.

The anatomy of the forearm can be best understood if viewed in layers. The most superficial layer contains the palmaris longus, flexor carpi radialis, flexor carpi ulnaris, and pronator teres (Fig. 4-13). These muscle units do not cross the wrist but are involved in wrist flexion and forearm pronation.

The second layer contains the flexor digitorum superficialis, which arises from two heads and separates into four tendons. The ring and long finger arise from the more superficial muscle belly, and the tendons are more superficial than the tendons of the index and little fingers in the carpal canal (Fig. 4-14). After exiting the carpal canal, the tendons diverge to their respective digits volar to the flexor digitorum profundus (FDP) tendon. The tendon flattens and splits into two slips, which encompass the FDP tendon, pass dorsal to it, and reunite to form a bed for the FDP tendon until it inserts in the proximal one-half of the middle phalanx. This area of division is commonly called the "chiasma of Camper."

The third layer of the forearm consists of the flexor digitorum

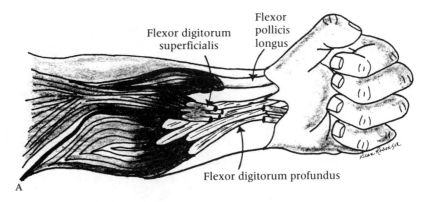

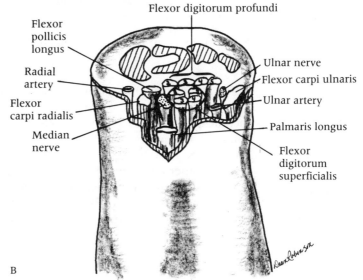

Fig. 4-14. A. Flexor musculature, middle and deep groups. *B.* Cross-sectional anatomy of the wrist.

profundus and the flexor pollicis longus. The conjoined FDP muscle mass separates into four tendons that course dorsal to the flexor digitorum superficialis tendon and penetrate it at the chiasma of Camper; it then inserts at the base of the distal phalanx. The flexor pollicis longus is located in the radial aspect of the carpal canal, travels through the thenar muscles in a fibroosseous canal, and inserts in the distal phalanx of the thumb.

The fourth and deepest layer of the volar forearm contains the pronator quadratus and is not usually important for acute tendon repairs.

Dorsal Forearm Compartment

The "extrinsic system" of the extensor system comprises muscle bellies originating in the proximal two-thirds of the dorsal compartment of the forearm and their tendonous extensions that insert into the wrist or digits. The tendons gain entrance to the hand through a series of fibroosseous canals overlying the wrist and are covered by the extensor retinaculum.

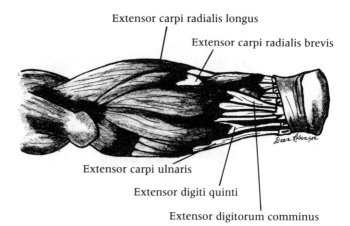

Extensor carpi radialis longus

Extensor carpi radialis brevis

Extensor carpi ulnaris

Extensor digiti quinti

Extensor digitorum comminus

Fig. 4-15. Extensor musculature, superficial group.

The "extrinsic" extensor tendons can be divided into the "superficial" and "deep" muscle groups. The "superficial" group includes the wrist extensors (ECRB, ERCL, extensor carpi ulnaris), common finger extensors (extensor digiti), and the extensor digiti minimi and arise from the distal humerus and the lateral epicondyle of the humerus. The "deep" muscle group includes the extensor pollicis longus and brevis, (EPL, EPB), abductor pollicis longus (APL), extensor indicis (EI), and supinator muscles. The supinator arises from the humerus, and the EPL, EPB, EI, and APL originate from the radius, ulna, and interosseous membrane (Figs. 4-15 and 4-16).

The deep fascia of the extensor surface of the forearm is thick over the wrist joint and forms the extensor retinaculum. Vertical septa from this dorsal carpal ligament connect to the radius and ulna creating six fibroosseous canals (Fig. 4-17). These fascial constraints contain the extensor tendons and their synovial sheaths. The retinaculum functions to prevent bowstringing of the tendons across the wrist. The first compartment contains the abductor pollicis longus and extensor pollicis brevis, the second the ERCB and ECRL, the third the extensor pollicis longus, the fourth the extensor digiti and indicis, the fifth the extensor digiti minimi, and the sixth the extensor carpi ulnaris.

Intrinsic System

The four dorsal interossei muscles are the abductors of the fingers and are centered around the axis of the middle finger (Fig. 4-18). The three volar interossei muscles are adductors of the fingers around the same axis of the middle finger. They cause flexion and adduction of the proximal phalanx and extend the PIP and DIP joints. The interossei muscles are usually innervated by the ulnar nerve. The lumbrical muscles arise from the profundus tendons in the palm, pass volar to the transverse metacarpal ligament, and join the radial lateral bands at the middle of the proximal phalanx. They

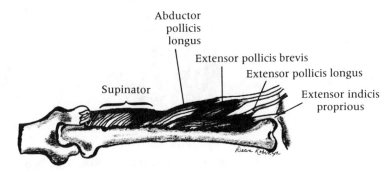

Fig. 4-16. Extensor musculature, deep group.

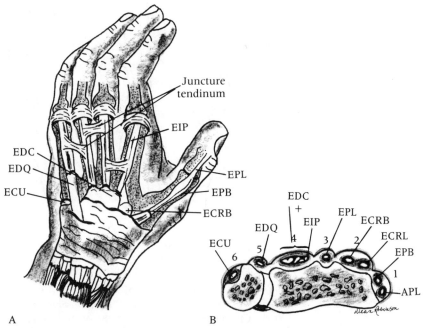

A   B

Fig. 4-17. A. Extensor retinaculum consist of six fibroosseous canals and helps prevent bowstringing. *B.* Cross-sectional area of the retinaculum at the level of the wrist.

cause flexion at the metacarpophalangeal (MCP) joint and extension at the PIP and DIP joints.

Bones and Joints

The skeleton of the hand consists of 27 bones that can be grouped into three main categories: 8 carpal, 5 metacarpal, and 14 phalangeal bones (Fig. 4-19). Each digit has one metacarpal and three phalangeal bones, except the thumb, which has two phalanges.

Carpal Bones
The carpus is composed of two rows: (1) the proximal row, composed of the scaphoid, lunate, triquetrum, and pisiform bones;

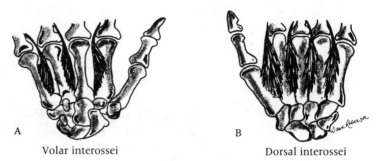

A   B
Volar interossei   Dorsal interossei

Fig. 4-18. A. Three palmar interossei. *B.* Four dorsal interossei.

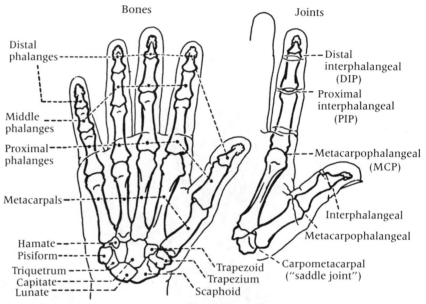

Fig. 4-19. Osseous skeleton of the hand and wrist. (From American Society of the Hand. *The Hand: Examination and Diagnosis,* 2nd ed. New York: Churchill Livingstone, 1978. With permission.)

and (2) the distal row, composed of the trapezium, trapezoid, capitate, and hamate. The carpal bones are covered by cartilage over most of their surfaces but have roughened areas on the volar and dorsal surfaces for ligamentous attachments and vascular pedicles. Wrist flexion and extension, as well as radial and ulnar deviation, are created by intercarpal and radiocarpal motion.

Metacarpal Bones

Each digit has a metacarpal bone that connects the digits to the wrist. The index and long finger metacarpals are firmly attached to the distal carpal row and form the "fixed" unit of the hand. Digital and hand motions are centered around this "fixed" segment. The metacarpals to the thumb, ring, and little fingers are part of the "mobile" unit and are suspended by ligaments to this unit.

Phalangeal Bones
Each finger, except the thumb, is composed of three phalangeal bones: proximal, middle, and distal. The thumb has only a proximal and a distal phalanx.

EVALUATION

The primary goals of the emergency room evaluation are to accomplish the following.

1. To evaluate comprehensively and precisely the structures injured
2. To determine if the patient's intervention requires the facilities of an operating room
3. To determine whether the patient's injury must be dealt with immediately or semielectively
4. To offer the patient information regarding the severity of the injury, short- and long-term management goals, and the expected long-term prognosis
5. To offer the patient and family assurance that the injury is being dealt with by an experienced and competent surgeon

After introducing yourself to the patient, a comprehensive history concerning the significant points related to the hand injury and an abbreviated general medical history are obtained from the patient while exposing and examining the extremity. Asking the patient how the hand was injured usually elicits a general statement about the mechanism of injury, the part of the extremity injured, and the time of occurrence. It is important to ask specific questions until the injury is completely understood.

1. *When?* How much time has elapsed since the injury? Relative contamination is usually low during the first 6 hours after injury, the "golden period." After this time, the growth of staphylococci in the wound is exponential. Muscle ischemia becomes more irreversible as the ischemia time approaches 6 hours, and the edema of the hand increases with passage of time after the injury.
2. *Where?* What was the environment like at the site of the injury? Was the patient working in a manure pile or in a sterile environment? What is the expected level of contamination, and what are the most likely organisms?
3. *How?* Was the mechanism of injury crushing or tearing, or was it a clean laceration? What was the position of the hand when the injury occurred? Was there an associated thermal injury? How traumatized is the remaining skin and soft tissue?
4. *Treatment given?* What type of first aid has been received thus far, and how have the amputated parts been preserved? Did the referring institution irrigate the wound? Is the patient's tetanus immunization up to date? Was a tourniquet placed? The less time the tissue is ischemic or contaminated, the better are the chances the patient will heal uneventfully.

5. *Other injuries?* Remember — rarely is an upper extremity injury life-threatening, but frequently it is the most obvious injury. Ensure that the patient is adequately evaluated for multisystem injury by a qualified professional. Successful replantation of a digit on a patient who dies of internal bleeding is less than desirable!

A brief general medical history should be obtained to guide the choice of anesthetic and offer necessary medical support. A history of diabetes mellitus, seizures, immunosuppression, steroid support, and drug allergies should be elicited and appropriate precautions taken.

It is important to remove all jewelry, tourniquets, and constricting clothing from the involved extremity. If it is determined that the patient requires the services of the operating room, exposing the injury completely in the emergency room can be avoided. Thus patients with substantial crush or explosion injuries need not be exposed to the pain and possible contamination associated with emergency room inspection. Motion, sensation, and vascularity can usually be accurately evaluated without removing the entire dressing. The outer dressings are trimmed down, and inner dressings are soaked off if necessary. Hydrogen peroxide may be helpful for loosening coagulated blood. No harmful detergent or astringent should be used on the wounds.

Once the extremity is exposed and placed on sterile towels, it is thoroughly evaluated. Inspection of the injured extremity can give the examiner a general overview of the extent of the injury and the extremity's vascular status. Obvious fractures, soft tissue losses, and the color and temperature of the extremity are noted. The neurologic status, presence or absence of tendon function, and range of motion of the joints are recorded. The degree of contamination and crush is ascertained, and radiographic evaluation for fractures is performed.

Except for superficial wounds, probing the wound in the emergency room is ill-advised. Most decisions on the need for operative exploration can be based on the results of a thorough physical examination. The risk of contamination and the pain associated with probing are usually not warranted.

Radiographs should be obtained for all but the most trivial hand injuries to elucidate the presence of any associated fractures or foreign bodies. Anteroposterior and lateral views are usually sufficient. Additional or special views may be ordered based on specific physical findings. Photographs should be obtained prior to definitive therapy for medicolegal purposes.

EXAMINATION
It is preferable to perform the physical examination on the uninjured, or less severely injured, hand first. This technique allows the patient to understand exactly what is expected of him or her and usually calms the patient significantly. The patient probably also

benefits psychologically from seeing the amount of normal hand function still available.

After inspecting the hand for color or temperature changes, a preliminary study of *sensation* is performed. Light touch is tested with the examiner's fingertip or cottonballs. The patient is asked to compare the sensation of the uninvolved hand or digit with the one suspected of injury. This method is much more sensitive than testing two point discrimination with a paper clip or other device. Patients are able to pick up relatively small differences in light touch testing. Systematic testing of the sensory dermatomes of the median, ulnar, and radial nerve are tested and recorded (see Fig. 4-11).

Vascularity is then tested by checking capillary refill and pulp turgor of each digit. The pulse of the radial and ulnar arteries is tested and a Doppler study is utilized if necessary. An Allen test is performed, and the patency of each artery is confirmed (Fig. 4-20). Doppler evaluation of the digital arteries and comparing pulse oximetery results of involved and uninvolved digits has also been a valuable adjunct. As a last resort, one can pinprick the pulp of the fingertip in an attempt to obtain bright red blood, a sign of adequate inflow.

If the shoulder was potentially injured, appropriate *range of motion* and *strength* are tested; otherwise, the routine examination begins with flexion, extension, pronation, and supination at the elbow. Measurements are recorded as the examination progresses and are later compared to those of the opposite extremity. Strength is tested only if a more proximal injury is suspected.

Wrist flexion and extension, strength, and range of motion are tested. The examiner asks the patient to extend the wrist against resistance in radial deviation (ECRL), in ulnar deviation (extensor carpi ulnaris, (ECU), and in the midline (ECRB) — palpating for the intact tendons at their metacarpal base insertions: ECRL, second; ECRB, third; and ECU, fifth (see Fig. 4-15). The patient then flexes the wrist against resistance, and the flexor carpi ulnaris and radialis are palpated (see Fig. 4-13). These tendons may be difficult to palpate in obese, edematous, or charred patients.

Flexor Tendons

There are four basic components to the examination of the flexor tendons of the digits: active motion, observation at rest, tenodesis effect, and the "squeeze test." (For an in-depth discussion, see Chapter 8.)

1. *Active motion tests.* In the awake, cooperative patient special maneuvers can be used to separate and test the functions of the flexor digiti profundus and superficialis (FDP, FDS) independently. This test is the most informative part of the flexor examination. By blocking and allowing only DIP flexion, one can test sequentially the FDP functions of each digit (Fig. 4-21). Next, one restrains the FDS of all other digits by holding the digits in extension and asking the

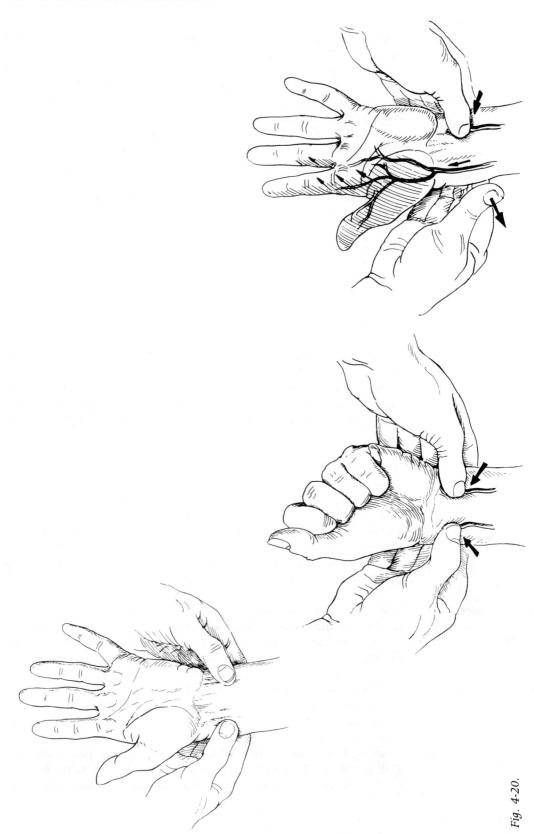

Fig. 4-20.

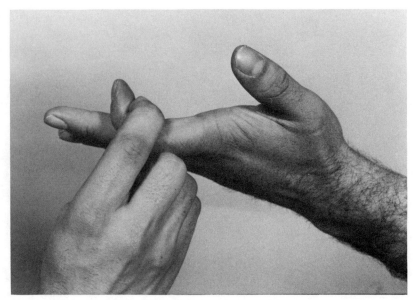

Fig. 4-21. Flexor digitorum profundus (FDP) function is assessed by isolated flexion at the DIP joint.

patient to flex the unrestrained digit. Full flexion at the PIP joint demonstrates an intact FDS tendon (Fig. 4-22). These maneuvers are done against light resistance; if pain is elicited, one should be suspicious that there is partial laceration of the involved tendon.

2. *Observation at rest.* One observes the cascade of the digits with the patient relaxed or under anesthesia. There should be a normal progression of increasing flexion as one proceeds from the index to the little finger. One finger in the extended position with an otherwise normal cascade is suspicious for a flexor tendon injury.

3. *Squeeze test.* If the injury is in the distal forearm one can test

◀ *Fig. 4-20.* Allen's test is useful for determining the patency of the radial and ulnar arteries. (From R. Chase. Allen's test. In *Atlas of Hand Surgery,* Vol. 1. Philadelphia: Saunders, 1973. With permission.)

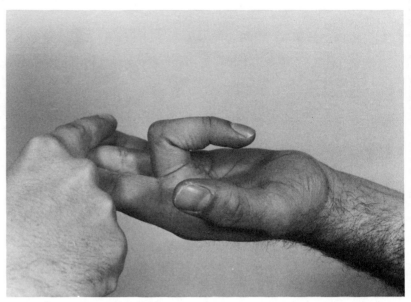

Fig. 4-22. Testing of the indicis proprius tendon. (From R. Tubiana. *Examination of the Hand and Upper Limb.* Philadelphia: Saunders, 1984. With permission.)

flexion of intact flexor tendons by placing pressure on the volar forearm proximal to the level of injury. Intact musculotendon units cause finger flexion. Partial lacerations give false-negative results.

Tenodesis effect. Gentle flexion and extension at the wrist should make all the fingers flex and extend in a normal cascade fashion. Again, fingers with disrupted flexor tendons remain in an extended position.

Extensor Tendons

There are three basic components to the examination of the extensor tendons of the digits: active motion, observation at rest, and the tenodesis effect. (For an in-depth discussion, see Chapter 9.)

1. *Active motion tests:* In the awake, cooperative patient special maneuvers can be used to separate and test the functions of each of the individual extensor muscle units independently. They constitute the most informative part of the extensor examination and include having the patient extend all fingers (extensor digiti), only the index and little fingers (extensor indicis and extensor digiti minimi), and the thumb. The examiner first dorsiflexes the patient's wrist to eliminate the automatic MCP extension, which occurs by a tenodesis effect. The patient then extends the proximal phalanges and is tested for any evidence of an extension lag. This test for the extensor digitorum communis is repeated again with light resistance on the dorsal proximal phalanx. An additional useful test, described by Chamay [1], involves placing the patient's hand flat on the table and sequentially having the patient lift each finger from the table. This

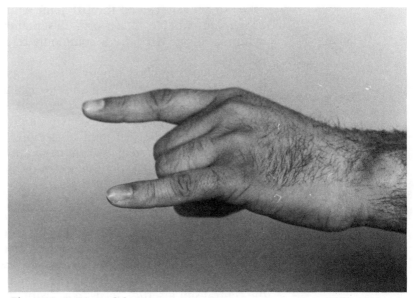

Fig. 4-23. Testing of the extensor proprious tendons. The patient immobilizes the extensor digitorum communis by immobilizing the third and fourth digits in flexion, and independently extends the index and little fingers.

motion can be performed only by the extrinsic extensors, not the intrinsic muscles.

The independent tendons of the index (extensor indicis) and little (extensor digiti minimi) fingers are tested by flexing completely the middle and ring fingers' MCP joints to eliminate the action of their extensor digiti contribution. The patient then extends the index and little fingers against light resistance (Fig. 4-23). These maneuvers are done against light resistance. Observe while palpating the extensor tendon being tested. This is possible because of the relatively thin dorsal skin covering.

To test the integrity of the central slips, the patient's fingers are placed with the PIP joints flexed at 90 degrees over the side of a table, and active extension of the middle phalanx is then tested. If the central slip is intact, the middle phalanx extends with a flail DIP joint. If the central slip is transected, extension is performed by force transmitted through the lateral bands, thus causing hyperextension of the DIP joint and absence or weak extension force on the middle phalanx at the PIP joint. If there is complete dorsal apparatus incompetence, the unrestrained action of the flexor digitorum sublimus causes flexion of the middle phalanx, the flexor profundus loses relative length, and the origin of the lumbrical is retracted. The retraction of the lumbrical muscle causes tension on the lateral bands and subsequent extension of the distal phalanx. This deformity is commonly referred to as the *buttonhole* or *boutonnière deformity*.

To test the integrity of the terminal extensor tendon, the patient is asked to actively extend the DIP joint while stabilizing the middle phalanx. If unable to perform this maneuver, the fixed flexion deformity of the DIP joint is commonly referred to as a *mallet finger deformity*.

The extensor pollicis longus is tested by active extension of the interphalangeal joint of the thumb against light resistance and effecting retropulsion of the column of the thumb. The extensor pollicis brevis is tested by active extension of the thumb metacarpal with the interphalangeal joint in flexion. The patient is asked to move the thumb in radial abduction, and the tension of the abductor pollicis longus is felt on the extensor border of the anatomic snuffbox.

2. *Observation at rest.* One observes the cascade of the digits with the patient relaxed or under anesthesia. There should be a normal progression of increasing flexion as one proceeds from the index to the little finger. The joint of the finger involved with an extensor tendon injury may have slightly increased flexion when compared to the other fingers at rest. Injury to the extensor tendon proximal to the central slip insertion leads to a flexion deformity of the PIP joint and hyperextension of the DIP joint. If the DIP joint is in a fixed flexed position, injury to the distal extensor tendon should be considered.

3. *Tenodesis effect.* Gentle flexion and extension at the wrist should make all the fingers flex and extend in a normal cascade fashion. Again, fingers with disrupted extensor tendons remain in a relatively flexed position when the other digits are extended.

The intrinsic muscles are tested by having the patient abduct and adduct the digits around the axis of the third finger. Muscle strength can be elucidated by testing against light resistance. Opposition of the thumb is also tested at this time by asking the patient to oppose the thumb and little finger.

INTERVENTION

After the examiner has performed the history and physical examination, it is time to evaluate the extent of the injury, timing of the intervention, and location at which the intervention is to take place.

For any injury to the upper extremity the injury is evaluated by "components," and a mental "shopping list" is made of the systems that are intact or injured. The injury is categorized into the following systems: (1) soft tissue; (2) skeletal; (3) vascular; (4) nerves; and (5) motor function. All aspects of the injury are addressed and dealt with effectively if each of these components is considered when planning the operative intervention and subsequent reconstruction. The chance of salvage and good function decreases with the more components injured.

This system improves the thoroughness of communication between the examiner and the consulting physicians. Excluding vascular injuries, most single-component injuries can be dealt with on a semielective basis. Tissue ischemia or compartment syndromes must be dealt with immediately and in the operating room.

Most isolated soft tissue injuries can be dealt with in the emergency room with adequate irrigation and débridement. Injuries with significant contamination or those that are produced by considerable amounts of tearing, crushing, exploding, or combustive forces have devitalized tissue associated with necrosis, edema, and venous and arterial thromboses. These wounds fare best with early operative irrigation and débridement, splinting, and reexploration within 24 to 48 hours. Exposed joints or neurovascular bundles also require early intervention for soft tissue coverage. For further detail on the management of soft tissue injuries see Chapter 11.

Isolated skeletal injuries can be splinted and treated during the first 12 to 36 hours when no neurovascular compromise is present. Closed reduction may be performed in the emergency room and may provide definitive treatment. Close follow-up is mandatory. For details on the treatment of skeletal injuries see Chapter 7.

Isolated nervous injuries do require operative repair with magnification but do not require immediate attention. There is little evidence that repair at any time during the first 7 days after injury alters eventual outcome. The patient is closely scrutinized for concomitant vascular injury. For details on the treatment of nerve injuries see Chapter 10.

Isolated extensor or flexor tendon injuries do not require immediate attention. There is little evidence that repair at any time during the first 7 days after injury alters eventual outcome. It is imperative that the skin be closed primarily after adequate irrigation. All of these injuries, except for partial extensor lacerations, require operative intervention and repair with magnification to obtain the best functional results. For further details on the treatment of tendon injuries see Chapters 8 and 9.

Multiple system injuries must be evaluated by trained hand surgeons, and decisions regarding the timing and location of interventions can be made based on their experience. If operative intervention is required, the involved extremity is splinted and elevated. The patient and family should be told of the proposed procedure, the length of recovery, and a general idea of the overall prognosis of a functional extremity.

REFERENCE

1. Chamay, J. C. A. Extensor tendon lesions of the dorsum of the hand and wrist. In C. Verdan (ed.), *Tendon Surgery of the Hand.* Edinburgh: Churchill Livingstone, 1979, p. 129.

Commentary on Chapter 4

James Hunter

This chapter excellently reviews the essentials for evaluating the upper extremity after injury. A few points need to be underscored to heighten the reader's awareness as he or she proceeds toward early diagnosis and treatment of the injured hand and upper extremity.

When reviewing emergency room records of hand injuries for legal depositions, I have often wished that the busy nurse or doctor could have slowed the pace for a moment and been more descriptive of the circumstances surrounding the injury. The next echelon of care caught up in the details of management must read quickly and often presume that what they are reading is all the information that was available. There are times, however, when some significant information has been overlooked.

For example, consider the history of a 26-year-old housewife who was seen in the accident ward. Her history described a crushing injury to the right index finger sustained by closing a door on her hand 1 day before this examination. Because of apparent vascular occlusion at the base of the right index finger she was taken to the operating room. Infection was found later and the organism identified as a β-hemolytic streptococcus. The site required extensive incision and drainage. This acute problem eventually called for transferring the patient to another hospital where further treatments failed and amputation of the finger became necessary.

A legal question arose based on the poor result — someone must be at fault. Later, in another hospital, the patient provided the additional information that the pulp of the index finger had been burned on a hot lightbulb earlier in the week, which explained the blister on the top of the finger that had initially been considered part of the crushing injury. Reviewing the overall problem, one could identify that this blister was a probable site of tissue necrosis and a portal of entry for a streptococcal infection. The patient had either overlooked, minimized, or denied an earlier injury. Perhaps at the time of the initial evaluation, additional prodding, different questions, or different approaches to the questioning would have elicited this information and have altered the future treatment and result.

The lesson here is to ask questions of the injured person that may even get personal regarding the activities of daily life. You may be rewarded with important information that may alter treatment. For example, the weekend carpenter with the saw injury may be a professional pianist. In addition, as stressed by Dr. Greco, ask and inquire into the details of the injury, e.g., the mechanism, the location of injury, and what happened to the total person during the injury process.

Traction injuries with delayed sequelae in the peripheral nerves and brachial plexus in the upper extremity may be secondary to injury to the hand and wrist. For example, with a crushing injury to the hand in a machine, sudden extreme forces may be applied by the patient or coworkers when trying to remove the patient from the offending machinery. The same situation may arise as a restrained or unrestrained driver holds the steering wheel or strikes the dashboard of the car with a force that is difficult to estimate. The brachial plexus may be injured owing to blunt contusions or whiplash forces produced by stretching or traction. This force may also be projected over the length of the extremity into the medial, ulnar, and radial nerves. Dislocations of joints and fractures in the hand and wrist may be the obvious treatable injury, but a whiplash injury in the cervical spine may be the inducer of a more serious future brachial plexus thoracic outlet syndrome.

The early findings from a peripheral nerve traction injury may be minimal or masked by other injuries, such as lacerations or fractures in the hand and wrist. Patients with sprains are often treated with support collars to the neck and splints to the arms and hands. Contused spastic muscles move the joints into a protected position and reduce symptoms from early nerve injury. The patients may simply say it hurts, or "I guess I bruised my shoulder." *Early examination, however, can raise a warning flag that peripheral nerve injury should be looked into in the future.*

Tardy neuropathies and palsies of the peripheral nerve and the brachial plexus (thoracic outlet syndrome) are increasing dramatically in the general population. This chronic disabling problem often occurs 1 to 3 years after the initial injury and poses a complex diagnostic situation to the neurologist or hand surgeon. Information gained from the early examination may be invaluable for the future prognosis of a nerve injury.

In addition to the brachial plexus and cervical spine, key compressive sites in the upper extremity are the ulnar nerve at the cubital compartment of the elbow, the radial nerve on the proximal dorsum of the forearm, and median nerve in the carpal compartment of the wrist, and the ulnar nerve in the pisiform canal at the wrist.

Crushing traction injuries may cause arterial injury and muscle compartment necrosis. Two locations remain areas of special concern: The first is just distal to the elbow, where the common ulnar artery gives off the anterior and posterior interosseous arteries. The anatomic arrangement here permits the radial artery to be free from compression, and a full radial pulse may exist when there is impending congestion and soft tissue depth in the flexor muscle forearm compartment. Congenital variations of the arterial anatomy to the thumb may be present, and on occasion an injury to the radial artery places ultimate survival of the injured thumb in jeopardy.

Second, peripheral nerve injury may produce paresis, although paresis may also be a clue to underlying acute compartment syndrome. Peripheral pulses and capillary filling are normally intact, which poses to the early examining physician a difficult diagnosis: Is it arterial compartment syndrome occlusion or neuropraxia?

Symptoms of compartment syndrome include pain that is out of proportion to that expected for the injuries sustained, increasing use of analgesics, and stress pain referred to the forearm compartment with passive motion of the digits. A careful sensory examination and review of paresis may be the clue to incipient compartment syndrome or more proximal nerve injury.

Remove all bandages before completing the initial examination. A tight bandage over the extremity compartment may cause a pressure rise of as much as 25 mm Hg within the compartment. Inexperienced application of an elastic-type bandage, for example, can make a tight compartment problem more severe. A tight, continuous hand bandage can produce localized Volkmann's necrosis to the first dorsal interosseous muscle. Bivalving the cast or opening the circumferential bandage must include every turn of the material.

For acute hand and wrist injuries, always consider obtaining a radiograph of the hand. Penetration by sharp objects such as nails, glass, and wood may leave little evidence on the skin but produce glaring silhouettes on the radiograph. The other hand should also be radiographed for comparison, especially when a fracture-dislocation around a finger joint or the wrist is suspected. This practice permits the untrained eye to quickly identify an avulsion fracture in the finger joint or a carpal dislocation.

Finally, examine the hand and upper extremity with respect and concern, showing appreciation of the hidden fears of patients that they may not be able to perform their lifetime work again. The skills of the musician or the cabinetmaker, for example, may be lost forever.

The human hand is a wondrously constructed anatomic and engineering marvel. Throughout history strong, silent, eloquent, beautiful hands have been linked with art and religion. When clasped, they may represent concern, worry, or faith; and when in a fist they may represent defiance and anger. Take some extra moments during the initial examination to ask and determine personal factors. It will be rewarding to all concerned.

Commentary on Chapter 4

James H. Herndon

The initial evaluation of the injured hand is important. Often the injuries are occult and not diagnosed immediately, so they may be missed for some length of time. Permanent loss of function may result and may be the only deficit a patient is left with once he or she has recovered from other, "more serious" injuries.

Someone trained and skilled in hand surgery should assess the hand injury and plan appropriate treatment immediately and during the patient's hospital stay.

1. *Skin*. Volar creases at the wrist, MCP joints, PIP joints, and DIP joints are important for allowing full flexion of those joints by overlapping the skin, preventing it from bunching up and therefore impairing motion.

2. *Vascular supply*. It is important with volar approaches to the wrist to remember that a volar branch from the radial artery passes between the distal pole of the scaphoid and the trapezium. It can be ligated, allowing the surgeon to mobilize the radial artery for exposures in this area especially for management of trauma or trapezium resection arthroplasty. The digital arteries lie volar to the digital nerves, distally in the palm; but before entering the finger they cross, so that each artery lies dorsal to the nerve as these structures course throughout the digit.

3. *Nerve*. The dorsal ulnar nerve, which is a sensory nerve, arises in the distal forearm and can be found crossing to the dorsum of the hand approximately 1 cm distal to the ulnar styloid process. It is important to identify this nerve as well as the radial sensory nerve with approaches about the wrist and hand in order to avoid painful neuromas. The radial nerve supplies innervation over the dorsal radial one-half of the hand. Occasionally, it provides some sensation to the more volar aspects of the thumb and index finger.

4. *Examination*. If an isolated digit is injured, it is important to obtain two radiographic views — anteroposterior and lateral — of the digit itself. Oblique or lateral views of the hand with the digits overlapping may obscure a fracture, subluxation, or dislocation.

When examining sensibility, I prefer two-point discrimination, which provides an accurate, reproducible baseline to which future examinations may be referred. When doing the Allen test it is well to remember that this test was originally described for use at the wrist for occlusions of the radial or ulnar artery. It may also be applied to each digit individually to determine patency of the radial or ulnar digital artery.

When examining the extensor tendons, it is sometimes difficult to determine whether the patient is extending a digit with the extrinsic or the intrinsic muscle tendon units. One can illuminate the intrinsic units by having the patient flex his or her PIP joints and then actively flex and extend the MCP joints. Any active extension of these joints with the PIP joints flexed is accomplished by means of the extrinsic extensor muscle tendon units.

When examining the extensor pollicis longus tendon, remember that the abductor pollicis brevis and adductor pollicis extend into the extensor mechanism, thereby providing active extension of the DIP joint. To assess the intact extensor pollicis longus, one must see active extension of the entire thumb while palpating the tendon and providing a resistive force.

5. *Intervention.* Severe bleeding of the hand can usually be managed by a compressive dressing and elevation or use of a tourniquet on the upper arm. It is important not to blindly use a hemostat to try and control an arterial bleeder. It is totally unnecessary for controlled bleeding; and under such circumstances, it is not uncommon to injure one of the important nearby nerves with such action.

5 FINGERTIP INJURIES

Kenneth C. Shestak

The fingertip is a highly specialized, indispensable part of the normal digit. Its architecture allows the performance of ordinary and complex tasks of everyday living, completes the grasps in prehension, and confers an appearance to the digit that is unique to primates.

Fingertip injuries constitute a significant percentage of surgical visits to the emergency room and together with injuries to the nail bed are the most common hand injuries. The distal aspect of the digit is the most exposed part of the hand in almost every type of work, and injuries to it can happen at almost any time; they are estimated to be responsible for more loss of time from work than any other single injury.

Because these injuries are so common, the anatomy so unique, and the sequela from the injury potentially serious, i.e., skin loss, poor healing, painful scars, deformities of the nail or distal phalanx, and ultimately impaired function of the injured digit, proper treatment is essential. An understanding of these injuries and the approach to treatment is important not only for hand surgeons and general surgeons but for all physicians who work in emergency rooms.

ANATOMY

The fingertip is usually defined as everything distal to the insertion of the extensor and flexor tendons at the distal interphalangeal (DIP) joint. It is composed of the bony distal phalanx, the fingernail/fingernail bed complex, and a covering of skin and subcutaneous fat that contains a high concentration of nerve fiber endings. The skin is attached to the underlying phalanx by vertically oriented, tough fibrous septae (Fig. 5-1). The fingernail is an important part of the digit because it not only gives a characteristic cosmetic appearance to the fingertip, it also stabilizes the soft tissues and maximizes sensory function, allowing the hand to perform many tasks that require well developed tactile function, such as picking up and manipulating small objects.

The skin cover of the pulp has a specialized epidermis that is sensitive and resistant to rubbing and friction. It is thick and durable,

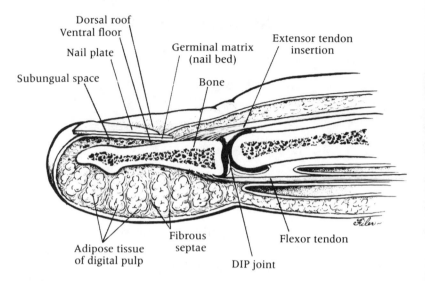

Fig. 5-1. Anatomy of the fingertip and nail.

and its convex orientation toward the nail maximizes the contact surface and touch function. This surface is cushioned by a buffer of fat that is compartmentalized by fibrous septae (Fig. 5-1). These septae anchor the skin to the bony distal phalanx; they also contribute to tip stability for grasping objects, limit the pliability of the skin, and have special significance for surgical treatment of various conditions, as discussed later. The surface of the skin on the palmar aspect of the digit is hairless, nonpigmented, and marked by digital rugae (fingerprints), which are a system of creases and papillary crests in the dermis. The fine creases allow better contact, and the ridges facilitate prehension. These rugae are specific for each individual, differing from one digit to another and remaining unchanged throughout life.

The dorsal skin is located on the sides and proximal part of the nail. The side folds are called the perionychia and the fold proximal to the nail is the eponychium (Fig. 5-2).

The fingernail, or nail plate, lies on top of the nail bed. One full length of nail growth takes approximately 100 days, growing slightly more than 0.1 mm per day. There is a delay in nail growth for approximately 20 days following an injury; and this delay is followed by an increase in nail formation for the next 50 days, causing a bulge as the nail grows out. It takes three to four full growths of nail for the nail to achieve maximum improvement after injury.

Contribution to the volume of the nail plate is from three sources: The dorsal roof of the eponychial fold, the ventral floor of the eponychial fold (germinal matrix or lunula), and nail bed distal to the lunula. The greatest contribution is from the ventral floor or germinal matrix, which provides up to 90 percent of the volume of

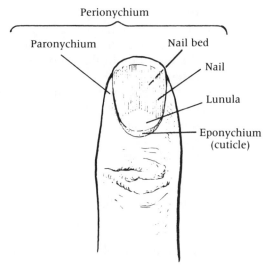

Fig. 5-2. Anatomy of the nail and perionychium. Dorsal view of the fingertip.

the nail. The nail is flat and grows distally because of pressure from new cells being produced in the nail fold, which forces growth in a distal direction. Close examination of the nail plate reveals many fine longitudinal ribs that contribute to the nail plate's adherence to the underlying nail bed.

Normal nail growth therefore requires a normal nail bed. This nail bed comprises all of the soft tissue underneath the nail and, as noted, is composed of the germinal matrix proximally and sterile matrix distally. The germinal matrix arises underneath the nail fold, and part of it is the white arc-shaped area called the lunula seen just distal to the fold. The nail bed is composed of fibrous tissue of variable thickness that derives its blood supply from terminal branches of the common volar digital artery, which passes just above the periosteum of the distal phalanx to nourish it. The veins in the nail bed are small and coalesce in the skin proximal to the nail fold; they remain small until they reach the level of the DIP joint. This situation makes microsurgical repair of the veins distal to the DIP joint nearly impossible. The abundant blood vessels and nerves of the nail bed coalesce distally in specific areas to produce the glomus, which is a thermo-regulating organ; and this organ contributes to modulation of the peripheral circulation.

The flat, smooth surface of the nail bed allows the overlying nail plate to grow out normally. Any injuries to this structure must be accurately and completely repaired to best ensure normal nail growth.

The distal phalanx extends from the DIP joint to approximately the mid-portion of the fingernail bed. It is composed of hard, cortical bone with a broad proximal metaphysis and narrow diaphysis, which is prolonged by a terminal cap often referred to as the "distal tuft." The stability of the fingertip results from both the bony phalanx and the contribution of the fingernail. The density and amount of cortical bone constituting the distal phalanx accounts for the extended healing time often noted with distal phalangeal fractures.

An understanding of the anatomic relations of the various parts of the fingertip is essential for appreciating the severity of various injuries and for individualizing treatment. The following sections deal with injuries to each of these parts and offer suggestions as to their treatment.

EVALUATION

Injuries to the fingertip can result from lacerations or punctures, but they most commonly involve a crushing mechanism. In decreasing frequency, the injury involves the middle finger followed by the ring, index, and small fingers, and the thumb. Such injuries usually occur in males (75 percent) between 4 and 30 years of age. Right and left hands are affected with equal frequency. The usual injury involves not only the skin and underlying soft tissue but also the nail plate and underlying nail bed. Of course, all structures of the fingertip can be involved when the injury takes the form of an open fracture or amputation.

A correct diagnosis of any condition in medicine is essential for proper treatment. It is especially true for fingertip injuries, and it requires a complete history, careful physical examination, and most often a radiographic evaluation of the digit. The physician seeing such a patient must ascertain the exact time and mechanism of injury, hand dominance and occupation of the patient, alterations of sensation, the presence and character of the pain, and any history of previous injuries to that hand or digit and their sequelae. In addition, information about the patient's general medical condition, medications, allergies, tetanus status, and time of last food intake is important. The injured digit(s) is examined for vascularity, obvious deformity (Is part of the digit missing, or is there a subungual hematoma?), and abnormalities of sensation or joint motion. Because there is a high incidence of associated bone injury, a radiograph of the injured part often provides important information.

Classification of Soft Tissue Injuries

In medicine, classifications are useful for selecting specific treatment plans and evaluating the outcomes of treatment. Most classifications of fingertip injuries have been based on the mechanism and level of injury. Except for simple lacerations, many of these wounds are amputations of some degree. A particularly useful classification of these injuries was proposed by Allen [1]. It separates amputation injuries into four types based on the level of amputation, i.e., through the tissue involved.

Type I injuries involve only the skin and the pulp of the distal digit.
Type II injuries involve the pulp and nail bed.

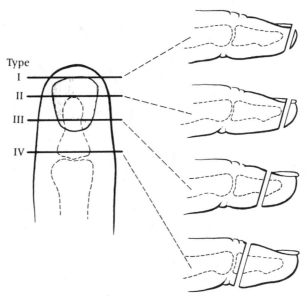

Fig. 5-3. Allen's classification of fingertip injuries.

Type III injuries involve loss of part of the terminal phalanx.
Type IV injuries are amputations proximal to the lunula (Fig. 5-3).
These injuries can be either transverse, i.e., at right angles to the
long axis of the digit, or oblique. If oblique, they can be oblique
dorsal (more tissue on the palmar than the dorsal side) or oblique
volar (more tissue on the dorsal side) (Fig. 5-4).

**Operative
Treatment**

The general principles involved in all reconstructive procedures for
the hand apply to fingertip injuries as well. A high priority is the
restoration of skin cover to protect underlying bone, tendon, and
nerve structures. Other priorities are to maintain or maximize
sensibility, preserve digit length (especially in the thumb), and
minimize cosmetic deformity. First and foremost, the hand is a
functional organ. Because it is so highly visible, though, the appearance of the reconstructed digit should be as normal as possible.

Injuries to the soft tissue can present either as lacerations without
loss of tissue or as partial or complete amputations with varying
degrees of tissue loss. In the absence of tissue loss or associated
injuries, lacerations should be cleaned, irrigated, débrided as necessary, and suture-repaired with accurate coaptation of the wound
edges. They can almost always be treated in the emergency room,
preferably in a clean, well-lit area, under digital block anesthesia and
utilizing a digital tourniquet.

Most of these injuries can be treated with regional anesthesia in
the form of a digital block. Such a block is most commonly
accomplished by injecting 1% or 2% lidocaine (Xylocaine) *without*
epinephrine around the digital nerves of the finger at the level of the
distal palmar crease or by placement into the web space. For

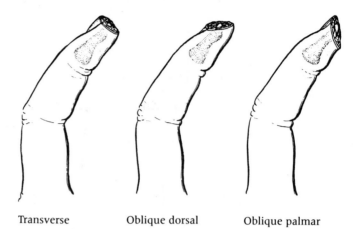

Transverse   Oblique dorsal   Oblique palmar

Fig. 5-4. Planes of angulation of fingertip amputations.

complete anesthesia of the digit, it is important to inject dorsally over the extensor hood in order to block the dorsal branches of the radial nerve. Approximately 2 hours of anesthesia results from this technique. Substitution of 0.5% bupivacaine for lidocaine lengthens the duration of the anesthetic effect to between 6 and 8 hours. Such a prolongation of pain relief may be helpful in patients who have sustained crush injuries with a phalangeal fracture or those with a subungual hematoma.

A digital tourniquet is easily constructed by placing a gauze sponge around the proximal aspect of the digit and wrapping a 1 inch Penrose drain around it. Just enough tension to keep the digit exsanguinated is maintained in the Penrose drain using a hemostat. To avoid injury to the digital vessels or nerves, it is imperative that the tourniquet not be *too* tight. After satisfactory anesthesia is achieved, the wound is cleansed with an antiseptic solution (e.g., Betadine or Hibiclens) and then is irrigated with either 0.9% normal saline or Ringer's lactate solution. The optimal pressure for wound irrigation to maximize mechanical removal of the contamination and minimize tissue injury is 7 pounds per square inch. This pressure is best achieved using a 30-ml syringe and an 18-gauge needle for irrigation.

Lacerations most often occur on the volar aspect of the digit. If there is evidence of sensory loss in the fingertip, the digital nerve underneath the laceration should be explored in the operating room. It is often possible to perform microscopic repair of the nerves, especially if the nerve injury is proximal to the eponychial fold. Such a repair offers the best chance for the return of sensation and is the optimal method for avoiding formation of a neuroma.

The lacerations should be accurately approximated using standard suture technique. This step is most commonly done utilizing a 5-0 or 6-0 monofilamentous suture (Prolene or nylon) on a small needle (P-1 or P-3). The need for antibiotics should be determined and, when appropriate, prescribed. A splint for the fingertip is often

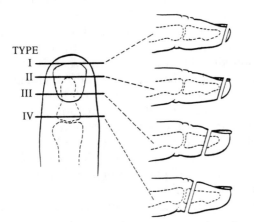

Treatment options

Nonoperative wound management
Skin graft

Composite graft
Flap closure
Skin graft
Nonoperative wound management

Flap coverage
Composite graft
Closure of amputation

Replantation
Closure of amputation

Fig. 5-5. Treatment options based on Allen's classification of fingertip injuries.

helpful for protecting the wound and can be left in place for 10 to 14 days. Sutures are customarily removed at 2 weeks after the injury.

Particular attention should be given to accurate alignment of the perionychial fold or the eponychial fold. In these cases it may be necessary to remove the fingernail to completely assess the injury and to provide the best repair. Replacement of this fingernail then splints the "potential space" underneath the folds. Again, sutures are removed at 14 days after surgery. In young children it is possible to use absorbable sutures of either chromic catgut or polyglycolic acid. This method obviates the additional trauma of suture removal.

When there is evidence of soft tissue loss (amputated tissue), i.e., when the wound cannot be repaired primarily, reconstruction of the injured fingertip must be undertaken. The choice of method depends on a multiplicity of factors including, for instance, the location of the injury, the amount of skin and subcutaneous tissue missing, the level and obliquity of the wound (Fig. 5-4), associated injuries to the fingernail, nail bed, or bone, injuries to adjacent digits, and the age and occupation of the patient. Allen's classification may be useful for selecting the treatment for patients with amputation injuries (Fig. 5-5).

Type I and many type II injuries are best treated by allowing healing to occur by secondary intention if the wound size is less than 1 cm^2. This choice is especially appropriate for children, who have remarkable healing potential. This "conservative" method has been shown to provide good sensation (measured by two-point discrimination) and offers an excellent cosmetic outcome. The main disadvantage is that it may take 4 to 8 weeks for complete healing.

Other methods of treatment used when preserving length is a primary concern are skin grafting, either full- or split-thickness grafts, the advancement of tissue from the injured digit as a skin flap (a V-Y advancement flap), the transfer of tissue from an adjacent digit or from the palm as in a cross-finger flap or thenar flap, and a pedicle flap transfer from a remote site. These methods are best suited to Allen's type II and III injuries. It is often possible to shorten the digit by resecting bone (cutting back the distal end of the bone) and then approximating the soft tissue over this shortened phalanx. This treatment is indicated when the entire nail/nail bed complex is lost or destroyed, i.e., Allen's type IV injuries. It is usually a straightforward method for obtaining wound closure, but care must be taken to perform an adequate neurectomy so as to place the nerve endings out of the wound, thereby minimizing the chance of postoperative neuroma formation. It should not be used in the thumb, where length is of paramount importance, and it is used with caution in the index finger.

Because it is important to have an adequate soft tissue bed for (1) skin grafting or (2) allowing healing to proceed by secondary intention, these methods are best employed for type I and II injuries. For injuries with substantial loss of skin and pulp tissue and perhaps bone, coverage with flap tissue may be a better option. For amputations proximal to the level of the lunula (type IV), the possibilities are microvascular reattachment or shortening and closure of the wound. Replantation is possible if the mechanism of injury is a sharp cut (guillotine type) rather than a crush and the level of amputation lies midway between the eponychial fold and the DIP joint. Microvascular expertise is required for successful anastomoses of these small vessels, but replantation at or just distal to the level of the trifurcation of the neurovascular bundle is possible. For amputations distal to this level, attempts at replacing the amputation as a composite graft are reasonable if the patient is less than 3 years old. Such grafts have a poor take when utilized in the adult population. The best potential for healing and graft take is in cases where the replaced part does not exceed 8 mm in length. This composite tissue provides a biologic dressing; and even if it does not completely survive, some of the more proximal portion of it may do so and add bulk to the fingertip.

NAIL BED INJURIES   The most common types of nail bed injury are simple lacerations, followed by stellate lacerations, crushes, and avulsions, in decreasing frequency. The middle one-third of the nail bed is most frequently injured, followed closely by the distal one-third. Distal phalangeal fractures occur in approximately 50 percent of all nail bed injuries. The usual injury includes some element of a crushing mechanism, which accounts for the large number of nonlinear nail bed injuries that are seen. The simple laceration is usually the result of a localized blow to the fingernail, causing a bend in the nail and a relatively straight type of laceration.

Treatment of the patient with a fingertip injury requires careful examination of the nail bed after establishing satisfactory anesthesia. Inspection of the nail bed and radiographic evaluation of the digit are necessary to rule out an underlying fracture. Careful, accurate repair is essential to avoid posttraumatic deformity of the fingernails following these injuries.

The treatment of fingernail injuries involves removal of the entire nail and exploration of all portions of the laceration. Once again, the hand should be surgically prepared with an antiseptic solution, and a digital tourniquet is used to allow accurate assessment of the injury. The nail can be removed from the nail bed with either a blunt-tipped periosteal elevator (Freer) or a fine hemostat. It must be done *without* traumatizing the uninjured portions of the nailbed. The nailbed should be evaluated using loupe magnification, with the extent of the lacerations and the amount of nail bed deficit determined. The wound should be irrigated and highly conservative débridement carried out as necessary. Nail bed repair should then be done utilizing a 7-0 chromic catgut suture on a fine needle. This procedure allows minimal trauma to the nail bed. After repair of the nail bed wound, the fingernail can be replaced on top of it to provide splinting and protection. A small hole may be placed in the nail to allow drainage of any blood that collects around the repaired laceration.

This method of repair is appropriate for almost all types of nail bed injury. Stellate lacerations have many more tissue fragments, but often they can be accurately approximated. Crushing lacerations are more severe than either of the other two types. It is important that all of the fragments in this type of injury be approximated as accurately as possible. Any fragments attached by fine strands to the underlying nail bed tissues should be replaced, and those fragments that have been avulsed can be placed back down as tissue grafts. Once again, the nail is replaced to provide splinting. If it is not possible to use the nail, a piece of Xeroform or Adaptic or the metal foil of a suture package may be used. This step is followed by application of a soft dressing and a splint.

When the nail and nail bed have been avulsed, every effort should be made to find the avulsed fragment. If it is found, it can be put back in place as a free graft. In these situations the nail bed often remains attached to the fingernail. It is necessary to "free up" only the edges of the nail bed to allow suturing to the remaining bed. The remainder of the nail bed should be left attached to the nail plate. If the avulsed fragment is not available, other treatment options include healing by secondary intention, split-thickness skin grafts, reverse dermal grafts, or full-thickness nail bed grafts (from a toe). Most authors believe that a full-thickness nail bed graft provides the best replacement for avulsed nail bed tissue. Such a graft may be harvested from a toenail.

Fractures with Lacerations

It is estimated that approximately 50 percent of nail bed injuries have an accompanying fracture of the tuft of the distal phalanx. It is important that tuft fractures be accurately reduced because if the bone underneath the nail is not properly aligned it is impossible to obtain a flat, normal nail bed. In most cases replacement of the nail after repair of the nail bed injury helps maintain the reduction by splinting the fracture. If it does not, a longitudinal smooth K-wire passed through the tip of the finger allows maintenance of the fracture reduction.

Subungual Hematoma

The nail bed is a highly vascular structure that bleeds when injured. Often after significant trauma the nail is not broken or dislodged, but the injury is sufficient to produce a collection of blood underneath the nail. This "subungual hematoma" usually produces severe pain. The pain can be significantly reduced with decompression of the hematoma by placing a small hole in the fingernail itself. Judgment must be exercised when there is a bony fracture in association with the hematoma. Contamination of such a hematoma may produce the undesirable sequela of an infected fracture. A hand-held ophthalmic cautery, 18-gauge needle, or heated paperclip are useful instruments with which to put a hole in the nail to drain the hematoma.

FRACTURES

Fractures of the distal phalanx are either open or closed fractures, and they can be either nondisplaced or displaced. For all bones the cardinal principles of fracture treatment are reduction of the displaced fracture with restoration of satisfactory alignment and then immobilization. For the most part, closed fractures of the terminal phalanx are either nondisplaced or minimally displaced and can usually be treated with protective splinting for a period of 10 to 14 days, allowing the pain to subside. The time needed for radiographic union or healing of these injuries is often prolonged, sometimes taking months.

Depending on the degree of instability, internal fixation with one or two parallel pins or K-wires may be required. These pins are usually advanced past the DIP joint and left in place for 4 weeks. At that point they can be removed, and the patient can be begun on motion.

Open fractures should be treated with a combination of wound irrigation, fracture reduction, and immobilization. It is important to irrigate these fractures and to treat them with a course of antibiotic therapy. The soft tissue over the fracture is repaired (either skin or nail bed); and, as previously mentioned, replacement of the fingernail often provides splinting of the fracture from the dorsal side.

INFECTION

Infections of the fingertip are common and are typically *Staphylococcus aureus* bacterial infections, although viral infections also occur. *S. aureus* is the most common bacterium producing such infections, which can occur either in the subcutaneous tissue of the finger, where they are most common on the dorsal side, or in the deeper pulp space of the fingertip. An infection that involves the folds along the fingernail produces a characteristic infection of the perionychial fold and is referred to as a paronychial infection. If the infection involves the fold over the proximal portion of the fingernail, it is termed an eponychial infection. Infections of the deep pulp space of the finger may produce significant discomfort. As previously outlined, the pulp of the finger consists of fat compartmentalized by multiple fibrosepta. When infection involves these septa, there is an expansion of the compartments because of the accompanying swelling, which sets up a localized compartment syndrome with pain produced by ischemia of the fingertip. Surgical decompression is most often required to treat this problem.

Infections of the fingertip can frequently be treated with a combination of warm soaks and antibiotic therapy. The patient is usually put on warm water soaks three times a day and treated with a staphylocidal antibiotic (semisynthetic penicillin or cephalosporin). It is important to examine these patients serially; and when there is evidence of a localized abscess, surgical drainage should be undertaken. The perionychial or eponychial folds can be drained by a variety of incisions. (See Chapter 10.)

The presence of a pulp space infection almost always requires surgical decompression because of the ischemic wound environment, as described above. The incisions employed are those made either along the mid-axis of the digit on one or both sides, or over the volar aspect of the fingertip. It is important not to perform a fishmouth-type incision, which can cause retraction of the soft tissues of the fingertip and persistent pain of the fingertip.

REFERENCE

1. Allen, M.J. Conservative management of finger tip injuries in adults, *Hand* 12(3): 257–265, 1980.

Commentary on Chapter 5

Robert C. Russell

Fingertip/nail bed injuries are the most frequent result of upper extremity trauma. Definitive treatment of complex injuries requiring local or distal flap coverage and nail bed reconstruction are best performed by a qualified hand surgeon in the operating room under general or regional block anesthesia. Simpler, more common injuries, however, can be repaired using a digital block and a Penrose drain finger tourniquet in the emergency room. Family practice physicians, emergency room physicians, and surgical house officers must be able to evaluate these injuries to determine if special treatment is required. They should have a knowledge of the regional anatomy, know how to do a basic hand examination, and after the history and physical examination be able to treat or triage the patient.

There are some aspects of this chapter that should be stressed and others with which I disagree. First, I believe all fingertip injuries should be radiographed with posteroanterior and lateral views. It is surprising what is revealed on these films — from undiagnosed fractures and foreign bodies to giant cell tumors and bone cysts. A discussion of fingertip amputation types is theoretically good, but almost none fits exactly into only one type. It is better to assess the degree of tissue injury and loss for each individual defect and then determine the most efficient and functional repair, considering such socioeconomic factors as age, sex, occupation, and medical history.

The glabrous skin and subcutaneous tissue on the volar hand surface is highly specialized for grasp and sensibility and is best replaced by similar tissue. When flap coverage is indicated, I prefer to use local V-Y or volar advancement flaps whenever possible.

A convenient method to irrigate small wounds in the emergency room, including fingertip injuries, is with a gas-sterilized plastic spray bottle, which can be purchased in any hardware store. The nozzle can be adjusted to produce a fine mist or a concentrated saline stream, and the bottle can be resterilized for the next case.

Subungual hematomas usually indicate a nail bed laceration and are inadequately treated by simply burning a hole in them. I remove the nail in all such cases and anatomically repair the nail bed with

7-0 chromic sutures using loupe magnification. The nail with a drain hole or a Silastic sheet, if the nail is missing or destroyed, is replaced in the nail fold to keep it open and to act as a stent. Sterile matrix avulsion injuries should be repaired at the time of injury with a split nail bed graft from adjacent uninjured nailbed or a split toenail graft. Allowing nail bed avulsion injuries to heal by secondary intention or using standard or reversed dermal skin grafts is not adequate treatment and causes the future nail plate to lift away from the area of scar or skin graft, producing permanent nail deformity. Nonadherent, irregular, or split nail deformities are difficult to correct at a later date and can be avoided by precise surgical repair at the time of the acute injury.

Small superficial areas of skin loss without exposed bone and especially in children can be allowed to heal by secondary intention; this method provides good contour and functional results. Larger areas of skin or distal nail bed and hyponychium avulsion injuries can also heal by secondary intention, but this method can produce stiff, hard, often sensitive fingertips that are prone to cold intolerance. It is better to replace the avulsed skin and distal nail bed as a full-thickness skin graft or use a split-thickness skin graft from the hypothenar eminence for volar injuries without exposed bone. The patient returns to work sooner and usually obtains a more functional result. We use composite tip replacement grafts for amputations distal to the lunula in patients up to 6 years of age.

I do not use parallel K wires but prefer crossed wires to hold unstable phalangeal fractures. Cellulitis of the fingertip or paronychium might be successfully treated by "warm soaks" and antibiotics, but these cases usually have a closed space infection of the proximal nail fold that "runs around" the perionychium. This problem should be treated by partial or complete removal of the proximal nail plate out of the eponychial fold to drain this closed space. It is not necessary to cut the skin for drainage in this area. Pulp space infections, or felons, should be incised and drained over the abscess and never through mid-axial incisions, which can result in skin loss between the incision site and the thinned skin over the point of the abscess.

6 REVASCULARIZATION, REPLANTATION, AND AMPUTATION

Haven J. Barlow
Sai S. Ramasastry

The traumatic amputation of an extremity, or part of it, constitutes a surgical emergency. Owing to the pioneering efforts of Lapchinsky [1], Snyder et al. [2], Jacobsen and Suarez [3], Kleinert et al. [4], Buncke and Schulz [5], Komatsu and Tamai [6], and others, successful revascularization and reattachment of amputated digits in centers throughout the world are approaching success rates of up to 95 percent [7–11]. However, success can no longer be measured by tissue survival alone [12]. Successful replantation includes functional recovery and the ultimate benefit to the patient in his or her use of the extremity for daily activities. The points to be considered in replantation/revascularization surgery therefore are (1) restoration of joint motion; (2) sensory recovery; (3) presence or absence of pain; and (4) the final cosmetic appearance [12–16]. Hence the decision to reattach the amputated part must be made with knowledge of the likely outcome of the various repairs.

TERMINOLOGY

An understanding of the terminology used in traumatology and microvascular surgery is important for establishing good communication between medical personnel [17]. *Complete amputation* is where the part is severed completely from the body with no attaching structures (Fig. 6-1). *Replantation* is reattachment of a completely amputated part. *Incomplete amputation* is the severed and devascularized part that remains attached by some connecting structures or tissue, albeit a single nerve, tendon, or soft tissue bridge (Fig. 6-1). *Revascularization* is restoration of the vascular supply to an incompletely amputated part. Frequently the distinction between revascularization and replantation is small. However, intact structures can lead to better functional results.

Cold ischemia is the period between the preparation of the amputated part on ice to the time when cooling is discontinued. Cooling helps reduce the anaerobic metabolism and protect the part. *Warm ischemia* is the time period from when the cooling is discontinued to the restoration of arterial inflow to the replanted part. During replantation surgery it is imperative to keep the total ischemia time to a minimum, especially the warm ischemia period.

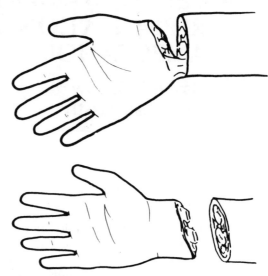

Fig. 6-1. Complete and incomplete amputations. (From S. Tamai. Replantation of upper arm and forearm. In *Symposium on Clinical Frontiers in Reconstructive Microsurgery, Plastic Surgical Education Foundation.* Vol. 24, p. 43. St. Louis: Mosby, 1984. With permission.)

PATIENT EVALUATION

Successful replantation begins by stabilizing the patient in the field and promptly transporting him or her to a replantation center. Emergency technicians should be sure that all amputated parts are retrieved from the field and properly packaged for transportation. The amputated parts are kept cool by wrapping them in moist saline gauze, placing them in a sealed plastic bag, and immersing them in an iced-saline container (Fig. 6-2) [14,18]. Maceration caused by immersion is not a problem; however, freezing (frostbite) of the part can be a problem if there is direct contact of the part with ice. If a plastic bag is not available, a moistened towel can be used to separate the part from the ice. If gross organic contamination has occurred, one should irrigate the tissue gently with tap water or saline. Under no circumstances should the tissue be submerged in fluids, particularly antiseptics, because they can cause cellular damage. Hemorrhaging vessels should be controlled by direct pressure (Fig. 6-2). The use of tourniquets is discouraged, and clamping of vessels must be avoided.

In the emergency room, the history should ascertain the patient's medical problems and the mechanism of injury. The patient is thoroughly evaluated and life-threatening problems are then addressed. Special attention should be paid to adequate volume replacement from major blood loss, especially in proximal limb amputations. Appropriate laboratory tests should include a complete blood count, prothrombin time, activated partial thromboplastin time, blood urea nitrogen, creatinine, electrolytes, and type and crossmatch for two to six units of packed cells. Radiographs of the distal stump, the amputated parts, and the chest should be obtained.

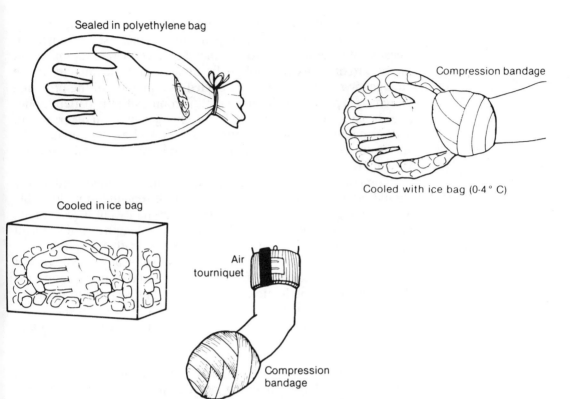

Fig. 6-2. Primary care of the amputated part and the proximal stump for transportation. (From L. R. Staub and B. D. Wilson. *Clinical Trends in Orthopedics.* New York: Thieme Medical Publishers, 1982. With permission.)

Tetanus prophylaxis, intravenous antibiotics, and rectal aspirin (10 grains) are administered. If necessary, arrangements are made for transportation to a replantation center. It is the duty of the emergency room physician to oversee coordinated, timely, efficient stabilization and transportation of the patient.

The decision as to limb viability and the potential for replantation should be made by the replantation team. It is tempting not to refer the patient to the replantation center when the salvageability of the extremity is in doubt, especially when large geographic areas are involved. *It is, however, far better that an inappropriate patient be referred for replantation than an appropriate patient not be referred.*

The replantation team should be notified immediately of the impending arrival of a potential replant. One should try to obtain from the referring physician, if possible, information about the mechanism of injury, the extent of the injury, the patient's overall general condition, and measures of resuscitation that have been taken. It is also essential to ensure that the amputated parts have been properly packaged. It is the responsibility of the replantation team to see that the patient is prepared for surgery and arrives in the operating room in a timely and expeditious manner.

Complete evaluation of the patient and the hand are performed on arrival of the patient at the replantation center (see Chapter 4). Because of patient discomfort or inability to cooperate, examination of the proximal extremity can be difficult and incomplete in the emergency room. Therefore a detailed examination of the proximal extremity is performed in the operating room with the patient under anesthesia. One can, however, in the emergency room determine to a great degree the extent of the injury as well as the potential for successful replantation by examining the amputated part and reviewing the patient's radiographs.

Upon completion of the initial evaluation, the patient and family should be informed of the following: (1) if replantation is possible and what digits are to be replanted; (2) the chances of success of the replant (50–90 percent); (3) that it is a lengthy and difficult operative procedure; (4) the prolonged postoperative hospitalization necessary (about 2 weeks); (5) additional surgical procedures that may be necessary to restore function to the part if it survives; and (6) the prolonged rehabilitation period (5–6 months) prior to return to work. Overall, the patient and family need to be assured that every effort will be made to restore the injured extremity to a useful and functioning condition.

Anesthesia and operating room personnel need to be advised of the approximate time of patient arrival and the need for any special instruments and the operating microscope ($\times 20$ magnification). Unreasonable delays in taking the person to the operating room can be avoided by readjusting the surgery schedule or calling in extra personnel.

**CLASSIFICATION:
ZONES OF INJURY**

Six zones of injury in the hand have been defined by Daniel and Terzis in an effort to assess the prognosis following replantation [19].

Zone 1: the area beyond the germinal matrix of the nail. Microvascular anastomosis is not possible in this area. Therefore the amputated part is attached as a composite graft, especially in children.

Zone II: the area between the germinal matrix and the distal interphalangeal (DIP) joint. The digital arteries measure 0.5 to 1.0 mm in diameter and can be anastomosed with 11-0 sutures. Venous anastomosis is difficult to impossible in these patients. At least 4 mm of dorsal skin proximal to the nail plate is needed on the amputated digit for realistic venous anastomosis to be possible. In the thumb, however, dorsal veins are somewhat larger and can be repaired with less difficulty.

Zone III: the area between the distal palmar crease and the DIP joint. It is the most common area for digital amputations.

Zone IV: the area of the hand between the line of the outstretched abducted thumb and the distal palmar crease.

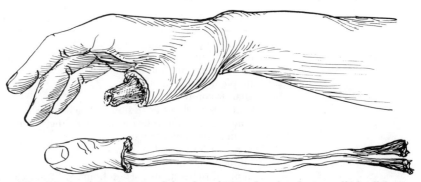

Fig. 6-3. Avulsion injury of the thumb. Tendon has been pulled off from its muscular attachment in the forearm and is hanging from the distal stump. (From R. A. Chase. *Atlas of Hand Surgery.* Philadelphia: Saunders, 1973. With permission.)

Zone V: the area between the distal wrist crease and the superficial palmar arch.
Zone VI: the area proximal to the distal wrist crease.

Zones III, IV, and V are well suited for microneurovascular repair.

MECHANISM/TYPE OF INJURY

The mechanism of injury is the single factor that determines the zone of injury. The zone of injury observed in guillotine-type amputations is small, and consequently the results after repair are favorable. With degloving or ring avulsion injuries, the soft tissue envelope may suggest limited damage; however, closer inspection usually reveals significant damage to the neurovascular bundles over a much greater distance. Avulsion injuries are often characterized by dangling nerves and tendons hanging from the distal amputated stump (Fig. 6-3). Conversely, the arteries have been torn from their vascular bed distally and can be identified on the proximal stump [20].

Crush injury produces the greatest zone of injury and damage to the neurovascular pedicle along the entire length of injury. After adequate débridement of devitalized tissue, large areas of soft tissue loss are usually encountered. It is no surprise that the poorest results in revascularization and replantation are found in this class of injuries. Rotatory machines often produce skip lacerations that result in multiple lacerations and injuries to the neurovascular bundles. Such injuries are associated with a poor prognosis for reconstruction [21].

REPLANTATION
Indications

All thumbs should be replanted (Table 6-1) [7,8,14,21–24]. Even a poorly mobile thumb can serve as an excellent post for opposition to the fingers. In addition to the thumb, all multiple-digit injuries as

Table 6-1. Indications for replantation of amputated parts

Do perform replantation.
Thumb amputation
Significant amputation in child
Multiple digit amputation
Partial or complete hand
Forearm and elbow (< 6 hours of ischemia)
Isolated digit distal to flexor digiti superficialis insertion
Do not perform replantation.
Severe crush or grinding injury
Multiple levels of injury
Prolonged ischemia time (> 6 hours with muscle mass)
Single digit proximal to PIP joint
Mentally unstable patient

well as amputation through the hand or wrist should be treated with reattachment. Replantation of amputated digits distal to the superficialis insertion typically gives excellent results. It must be stressed that all amputated parts in children should be reattached because of the excellent result that can be anticipated.

A proper history and physical examination of the injured extremity and amputated part help determine, to a great extent, the potential for successful replantation and restoration of function. Guillotine amputations and those with moderate crushing offer the best chance of survival. Moderate crush injuries form the largest group, and approximately 80 percent of them can be successfully replanted. Avulsion injuries present considerable problems. With multiple amputations the least damaged amputated part should be replanted on the most useful stumps to provide digits with better function than would be the case were the replantations placed in their true position (Fig. 6-4). The basic goal with mutilated hands should be the restoration of the thumb, web space, and, if possible, two other opposing digits.

The most important factor in the success rate of replantation is case selection. Patient motivation is important; the patient must have the desire and the capacity to participate in a long period of postoperative rehabilitation.

Contraindications   *Severe crush injuries, multiple-level amputations, and severely atherosclerotic vessels* are contraindications for replantation. A poor functional result is usually seen with single digit amputations at or proximal to the proximal interphalangeal (PIP) joint or flexor superficial insertion. Replantation of an index finger is generally thought to be contraindicated, as the patient can quickly bypass a poorly functioning index finger for the middle finger. Also, a single amputation of a digit on the ulnar side of the hand can greatly inhibit the power-gripping function of the adjacent digits. Therefore replantation of a single digit is not recommended. The exceptions to this rule are amputations distal to the PIP joint, all single digits in children, and zone 2 injuries in a highly motivated patient [25,26]. A strong

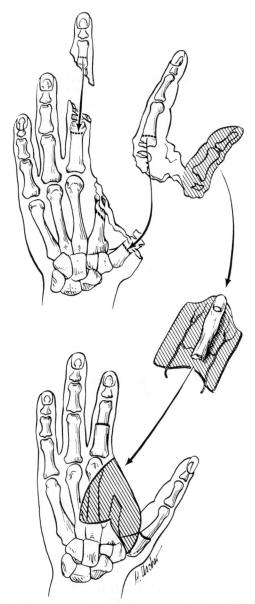

Fig. 6-4. With multiple digit injuries, the best digit is replanted on the least damaged or the most useful stump. (The index finger is replanted as a thumb, and the fileted thumb is revascularized as skin for the web space.) (From B. R. Brooks, ed. The hand. In *Rob and Smith's Operative Surgery*. St. Louis: Mosby, 1984. With permission.)

argument can also be made for reattachment of a ring finger in a female patient for cosmetic purposes.

Another contraindication for reattachment is a *prolonged ischemia time*. Tissue with muscle survives for about 6 hours without cooling and up to 12 hours if adequately cooled [15]. Ischemia time is

Table 6-2. Classification of ring avulsion injuries

Class I:	Circumferential injury with intact circulation. Nerve damage absent to minimal (usually temporary).
Class II:	Partial degloving. Revascularization and nerve repair usually necessary.
Class III:	Complete degloving or avulsion of soft tissue; revascularization and nerve repair required. Although revascularization, usually with interposition vein grafts, can restore circulation, restoration of function and adequate sensory return are unsatisfactory. Completion of amputation is recommended.

particularly important in amputations around the elbow and upper forearm. The muscle tissue breakdown following prolonged ischemia, with its resulting fibrosis and contracture, leads to poor functional results, even after revascularization. Replantation of upper arm amputations is generally contraindicated owing to the extensive muscle atrophy seen after the period required for nerve regeneration.

The *patient's age* deserves careful consideration. Because of the inevitable joint stiffness and slower regeneration of nerves in the older patient, many believe that replantation should be limited to those under 50 years of age. Severe atherosclerotic changes in the older patient population reduce the chances of successful replantation. However, excellent results have been obtained in highly motivated older patients. Therefore the patient's age alone should not be an absolute contraindication.

Mental instability is often stated as a relative contraindication for replantation. Caution must be taken in cases manifested by aggressive, self-abusive acts. A psychiatric consult is helpful for determining the prognosis in such patients. The patients should be evaluated as to their ability to participate in a rehabilitation program. An uncooperative patient is an unsuitable candidate for replantation because of a poor functional outcome. Admittedly, it is a difficult evaluation to make, even for the psychiatrist, as many of these patients are able to cooperate satisfactorily in a rehabilitation program.

With *severe crush* and *avulsion injuries* no attempt should be made to replant the avulsed digits if the vessels are torn out at an exceptionally distal level. Although revascularization can frequently be obtained for class II and III avulsion injuries with the utilization of vein grafts, the return of sensation is usually unsatisfactory and the functional results are poor (Table 6-2) [27,28]. However, avulsed thumbs should be replanted.

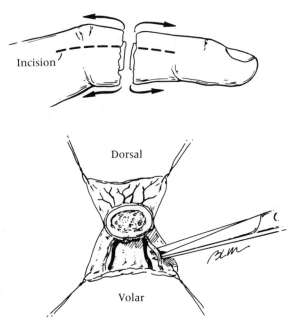

Fig. 6-5. Midlateral incisions are made slightly toward the dorsal side, and dorsal and volar skin flaps are reflected to locate and tag the arteries and veins. (From J. R. Urbaniak. Replantation. In D. P. Green, ed., *Operative Hand Surgery,* 2nd ed. New York: Churchill Livingstone, 1988. With permission.)

SURGICAL EVALUATION AND TECHNIQUES

Successful replantation or revascularization surgery usually involves a two-team approach. Even before the patient arrives in the operating room, the first team or at least one microvascular surgeon should take the *amputated part* to the operating room and start the initial débridement and microscopic identification of the neurovascular bundles. In the case of multiple digit amputations, the digits not being prepared should be kept in the refrigerator until they are ready to be utilized.

The operating room microscope is used to identify and tag arteries and nerves with sutures through bilateral mid-axial incisions [29] (Fig. 6-5). The dissection is carried out until normal vessels are encountered. The dorsal veins (two veins for every artery) should be prepared and tagged (Fig. 6-6). Identification of the veins distally saves time and facilitates localization of the corresponding proximal veins. Occasionally, the digital veins are best identified after arterial inflow has been restored. Tendons should be identified and tagged.

Skeletal shortening is performed only to débride necrotic edges and to stable opposition of bone ends; it should not be used to get the vessels together [30–32]. Double-ended 35-mm longitudinal Kirschner wires (K-wires) can be passed through the distal stump at this time (Fig. 6-7). Our preference is to make drill holes for interosseous wire fixation (Fig. 6-8). Bone shortening provides adequate length for

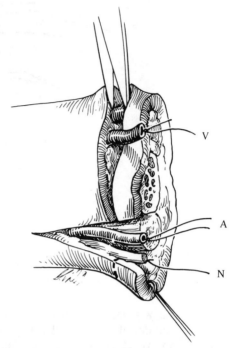

Fig. 6-6. Tagging of neurovascular bundles in the amputated part. A = artery; V = vein; N = nerve. (From B. R. Brooks, ed. The hand. In *Rob and Smith's Operative Surgery.* St. Louis: Mosby, 1984. With permission.)

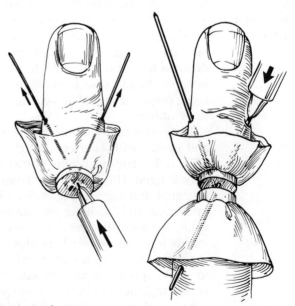

Fig. 6-7. K-wire technique. Crossed K-wires are inserted through the distal cut bone. The amputation fracture is reduced, and the K-wires are advanced proximally. (From B. R. Brooks, ed. The hand. In *Rob and Smith's Operative Surgery.* St. Louis: Mosby, 1984. With permission.)

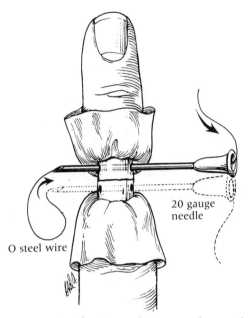

20 gauge
needle

O steel wire

Fig. 6-8. Intraosseous K-wire fixation technique. Holes are drilled using a 20-gauge hypodermic needle, and wires are passed through the holes. The amputation fracture is reduced, and the intraosseous wire is tightened. (From B. R. Brooks, ed. The hand. In *Rob and Smith's Operative Surgery.* St. Louis: Mosby, 1984. With permission.)

primary repair of tendon and neurovascular structures and facilitates soft tissue coverage. For thumb amputations, we prefer to shorten the bone on the detached part, so that a maximal amount of bone can be preserved on the stump to ensure good bone stock should the replantation fail. Generally, débridement of tendons and nerves should be conservative. At this time, a Kessler-type suture is passed into the distal flexor tendon stump for later tenorrhaphy (see Fig. 8-4).

It should be stressed that a part that is so irreversibly damaged that it cannot be replanted can be a valuable source of donor tissues for other injuries in the same or the opposite hand (Fig. 6-9). If the patient has multiple injuries, the amputated digits may be preserved at 4°C for about 24 hours and then replanted [33]. However, this technique is not possible with forearm or arm amputations.

The second microsurgical team accompanies the patient to the operating room. A Foley urinary catheter, warming blanket, venous access lines, and appropriate monitoring devices are necessary, as the procedures are long. General anesthesia is recommended for all replantations; however, regional anesthesia with long-acting axillary block is occasionally utilized [34]. The anesthesiologist should be asked to maintain a high hourly urine output and normal blood pressure, which reflect an adequate intravascular volume and normal core body temperature.

Preparation of the proximal stump should proceed generally in the same sequence as that of the amputated part and is usually performed

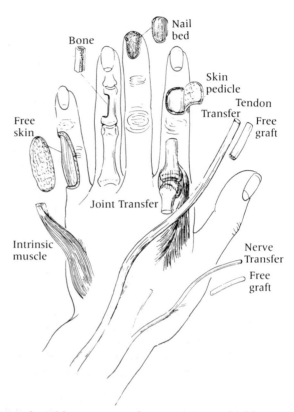

Fig. 6-9. Nonreplantable parts can often serve as a valuable source of donor tissues for other injuries in the hand. (From R. A. Chase. *Atlas of Hand Surgery.* Philadelphia: Saunders, 1973. With permission.)

simultaneously, if possible, with the preparation of the distal stump (Figs. 6-5–6-7). All devitalized tissue is débrided. The neurovascular bundles are identified and dissected back to normal tissue outside the zone of injury. Dorsal veins are identified in digital amputations. Adequate outflow from the proximal arteries is verified before the tourniquet is applied. Previously identified nerves and vessels are often difficult to find once reattachment has begun; therefore we strongly recommend tagging all neurovascular structures with a 7-0 suture. For distal forearm amputations it is helpful to identify the flexor tendons in groups to facilitate a rapid repair. The flexor pollicis longus tendon is frequently missed in distal forearm amputations because it often retracts proximally into its isolated sheath in the forearm; a separate incision to retrieve it may be needed. Interposition vein grafts and nerve grafts are often necessary and should be harvested at this point.

The *reattachment* of an amputated part follows a logical sequence as follows: (1) bony fixation; (2) extensor tendon repair; (3) flexor tendon repair; (4) venous anastomoses; (5) arterial anastomoses; (6) neurorrhaphy; and (7) soft tissue coverage

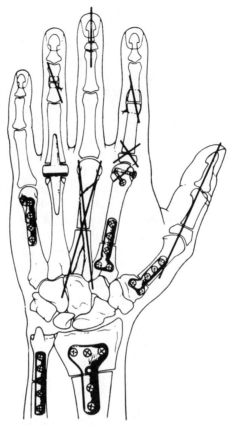

Fig. 6-10. Synopsis of the methods most widely used to achieve skeletal fixation during replantation surgery. (From V. E. Meyer. *Upper Extremity Replantation: Basic Principles, Surgical Technique, and Strategy.* New York: Churchill Livingstone, 1985. With permission.)

[10,11]. The larger and deeper structures are therefore repaired first, leaving the delicate microvascular anastomoses for last. Some microvascular surgeons prefer to do the arterial anastomoses first to limit ischemia time. However, this method can contribute to significant blood loss from the veins. Once blood flow has been restored through the arterial anastomoses, it is best not to reapply the tourniquet. Double bar venous clamps should be applied on the vein that is to be anastomosed first and single venous clamps on the other veins.

Bone fixation provides a stable framework for the replantation [30–32]. The technique of fixation depends on the level of the amputation and the type of fracture (Fig. 6-10). The best method is one that provides satisfactory bone stabilization for healing and allows initiation of early motion. In the hand and digits interosseous wiring with a longitudinal K-wire is our preferred method. K-wires in the oblique plane may cause injury to the vascular bundles and are better avoided. Proper anatomic alignment and correct rotation of the replanted part(s) should be ensured, especially with multidigit replantations. Some situations, however, dictate the use of a combination of techniques (Fig. 6-10), including external fixation. For amputations of the distal forearm and the long bones, compression plates provide the best internal fixation [35,36]. However, with contaminated wounds or severe blast injuries, external fixation devices may be necessary [37] (see Chapter 7). Amputations that cross joints are treated by shortening and primary arthrodesis in a position of function [38].

For arthrodesis at a joint level, interosseous wire and a single K-wire are used. Implant arthroplasty has been recommended in select cases of replantation of one or more fingers that have been clearly amputated through the PIP joint (e.g., in a pianist) [38].

The tendons are repaired as for any normal tendon laceration. The extensors are repaired with figure-of-eight 4-0 nylon sutures, and the flexor tendons are repaired using a modified Kessler technique and 4-0 and 6-0 nylon sutures (see Chapters 8 and 9).

Attention is now directed toward the *microvascular anastomoses.* Certain principles must be observed: (1) The anastomoses must be performed outside the zone of injury; (2) pulsatile arterial inflow must be established; (3) atraumatic microvascular technique is utilized; and (4) a tensionless repair is essential. Débridement of the arteries should be undertaken both proximally and distally until normal intima is encountered and brisk pulsatile arterial bleeding is verified proximally. Poor arterial inflow usually indicates inadequate proximal débridement of the injured arteries [39]. Fine platelet aggregates inside the lumen, fibrin strands, and intimal telescoping are sure signs of inadequate débridement that lead to vascular thrombosis. Inadequate débridement is therefore not an alternative for avoiding an interposition vein graft.

Shortening of the bony skeleton during fixation usually allows for a tension-free primary microvascular repair. In the event that sufficient skeletal shortening cannot be obtained for a tension-free primary vascular repair, we recommend interposition vein grafts [40]. Veins in the immediate proximity are of similar caliber and suitable for anastomosis. Veins in the same extremities should be chosen carefully for vein grafts so as not to compromise their use to salvage a venous thrombosis. Veins of the lower extremity are thicker and have characteristics of the arteries of the upper extremity. For this reason, we prefer to choose veins from the distal lower extremity for arterial interposition grafts. Opposite hand and forearm are also an excellent source for vein grafts.

If injury or débridement leaves the proximal stump with no available arterial outflow or venous inflow, an artery or vein can be transposed from an adjacent part of the digit [41]. This technique is particularly important with crushing or avulsion injuries. Alternatively, the superficial palmar arch can be divided and straightened to provide a distal arterial supply to an amputated digit.

We routinely prepare one lower extremity and the opposite hand

and forearm for potential vein grafts. One needs to advise the anesthetist of this intent so multiple intravenous punctures are not attempted in the opposite hand. The length of the vein graft is made approximately 20 percent shorter than the defect because veins have a tendency to elongate and dilate after reperfusion.

We recommend repairing one artery per digit during multiple digital amputations. However, always attempt to repair both digital arteries, if possible, when replanting one or two digits. We repair both ulnar and radial arteries in hand or forearm amputations.

Vascular spasm is a common problem encountered after reperfusion [42]. It is most effectively relieved by mechanical dilatation using a strong arterial inflow. Topical 20% lidocaine is also effective for relieving localized spasm in small vessels. Vascular spasm is occasionally triggered by a cold room. Room temperature should therefore be kept around 78°F. Warm compresses on the distal extremity and over the anastomoses may help reverse the spasm. After having established arterial inflow and satisfactory venous outflow, warm compresses are placed over the entire extremity and the patency of the vessels observed for about 20 minutes. Most microvascular failures can be recognized within this early period. This short period of observation provides a well deserved rest and a chance to identify and correct an impending vascular failure.

Almost universally, *failure after reperfusion* of a microvascular anastomoses can be attributed to one of two causes: (1) technical error at the anastomotic site; or (2) unrecognized vascular injury/inadequate débridement. The two-team approach pays its highest dividends at this time. Fatigue can contribute to judgment errors and technical mistakes. In the event of failure of microvascular anastomoses and cessation of flow, a well rested second microvascular team should evaluate the repair to detect problems that may have been missed. If the anastomosis occludes without obvious abnormality of the arterial wall, the anastomosis should be taken down and redone. Heparin (5000 units), as an intravenous bolus, is given prior to reestablishing the circulation and may prevent a recurrence of the thrombosis.

The use of the tourniquet is essential. With multiple digital replants, the tourniquet can be inflated and deflated multiple times without compromising the vascular repair, so long as the patient is heparinized [43].

Special considerations are necessary with *thumb replantation* [29, 32]. Because of the anatomic arrangement of the neurovascular pedicles on the volar surface of the thumb, positioning for microvascular anastomoses can be difficult. Excessive bone shortening in an attempt to attain primary nerve and vascular repair may sacrifice valuable functional length. A useful alternative is to anastomose an interposition vein graft to the ulnar digital artery of the thumb prior to skeletal fixation. The interposition graft then, at the appropriate time, is anastomosed well away from the thumb usually to the

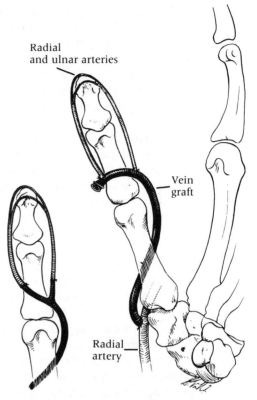

Fig. 6-11. Revascularization of the ulnar digital artery of the thumb with a vein graft to the radial artery in the anatomic snuffbox. (From H. E. Kleinert and J. B. Jupiter. Replantation — an overview. In L. R. Staub and B. D. Wilson, eds., *Trends in Orthopedics.* New York: Thieme-Stratton, 1982. With permission.)

princeps pollicis artery (end-to-end) or to the radial artery (end-to-side) in the anatomic snuffbox [44] (Fig. 6-11). Access to the venous anastomoses usually is not a problem.

Distal fingertip amputations also pose a unique problem [20,24]. The small size of the vessels makes the microvascular repair challenging. It may be difficult to find suitable veins, especially in close proximity to the nail bed. Although excellent results have been attained with reattachment of the part as a composite graft, in children microvascular repair provides the best results. Partial nail removal and application of heparin-soaked gauze has been successfully used as an alternative method of venous drainage [45]. Satisfactory revascularization can occasionally be obtained with microvascular anastomoses of an artery to a distal vein at this level if differentiation of arteries from veins becomes difficult [46]. Therefore at the distal tip two anastomoses, one arterial and one venous, are all that is necessary.

The *nerves* are then repaired with great care under the microscope using interrupted 9-0 sutures. For digital nerves, only two to three

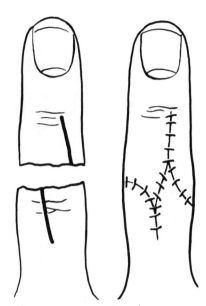

Fig. 6-12. Z-Plasty closure increases the length of the circumferential scar and facilitates a loose closure over the vessel repairs. (From B. R. Brooks, ed. The hand. In *Rob and Smith's Operative Surgery.* St. Louis: Mosby, 1984. With permission.)

sutures are necessary. Proximal nerve injuries need more sutures for coaptation. The long duration of ischemia does not seem to have an effect on the eventual quality of nerve regeneration [13]. Primary nerve repair or nerve grafting therefore should be carried out.

The *skin closure* should be tension-free. The mid-axial incisions should be carefully closed so as not to injure the vascular bundle underneath. Z-Plasties of the skin incisions may occasionally be utilized (Fig. 6-12). Sometimes primary closure of the skin wound is not possible because of excessive swelling from prolonged ischemia or trauma. Skin grafts may be used to provide a permanent or temporary coverage of wounds, even including the vascular pedicles. Local flaps or microvascular free flaps are preferable to cover exposed tendon, bone, or neurovascular bundles.

DRESSING THE WOUND

After satisfactory skin closure, the extremity is cleansed and a nonstick gauze is placed over the incisions followed by a generous layer of dry gauze held circumferentially with cast padding. A sugar-tong splint is then fashioned and extended beyond the finger-tips. The dressings should allow easy access to and exposure of the fingertips in order to evaluate perfusion, although they must also offer protection from exposure (Fig. 6-13). Application of a sponge dressing prior to placing the splint permits further swelling of the extremity without fear of compression of the dressings. The dressings are not changed for several days, but care is taken to prevent

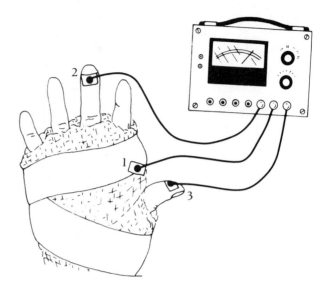

Fig. 6-13. Postoperative dressing leaving the fingertips exposed. Temperature probes — 1 (ambient temperature), 2 (control), and 3 (replanted digit) — for monitoring are in place. (From J. R. Urbaniak, Replantation of amputated hands and digits. In *AAOS Instructional Course Lectures.* St. Louis: Mosby, 1978.

constricting dressings from dried blood, which may interfere with venous return. The extremity should be elevated to relieve venous congestion.

POSTOPERATIVE CARE

The replanted digit or extremity should manifest a normal healthy pink color. Color changes in darkly pigmented patients are frequently of little or no help, and here the color of the nail bed should be closely inspected. Prolonged vascular refill with a pale digit is suggestive of arterial thrombosis. A congested, dusky blue digit is suggestive of venous thrombosis. Early venous thrombosis is demonstrated by a rapidly refilling, brightly pink digit. If such is noted, releasing some of the skin sutures may be all that is necessary. A gentle massage over the dorsum of the replant sometimes helps restore moderately compromised venous outflow. Skin turgor should be soft and supple. Induration or firmness is suggestive of vascular compromise. Puncture of the extremity with a 25-gauge needle is a useful diagnostic maneuver. Bright red blood following the needle stick indicates that the arterial anastomosis is probably satisfactory. Venous congestion can be appreciated by a dark-appearing blood. A pale digit with no bleeding on needle stick means arterial thrombosis.

Skin temperature can be monitored by skin probe and is helpful for monitoring the vascular anastomosis (Fig. 6-13) [47]. A temperature that falls below 30°F or more than 2°F lower than the temperature of a controlled, uninjured digit is highly suspicious of vascular compromise. The laser Doppler technique and the pulse oximeter have become reliable methods for continuously monitoring the viability of replants [48,49]. If oxygen saturation falls below 91 percent saturation, it is suggestive of vascular compromise. One should not hesitate to explore early if a change is noted in the clinical status of a replanted extremity or digit [50].

The greatest percentage of microvascular replant failures occurs within the first 48 hours, when swelling is at its maximum and external pressure along the anastomosis is the greatest. The patient should continue to be monitored for at least 5 to 8 days under the best of circumstances.

The extremity is kept elevated, and care is taken to avoid circumferential or compressive dressings on it. Antibiotics are usually continued for 24 hours to 5 days depending on the nature of the injury and potential contamination. The patient is maintained NPO for the first 12 hours so that he or she can be readily returned to the operating room for reexploration if indicated. The temperature of the room is kept elevated at 78°F; and, if necessary, a heating lamp is placed over the replanted extremity. No smoking is allowed by the patient or in the patient's room to negate the vasoactive effects of nicotine [51,52]. Stellate ganglion block can be useful for obtaining vasodilatation and pain relief [34].

Aspirin is given, 10 grains daily, for 30 days because of its antithrombogenic effects. The efficacy of low-molecular-weight dextran and heparin are controversial and unproved. Nevertheless, they are routinely utilized postoperatively by some microvascular surgeons with excellent results. Dextran at 25 ml per hour is usually given for 5 days and then discontinued. We recommend heparin therapy in situations where there is unusual technical difficulty or sluggish flow despite a technically good anastomosis, especially if the anastomosis has to be redone, and in cases where the tourniquet is inflated and deflated multiple times in the face of recent anastomosis [43,53]. Both dextran and heparin are capable of producing serious bleeding diatheses, and the patient should be carefully monitored for such complications. Dextran can also cause anaphylactic reactions.

COMPLICATIONS   Complications [54,55] include the following.

1. *Swelling* is common. Tight skin closure and tight circumferential dressings should be avoided.

2. *Venous congestion* is recognized by a temperature drop of the part and a flushed purple appearance with a rapid capillary refill. The pulp of a congested digit has increased turgor and a feeling of fullness. Significant bleeding from the wound edges due to venous hypertension is noteworthy.

Tight sutures and constricting bandages are released. Additional elevation and gentle milking along the dorsum of the digit toward the microvenous anastomoses may improve the venous outflow. Incisions in the distal pulp with dark bleeding confirms the diagnosis and may improve the circulation, as demonstrated by a change in the color of the digit. Vascular decompression can be accomplished by: (1) making an incision in the finger pulp or by removing the nail plate and treating the patient with local and systemic heparin [45,56]; and (2) the application of leeches [57]. The anticoagulation drug is readjusted. If there is no improvement in 2 to 3 hours, reoperation is desirable. Reoperation must not be delayed, as secondary thrombosis of the arterial anastomosis can result.

3. *Arterial occlusion* is the most common cause of failure [9]. The first sign of arterial insufficiency is a slowed capillary return. The replant becomes a mottled bluish color, the temperature of the replant falls, and the pulp develops an empty feel. Again, constricting bandages, tight sutures, and hematomas should be released. Early surgical intervention is usually necessary.

Revisional surgery to alleviate a deficiency in circulation is difficult. Anastomosis of unused vessels is more reliable than further surgery to the original anastomosis, as the fragile vessels are difficult to resuture and intimal changes that accompany thrombosis predispose to further clotting. A faulty anastomosis should be taken down and if necessary a vein graft interposed. One needs to avoid kinking and rotation of vein grafts.

4. *Postoperative bleeding* results from improper anticoagulation and untied dorsal veins. Correction or cessation of anticoagulation is necessary. If bleeding continues, reexploration is indicated.

5. *Infection* occurs rarely.

6. *Skin necrosis* is common on the dorsal surface of the digits. Localized skin necrosis is treated conservatively. Exposure of the venous anastomosis leads to a high risk of thrombosis. Gradual débridement with secondary healing, skin grafts, or local flaps may be necessary.

7. *Bone nonunion* occurs rarely [36].

REHABILITATION   The postreplantation digit presents a rehabilitative challenge [58]. Because both flexor and extensor mechanisms are involved, early therapy should use active exercises, avoiding vigorous passive exercises. Three weeks postoperatively, dynamic dorsal block splints are applied to provide stability and allow motion of the involved digits, tendon gliding, and range of motion.

The *success* of any replantation can be measured only by the functional restoration. An 80 percent or more viability rate should be achieved in any good replantation center [7–11]. Approximately 50 percent or more active range of motion is achieved in most patients. Nerve recovery is comparable to that of isolated nerve transection [13,20,59]. Cold intolerance is a definite problem but improves after 18 to 24 months. The cosmetic appearance following replantation along with the sensory recovery far supercedes the prosthesis.

Approximately 40 percent of the digits require secondary surgical procedures, including tenolysis, nerve graft, capsulectomy, tendon graft or transfer, pedicle flaps, and free flaps for tissue coverage [35].

Return to employment does not correlate with the mechanism of injury or the amputation level; it largely depends on individual motivation. The average time for return to work is approximately 6 months [8, 15].

MAJOR LIMB REPLANTATION

Major limb amputations often have significant crushing of tissues and can be associated with life-threatening injuries and hypotension due to blood loss. Hyperkalemia or myoglobinuria after revascularization and hypotension can cause acute renal failure. Hypothermia may also be a major problem [12, 21, 24, 35, 36, 60–62].

The statistical survival of the replanted part improves as one progresses from the palm to the proximal forearm and arm because of the large diameter of the injured arteries and veins; however, functional restoration becomes increasingly more difficult. Ischemia becomes a critical issue because of the muscle mass involved. The end result cannot be assessed for 12 to 24 months because of the prolonged period of recovery required.

Replanted amputations at the level of the palm, wrist, and distal forearm result in good hand function; however, good results are not always obtained with proximal limb amputations. Muscle necrosis and infection further add to the poor outcome [14, 35, 36].

Management

Cooling is essential, as it doubles the ischemia time and reduces the acidosis induced by the production of lactate. No time can be wasted because of ischemia time to the muscle mass. One should rule out major head, thoracoabdominal, and lower extremity injuries. The limb should not be replanted under the following conditions: if the limb has suffered multiple-level amputations, avulsion, or a crush injury; if there has been more than 6 to 12 hours of warm ischemia time; if there is poor mental status; if the patient is over 50 years old; or if there is other significant bodily injury.

Major limb replantations produce better functional results than any presently available prosthesis. In addition, retention of the limb is psychologically important to the patient.

Preparation of the Amputated Part

The proximal and distal parts should be prepared as quickly as possible to keep the ischemia time to a minimum. Arteries, veins, and nerves are tagged with 7-0 nylon to enable easier visualization under the microscope. Extensive muscle débridement on the detached part and the stump is essential to prevent myonecrosis and infection. An arterial shunt can be used to obtain rapid arterial inflow from the proximal vessel to the amputated part if the ischemia time has already been prolonged (4–6 hours) [63]. Arterial repair should always be performed prior to venous anastomosis.

Six-hole plates are used for the humerus and four-hole plates for forearm bones [35,36]. One should limit the periosteal stripping. External fixation is recommended for heavily contaminated wounds [37]. For amputations through the wrist, 45-mm, long K-wires are introduced through small stab incisions at the neck of the metacarpal, avoiding the dorsal veins and the MCP joints. The K-wires are driven into the metacarpal block if the radiocarpal joint is intact. This technique results in carpometacarpal arthrodesis. Proximal row carpectomy is occasionally necessary if the radiocarpal joint is badly injured. The wrist is immobilized in neutral position if wrist fusion is required.

The tourniquet is applied after the bone fixation is completed. Tendon repair is performed next using figure-of-eight sutures, provided it is possible to do it without interfering with vessel and nerve repair. In the mid-forearm, muscles are simply approximated with 3-0 chromic sutures in the myofascia. The major problem with mid-forearm amputation is to match the tendons in the distal segment with the muscle tendinous units in the proximal part.

We routinely use the microscope for anastomosing nerves and vessels. The microscope offers several advantages: the ability to determine if the intima has been damaged, the ability to use 8-0 and 9-0 sutures, and the avoidance of having to use adventitial flaps in the lumen. The arteries are addressed first and then the veins. Once again one should ensure good proximal pulsatile flow. Reestablishment of arterial inflow causes significant venous bleeding, which is controlled by vascular clamps. The anesthesiologist must be warned when the arterial clamps come off because toxic products are mobilized into the general circulation after revascularization. Our practice is to let the veins drain for a few minutes to prevent this problem. The veins are then anastomosed, followed by the nerves. We prefer epineural repair; if the nerve ends are severely crushed or avulsed, sural nerve cable grafts are used after débridement [59]. For proximal limb replantations fasciotomies of the flexor and extensor compartments are performed as required. Both radial and ulnar arteries are repaired to limit cold intolerance and for improved perfusion. If the underlying muscle is of good quality, a split-thickness skin graft is used for soft tissue coverage. Primary skin closure is preferred whenever possible.

Postoperative Management

A supportive bandage is applied leaving the fingers free. Residual iodine is cleared from the patient's nails to be able to check the color. Monitoring is carried out as for digital replants. We use acetylsalicylic acid 10 grains per day rectally or orally for 1 month and dextran 25 ml per hour for 5 days. Gentle passive finger movements are started early.

Functional results do not become clear for a minimum period of 18 to 24 months. Intrinsic muscle paralysis is the major problem with these replantations, particularly adduction contracture of the thumb, and requires proper splinting. It may be due to prolonged ischemia or lack of reinnervation. Only 40 percent of patients achieve good results [36,61,62]. Precision work usually cannot be undertaken by the replanted limb.

No reflow phenomenon is the term applied when all flow into the replanted part ceases, despite a well executed arterial repair that passes all patency tests, and venous return is sluggish or absent [64]. This problem has been attributed to production of free oxygen radicals secondary to prolonged warm ischemia, diffuse intravascular thrombosis, and loss of vascular integrity [65–67].

Replantation surgery may result in significant psychological problems, which are often similar to grieving [68]. It might be in the form of nightmares, flashbacks, and affective lability. Psychological problems may be potentiated by patient's concerns regarding his or her ability to return to work and other financial matters.

Fasciotomy

Fasciotomies are carried out without reservation if there are indications of compression or constriction to decompress the vessels and muscles and prevent myonecrosis and infection. The procedure should include both volar and dorsal compartments, thenar and hypothenar muscle masses, and the interossei. The fasciotomy incisions are dressed with Adaptic gauze dressings. The limbs must be examined in the operating room under regional or general anesthesia 48 hours later to evaluate the muscles and to débride any necrotic areas.

Summary

A replantation center with a well trained staff of microsurgeons and hand therapists can achieve a high level of success in most replantation patients. The ideal candidate for replantation is a young patient with a sharp, clean amputation distal to the insertion of the flexor digitorum superficialis tendon. However, careful selection is the key to achieving a functional digit that is useful to the patient.

When more than one digit is amputated, the ulnar side of the hand should be reconstructed first to restore the power grip and allow grasping of large objects. If the thumb is also amputated, it should be replanted first; but if the thumb is badly damaged, another digit should be transposed to the thumb position.

Amputation of one finger when accompanied by serious injury to other digits, though technically constituting "a single digit amputation," should be considered a "multiple finger injury."

AMPUTATIONS

Amputation of a digit or the whole hand may result from injury or be required following injury; or it may be indicated as a planned procedure in the patient with malignancy or ischemic gangrene. The large group of amputations, however, is caused by sharp cutting machinery or a rotary saw.

Most traumatic amputations affect the tip of the digit and are not

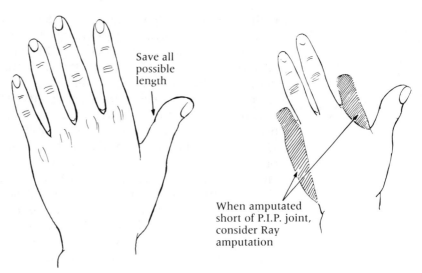

Fig. 6-14. Save as much length as possible during thumb amputations. When the amputation is short of the PIP joint in the index and little fingers, consider ray amputation. (From R. A. Chase. *Atlas of Hand Surgery*. Philadelphia: Saunders, 1973. With permission.)

discussed here (see Chapter 5). Single traumatic amputations at a more proximal level, associated with crushing, are best treated by shortening the bone and effecting primary skin closure to provide good quality sensate skin with excellent padding that is mobile over bone. Volar skin flaps provide the best skin. The tendons are cut and allowed to retract. The nerves are cut sharply at least 1 cm proximally and allowed to retract into the subcutaneous fat pad. For an amputation involving disarticulation of a joint, the condylar heads are trimmed to prevent a bulbous stump. When the thumb is involved, irrespective of whether other digits are involved, one should preserve as much length as possible. Several local advancement flaps are available to achieve adequate padding during the closure of amputation stumps (see Chapter 11). In the small child (under 2 years) the wound is cleaned and dressed in anticipation of excellent tissue regeneration. When the tissue is recovered, it can often be reattached, without revascularization, as a composite graft.

Amputation at any site in the hand should be treated with great care to allow primary healing. Good skin cover, normal sensation, and minimal scarring are the key. Painful neuroma of the digital nerve is one of the more common complications of digital amputation, and its treatment is difficult.

The level of amputation is of great practical importance [69,70]. In the thumb as much length as is permissible is preserved (Fig. 6-14). For other digits, amputation distal to the insertion of the superficialis tendon gives a useful stump. The stump is rarely of great functional benefit when proximal to the insertion of the superficialis tendon. Therefore for the index and little fingers a more proximal

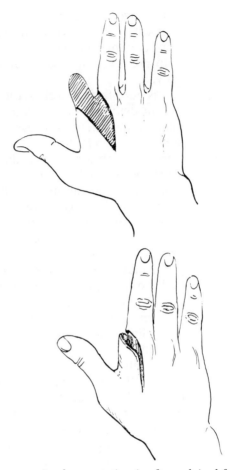

Fig. 6-15. A more proximal amputation is often advised for the index and little fingers. Oblique section through the metacarpal neck removes the unsightly projection of the metacarpal head. (From R. A. Chase. *Atlas of Hand Surgery.* Philadelphia: Saunders, 1973. With permission.)

amputation is often advised; an oblique section through the metacarpal neck removes the unsightly projection of the metacarpal head (Fig. 6-15) but preserves the attachment of the deep transverse ligament of the palm, thereby retaining the span of the palm. The first dorsal interosseous in the index and the abductor digiti minimi in the little finger are elevated subperiosteally before the bone is sectioned. The tendons are then sutured to the base of the proximal phalanx of the adjacent digit. This technique provides an excellent aesthetic appearance to the hand.

In the central digits (i.e., the long and ring fingers) the best site for amputation is beyond or at the PIP joint level. To prevent objects sliding through the defect left by the missing finger, always retain a small segment of the proximal phalanx. In the middle ray, particularly in the female, more proximal amputation through the neck of the metacarpal, complete ablation of the third ray, and moving the index finger over by reattaching the deep transverse palmar ligament provides excellent cosmetic results [71,72]. It is also possible to transfer either the second or the fifth ray to replace the missing ray with preservation of good function and with less noticeable deformity.

It is our practice to close the amputation stump initially and carry out the definitive ray resection as a delayed procedure several weeks later. Some patients, however, do not wish to go through any further surgery and prefer to keep the stump. Occasionally, patients become unhappy with a replanted digit or limb that is painful and hypersensitive, especially in the cold weather. Such patients may request amputation several months after all the scars are well healed [36].

When the hand is not replantable, disarticulation of the wrist and preservation of the triangular fibrocartilage to maintain stability of the distal radioulnar joint has the advantage of preserving full pronation and supination.

A painful stump is one of the common problems of hand injuries and is often difficult to manage [73]. Adherent free skin graft to the bony stump is a common cause. The stump needs revision by shortening the bone and providing a soft and supple skin cover with local advancement flaps.

Tender neuroma of one or both digital nerves in close contact to dense, adherent scar can be a source of severe pain [74,75]. Resection of the neuroma is justified and should be combined with burying the neuroma in a pad of fat or muscle or in bone. Capping the nerve with a silicone cap is often recommended as an alternative. Local infiltration of lidocaine, phenol, or alcohol, local percussion, and gentle tapping of the end of the stump on a firm surface produce only temporary and not so reliable results.

Occasionally there is no discernible local abnormality to account for the stump pain. The patient is often a tense and nervous individual. This causalgic type may be associated with litigation claims following an industrial injury. Analgesics, depressants, and sympathetic blockade may be useful. Some of these patients improve with time.

Lack of sensitivity over the fingertip can be distressing to some patients. This problem is seen occasionally after skin grafting techniques. Stump revision may be helpful. In most situations, no surgery is recommended, so long as the skin is soft, pliable, and nonadherent to bone.

REFERENCES

1. Lapchinsky, A. G. Recent results of experimental transplantation of preserved limbs and kidneys and possible use of this technique in clinical practice. *Ann. N.Y. Acad. Sci.* 87:539, 1960.
2. Snyder, C. C., et al. Extremity replantation. *Plast. Reconstr. Surg.* 26:251, 1960.
3. Jacobsen, J. H., and Suarez, E. L. Microsurgery in anastomosis of small vessels. *Surg. Forum* 2:243, 1960.

4. Kleinert, H. E., Kasdan, M. L., and Romero, J. L. Small blood vessel anastomosis for salvage of the severely injured upper extremity. *J. Bone Joint Surg.* [*Am.*] 45:788, 1963.
5. Buncke, H. J., Jr., and Schulz, W. P. Experimental digital amputation in replantation. *Plast. Reconstr. Surg.* 36:62, 1965.
6. Komatsu, S., and Tamai, S. Successful replantation of a completely cut-off thumb: case report. *Plast. Reconstr. Surg.* 42:374, 1968.
7. Morrison, W. A., O'Brien, B. M., and MacLeoad, A. M. Evaluation of digital replantation on a review of 100 cases. *Orthop. Clin. North Am.* 8:295, 1977.
8. Tamai, S. Digit replantation: analysis of 163 replantations in an eleven-year period. *Clin. Plast. Surg.* 5:195, 1978.
9. Tsai Tsu-Min. Experimental and clinical applications of microvascular surgery. *Ann. Surg.* 2:169, 1975.
10. O'Brien, B. McC., et al. Clinical replantation of digits. *Plast. Reconstr. Surg.* 52:491, 1973.
11. O'Brien B. McC., and MacLeoad, A. M. Replantation surgery. In R. J. Manchee and J. T. Hueston (eds.), *Transactions of the Sixth International Congress of Plastic and Reconstructive Surgery,* Paris, 1976.
12. Chen Chun Wei. American replant mission to China: replantation surgery in China. *Plast. Reconstr. Surg.* 52:476, 1973.
13. Morrison, W. A., et al. Long term nerve function in replantation surgery of the hands and digits. *Ann. Chir.* 29:1041, 1975.
14. Dobyns, J. H. (Seminar Chairman). Results of microsurgery in orthopedics. *Am. Acad. Orthop. Surg.* 665:1981.
15. Kleinert, H. E., Jablon, M., and Tsai, T. M. An overview or replantation and result of 347 replants in 245 patients. *J. Trauma* 20:390, 1980.
16. O'Brien, B. M., et al. Replantation and revascularization surgery in children. *Hand* 121:12, 1980.
17. Urbaniak, J. R. Replantation. In D. P. Green (ed.), *Operative Hand Surgery,* 2nd ed. New York: Churchill Livingstone, 1988. P. 1105.
18. Van Gresen, P. J., Seaber, A. V., and Urbaniak, J. R. Storage of amputated parts prior to replantation: an experimental study with rabbit ears. *J. Hand Surg.* [*Am.*] 8:60, 1983.
19. Daniel, R. K., and Terzis, J. K. *Reconstructive Microsurgery,* 1st ed. Boston: Little, Brown, 1977.
20. Van Beek, A. L., Kutz, J. E., and Zook, E. G. Importance of the ribbon sign, indicating unsuitability of the vessel in replanting a finger. *Plast. Reconstr. Surg.* 61:32, 1978.
21. MacLeod, A. M., O'Brien, B. McC., and Morrison, W. A. Digital replantation. In D. A. Campbell Reid and R. Tubiana (eds.), *Mutilating Injuries of the Hand.* New York: Churchill Livingstone, 1984.
22. Chen, Z. W., et al. Present indications and contraindications for replantation as reflected by long-term functional results. *Orthop. Clin. North Am.* 12:849, 1981.
23. Urbaniak, J. R. *Replantation of Amputated Hands and Digits.* AAOS Instructor Course Lecture, Vol. 27. St. Louis: Mosby, 1978. Pp. 15–26.
24. Urbaniak, J. R. Replantation of amputated parts in technique, results and indications. In *American Academy of Orthopedic Surgeons, Symposium on Microsurgery: Practical Use in Orthopedics.* St. Louis: Mosby, 1979. P. 64.
25. Urbaniak, J. R., et al. The results of replantation after amputation of a single finger. *J. Bone Joint Surg.* [*Am.*] 67:611, 1985.

26. May, J. W., Toth, B. A., and Gardener, M. Digital replantation distal to the proximal interphalangeal joint. *J. Hand Surg* 7:161, 1982.
27. Urbaniak, J. R., Evans, J. P., and Bright, D. S. Microvascular management of ring avulsion injuries. *J. Hand Surg.* 6:25, 1981.
28. Carroll, R. Ring injuries to the hand. *Clin. Orthop.* 104:175, 1981.
29. Nissenbaum, M. A surgical approach for replantation of complete digital amputations. *J. Hand Surg.* 5:58, 1980.
30. Lister, G. Intraosseous wiring of the digital skeleton. *J. Hand Surg.* 3:427, 1978.
31. Urbaniak, J. R., Hayes, M. G., and Bright, D. S. Management of bone in digital replantation: free vascularized and composite bone grafts. *Clin. Orthop.* 133:184, 1978.
32. Schlenker, J. D., Kleinert, H. E., and Tsai, T. M. Methods and results of replantation following traumatic amputation of the thumb in 64 patients. *J. Hand Surg.* 5:63, 1980.
33. May, J. W., Jr. Successful digital replantation after 28 hours of cold ischemia. *Plast. Reconstr. Surg.* 67:566, 1981.
34. Matsuda, M., Kato, N., and Hosoi, M. Continuous brachial plexus block for replantation in the upper extremity. *Hand* 14:129, 1982.
35. Ferreira, M. C., Marques, E. F., and Azze, R. J. Limb replantation. *Clin. Plast. Surg.* 5:211, 1978.
36. Tamai, S., et al. Major limb, hand and digital replantation. *World J. Surg.* 3:17, 1979.
37. Weiland, A. J., Robinson, H., and Futrell, J. External stabilization of a replanted upper extremity. *J. Trauma* 16:239, 1976.
38. Wray, R. C., Young, V. L., and Weeks, P. M. Flexible implant arthroplasty and finger replantation. *Plast. Reconstr. Surg.* 74:97, 1984.
39. Sanders, W. E. Principle of microvascular surgery. In D. P. Green (ed.), *Operative Hand Surgery,* 2nd ed. New York: Churchill Livingstone, 1988. Pp. 1049–1103.
40. Alpert, B. S., Buncke, H. J., and Brownstein, M. Replacement of damaged arteries and veins with vein grafts when replanting crushed, amputated fingers. *Plast. Reconstr. Surg.* 61:17, 1978.
41. Pho, R. W., Chacha, P. B., and Yeo, K. O. Rerouting vessels and nerves from other digits in replanting an avulsed and degloved thumb. *Plast. Reconstr. Surg.* 64:330, 1979.
42. Phelps, D. B., Rutherford, R. B., and Boswick, J. A., Jr. Control of vasospasm following trauma and microvascular surgery. *J. Hand Surg.* 4:109, 1979.
43. Tamai, S. Multiple digit replantation. In R. K. Daniel and J. K. Terzis (eds.), *Reconstructive Microsurgery.* Boston: Little, Brown, 1977. Pp. 172–176.
44. Kleinert, H. E., Tsai, T. M., and Jupiter, J. B. Replantation — an overview. In L. R. Straub and P. D. Wilson (eds.), *Clinical Trends in Orthopedics.* New York: Thieme-Stratton, 1982.
45. Gordon, L., et al. Partial nail plate removal after digital replantation as an alternative method of venous drainage. *J. Hand Surg.* [*Am.*] 10:360, 1985.
46. Smith, A. R., Sonneveld, G. F., and Vander Mullen, J. C. AV anastomosis as solution for absent venous drainage in replantation surgery. *Plast. Reconstr. Surg.* 71:525, 1983.
47. Stirratt, C. R., et al. Temperature monitoring in digital replantation. *J. Hand Surg.* 3:332, 1978.

48. Heden, P. G., et al. Laser Doppler surveillance of the circulation of free flap and replanted digits. *Microsurgery* 6:11, 1985.
49. Graham, B., Lauling, D. A., and Caffee, H. H. Pulse oximetry for vascular monitoring an upper extremity replantation surgery. *J. Hand Surg.* [*Am.*] 11:687, 1986.
50. Tupper, J. W. Vascular defects and salvage of failed vascular repairs. In *AAOS Symposium on Microsurgery. Practical Use in Orthopedics.* St. Louis, Mosby, 1979. P. 111.
51. Harris, G. D., Finseth, F., and Buncke, H. J. The hazards of cigarette smoking following digital replantation. *J. Microsurg.* 1:403, 1980.
52. Savin, C. L., Austin, J. C., and Nickel, W. O. Effect of smoking on digital blood flow velocity. *J.A.M.A.* 229:1329, 1974.
53. Rapoport, S., et al. Aggressive postoperative pharmacotherapy for vascular compromise of replanted digits. *A.J.R.* 144:1065, 1985.
54. Leung PC. Analysis of complications in digital replantations. *Hand* 14:25, 1982.
55. Strauch, B., et al. Problems and complications encountered in replantation surgery. *Hand Clin.* 2:389, 1986.
56. Sadahiro, T., and Endoh, H. Continuous blood letting for congestion in replantation of the amputated finger. *J. Hand Surg.* [*Br.*] 9:83, 1984.
57. Lim, C. L. Successful transfer of free microvascular superficial temporal artery flap with no obvious venous drainage: use of leeches for reducing venous congestion; a case report. *Microsurgery* 7(2):87, 1986.
58. Kader, P. B. Therapist's management of the replanted hand. *Hand Clin.* 2:179, 1986.
59. Wilgis, E. F. S., and Maxwell, G. P. Distal digital nerve grafts: clinical and anatomic studies. *J. Hand Surg.* 4:439, 1979.
60. Malt, R. A., and McKhann, C. F. Replantation of severed arms. *J.A.M.A.* 189:716, 1964.
61. Malt, R. A., Remensnyder, J. P., and Harris, W. H. Long term utility of replanted arms. *Ann. Surg.* 176:334, 1972.
62. Jaeger, S. H., Tsai, T., and Kleinert, H. E. Upper extremity replantation in children. *Orthop. Clin. North Am.* 12:897, 1981.
63. Nunley, J. A., Coman, L. A., and Urbaniak, J. R. Arterial shunting as an adjunct to major limb revascularization. *Ann. Surg.* 193:271, 1981.
64. May, J. W., et al. The no-flow phenomenon in experimental free flaps. *Plast. Reconstr. Surg.* 61:256, 1978.
65. Zdeblick, T. A., Schaeffer, J. Q., and Field, G. A. An ischemia induced model of revascularization failure of replanted limbs. *J. Hand Surg.* [*Am.*] 10:125, 1985.
66. Erickson, E., Anderson, W. A., and Reglogle, R. L. Effects of prolonged ischemia on muscle microcirculation in the cat. *Surg. Forum* 25:254, 1974.
67. Korthius, R. J., et al. The role of oxygen derived free radicals in ischemia induced increases in canine skeletal muscle vascular permeability. *Circ. Res.* 57:599, 1985.
68. Schweitzer, I., Rosenbaum, M. B., and Sharzer, L. A. Psychological reactions and processes following replantation surgery: a study of 50 patients. *Plast. Reconstr. Surg.* 76:97, 1985.
69. Chase, R. A. Functional levels of amputation of the hand. *Surg. Clin. North Am.* 40:415, 1960.
70. Swanson, A. B. Levels of amputation of fingers and hand: considerations for treatment. *Surg. Clin. North Am.* 44:1115, 1964.

71. Carroll, R. ·E. Transposition of the index finger to replace the middle finger. *Clin. Orthop.* 15:27, 1959.
72. Peaock, E. E., Jr. Metacarpal transfer following amputation of the central digit. *Plast. Reconstr. Surg.* 29:345, 1962.
73. Russell, W. R. Painful amputation stumps and phantom limbs. *Br. Med. J.* 1:1024, 1949.
74. Tupper, J. W., and Booth, Đ. M. Treatment of painful neuromas of sensory nerves in the hand: a comparison of traditional and newer methods. *J. Hand Surg.* 1:144, 1976.
75. Swanson, A. B., Boeve, N. R., and Lumsden, R. M. The prevention and treatment of amputation neuromata by silicone capping. *J. Hand Surg.* 2:70, 1977.

Commentary on Chapter 6

Harold E. Kleinert

This excellent chapter on replantation, revascularization, and amputation is inclusive of present day treatment. It will be useful to all physicians interested in this subject. My critique includes comments and procedural variants on replantation as practiced on the Hand Service at the University of Louisville School of Medicine.

A comment is necessary on the terminology "warm and cold ischemia": Warm ischemia, in my mind, is the total time a part is exposed to ambient temperatures following amputation. It includes (1) the time from amputation to cooling the part on ice, and (2) the time after removal from ice to restoring blood flow. Cold ischemia is the total length of time the part was cooled with ice.

It is possible to store amputated parts in cold storage for replantation after one has dealt with the life-threatening problems. The more proximal amputations contain more muscle tissue; hence the longer the cold storage, the more hazardous such replants become to the patient. Because of the larger muscle mass, there is a greater potential for myoglobinuria. Arterial repair can be accomplished prior to venous repair, thereby providing an opportunity of flushing metabolic products out of the replanted part.

We prefer a classification for amputation zones different from the one offered by Daniel and Terzis, particularly for their zone III. Their zone III lies between the distal palmar crease and the DIP joint. We think any finger replantation that can be done distal to the PIP joint is good, because that joint will function. The next zone would be the proximal phalanges, a difficult replantation zone because of flexor tendon repair in this area. With amputations through the proximal phalanx, where three tendons glide through the fibroosseous tunnel, consideration should be given to repairing only the profundus tendon. Our third zone is through the metacarpals, then the carpus, then the area proximal to the wrist. In Daniel and Terzis' zone II, which is between the germinal matrix and the DIP joint, venous repair can usually be accomplished, although it may require anastomosis of a volar vein. In these areas (zones I and II), the vessel repairs are often done prior to bone fixation in order to facilitate exposure for the microvascular repair. We have successfully replanted fingertips sharply amputated at the mid-nail level. Some of these replanted tips have survived on an arterial vessel alone, as an appropriate vein could not be located for repair.

Contrary to some reports, including one from Louisville, composite grafts have not done well in my personal experience, especially in adults. Rather than survive, most nonvascularized fingertips replaced as a composite graft function more as a dressing under which slow epithelialization of the stump occurs; the tip then appears healed as the thick, black eschar falls off.

With digital avulsion injuries, the skin is usually avulsed beginning over the proximal phalanx and is stripped distally where the complete amputation usually occurs through or proximal to the DIP joint. Such injuries usually require arthrodesis of the distal joint; but because the PIP joint and its attached tendons are intact, good functional results are expected. Avulsion injuries require interpositional vein grafts for both arterial and venous repair. The nerves are always repaired, and sometimes nerve grafts are required. We have published elsewhere good results on ring avulsion injury replantation [1].

We routinely use axillary block anesthesia for replantations because it has the advantage of providing a sympathetic blockade.

An alternative incision for replantation exposure is a volar zigzag incision and a midline dorsal incision on the finger. These incisions have less potential for causing devascularization of the dorsal skin when compared with bilateral midline finger incisions.

We prefer to shorten bone on the amputated part. We agree that during bone shortening it is not only important to preserve a maximum amount of bone but also to maintain joints, which means (according to the joint situation) it may be necessary to shorten more bone in the proximal stump than in the amputated portion in order to maintain intact joints.

The flexor tendon suture technique (Kessler) described in this chapter was first described by Kirchmayr, from Vienna, in the German scientific literature in 1917 [2]. That article included an accurate description (complete with diagram) of this tendon-grasping suture. We prefer a 4-0 Tycron to nylon as the tendon "core" suture, because nylon tends to stretch more than Tycron.

We use Dacron batting as a dressing because it lessens the likelihood of a dried blood dressing forming a constrictive band. The Dacron batting is more absorbent than cotton material and remains spongy. The postoperative management of metacarpal, wrist, and distal forearm replantations includes placing them in a light extensor crane brace by the third postoperative day. The metacarpophalangeal joints are held in partial flexion by the crane outrigger splint, which provides a light extensor assist for the PIP joints and protects the thin, smaller extensor tendon apparatus from being stretched by the stronger flexor tendons. The thumb is maintained in abduction, which allows the patient to perform finger flexion and extension and has added significantly to good or excellent results by reducing tendon adhesions. The metacarpal block protects against intrinsic muscle stretching so that a "claw hand" does not occur, and the light extensor assist protects the thin extensor mechanism. Our patients have not experienced ruptures of the flexor tendons, and most of these replantation cases have not required a second operation to obtain good function.

Postoperatively, we do not use a heating lamp over the replanted extremity, as it is likely to cause thrombosis. Low-molecular-weight dextran is employed on our service for major replantation, mainly to protect the kidneys from myoglobinuria. We believe that most replantation failures occur within the first 24 hours, and patients are kept NPO during this time.

Index and little finger ray amputation is usually done as a delayed procedure because leaving the metacarpal protects the palmar arch and makes a stronger hand if the patient does heavy work. If a patient does light work and desires a better appearance of the hand, ray resection is performed as a secondary procedure.

We often perform replantation in patients over age 50. Physiologic age is more important than chronologic age. In particular, I remember an 82-year-old man who had amputated his thumb in his woodworking shop. Since replantation he has enjoyed 5 years of good function of the replanted thumb and continues with his woodworking.

REFERENCE

1. Tsai, T. M., Munstein, C., DuBou, R., Wolff, T.W., Kutz, J. E., and Kleinert, H. E. Primary microsurgical repair of ring avulsion amputation injuries *J. Hand Surg.* 9A:68–72, 1984.
2. Kirchmayr, L. Zur technik der sehnennaht. *Zentralbl. Chir.* 44:27, 1917.

7 FRACTURES AND DISLOCATIONS IN THE HAND

Pat L. Aulicino

Fractures of the small bones of the hands account for one-third of all fractures. Because the hand is involved in almost 50 percent of all industrial accidents, these accidents can result in a significant economic impact on the patient and on society as a whole. Prompt and appropriate treatment can significantly decrease the disability and cost associated with these injuries.

The force that fractures a bone in the hand also produces significant soft-tissue injury. Associated skin, tendon, ligament, and neurovascular injuries are not uncommon. To rehabilitate the hand maximally, the skeleton must be appropriately stabilized. Although most fractures do not require internal fixation, unstable fractures and fractures that have significant associated soft tissue injury require rigid, anatomic fixation to restore early active motion. The sooner motion can be restored to the injured hand, the better the functional outcome will be. The primary reason for internal fixation is to obtain optimal functional return.

EVALUATION

As with all injuries, the history and physical examination are the cornerstones of diagnosis and all subsequent treatment. The mechanism of injury (e.g., crushing or twisting) and the time and place of injury are important.

Highly contaminated wounds, such as those that occur in a barnyard or an agricultural setting, should be adequately débrided and left open. Secondary fracture fixation and bone grafting after the wound has been rendered surgically clean help prevent serious complications.

Crushing injuries may result in compartment syndromes of the hand with subsequent necrosis of the intrinsic muscles if not treated promptly by fasciotomy. One must therefore treat the patient, not the radiograph. Once an adequate history has been obtained, the physical examination should involve inspection of the hand to determine the neurovascular status and rotational alignment of the digits. The alignment of the nail plates is an excellent guide. All digits

Table 7-1. Fracture terminology

Bone and facture pattern	Location	Fracture angulation
Bone	Base	Apex dorsal
Distal phalanx	Mid-shaft	Apex volar
Middle phalanx	Neck	
Proximal phalanx		
Metacarpal		
Fracture pattern	Intraarticular	Open vs. closed
Transverse	Extraarticular	
Oblique		
Spiral		
Comminuted		

should also converge on the scaphoid tuberosity when individually flexed actively or passively. The intrinsic flexor and extensor tendons as well as the intrinsic muscles of the hand should be examined as outlined in Chapter 4.

RADIOGRAPHIC EXAMINATION

Radiographs should always be taken in at least two planes at 90 degree angles to one another. True posteroanterior and lateral radiographs of the hand are absolutely necessary to adequately diagnose and treat fractures.

Special radiographs are required to evaluate the first metacarpal trapezial joint, the base of the fifth metacarpal hamate joint, and the metacarpal heads. These radiographs should be ordered if fractures are suspected in these areas.

The Brewerton view reveals occult fractures of the metacarpal head. The Roberts' hyperpronated view yields a true anteroposterior view of the thumb. The 15-degree pronated oblique view is necessary to demonstrate fractures and fracture-dislocations of the fifth metacarpal hamate area.

CLASSIFICATION

Once adequate radiographs are obtained, the fractures can be classified as stable or unstable. In general, *unstable fractures* are those that cannot be reduced closed; or if they can be reduced closed, they cannot be held in the reduced position without supplemental internal or percutaneous fixation.

A fracture is described according to its location in the bone, the direction of a fracture line, the direction of angulation, and the amount of comminution. Also, it is important to note whether the fracture is open or closed (Table 7-1). Once the fracture stability has been determined, a rational decision for closed or open reduction can be made.

OPEN FRACTURES   Cultures should be taken of all open fractures. Such fractures require surgical débridement and appropriate antibiotic coverage. The most overlooked open fracture in the hand is the distal phalangeal fracture. Sloan and associates [1] reported a prospective study of 85 patients with open distal phalanx fractures. There was a 30 percent infection rate in those not treated with antibiotics. Only 3 percent of the treated group developed an infection. Osteomyelitis of the distal phalanx is not uncommon and may result in shortening and possibly amputation of the fingertip. The presence of subungual hematoma with an associated underlying distal phalanx fracture should be considered an open fracture.

Open fractures often require internal fixation. The timing of that fixation depends on the degree of contamination and the associated soft tissue injury. The use of an external fixator should be considered in severely contaminated wounds or wounds with significant bone loss such as high velocity gunshot wounds. The external fixator maintains length, so that future bone grafting and buttress plate fixation can be performed after the tissues have been rendered surgically clean.

The type of antibiotic coverage used depends on the mechanism of injury and the degree of contamination. In general, first generation cephalosporins provide adequate coverage, as most osteomyelitis in the hand is due to *Staphylococcus aureus*. Wounds that are contaminated with soil require additional coverage for *Clostridium* and gram-negative organisms. Wounds from the human oral cavity, e.g., fight bite fractures of the metacarpal head, require both cephalosporin coverage and penicillin. *Eikinella corrodens*, a frequent inhabitant of the oral cavity, is resistant to cephalosporin antibiotics. Therefore once this organism has been identified and its sensitivity determined, the antibiotics are adjusted accordingly.

Tetanus prophylaxis is required for all open fractures unless there was a known complete immunization series and a booster within the last year.

An open fracture of the hand is a true surgical emergency. Débridement should be performed quickly and completely. Antibiotics are no substitute for adequate surgical débridement.

Because of the rich vascularity of the hand, type I and II open fractures may be closed primarily provided they have been adequately débrided and rendered surgically clean (Table 7-2). Internal fixation can be performed on these wounds at the same time as primary closure. Type II wounds should be left open, and internal fixation is usually not indicated for these injuries. The external fixator should be considered, or delayed internal fixation can be done at the time of delayed primary closure of skin grafting.

INDICATIONS FOR FRACTURE FIXATION   Indications for open reduction and internal fixation should always be considered relative, not absolute. However, certain fracture patterns require either internal fixation or percutaneous pinning for

Table 7-2. Open fracture classification

Type I
Puncture wound 1 cm or less and relatively clean
Inside-out puncture wound
No muscle contusion or soft tissue involvement
No crushing component
Type II
More than 1 cm laceration
Without extensive soft tissue damage, flaps, or avulsion
Minimal to moderate crushing component
Type III
Extensive damage to soft tissue
Muscle, skin, or neurovascular associated injury
High velocity or severe crushing injury

Source: R. B. Gustilo et al. *Orthopaedic Infection.* Philadelphia: Saunders, 1989.

optimum results. Unstable fractures, displaced intraarticular fractures, and fractures that cannot be reduced closed may require internal fixation. Fractures that are best treated by internal fixation are spiral proximal phalanx fractures, transverse fractures of the middle phalanx, and the multiply fractured hand. Fracture-dislocations of the first carpometacarpal joint such as a Bennett or Rolando fracture and fracture-dislocations of the fifth carpometacarpal joint also require either percutaneous or open reduction and internal fixation. Dorsal and volar fracture-dislocations of the proximal interphalangeal (PIP) joints as well as avulsion fractures that involve more than 15 to 20 percent of the articular surface (e.g., a bony gamekeeper's thumb or an avulsion of a metacarpal head collateral ligament) may also fall into this category. Grade I and II open fractures in the polytraumatized patient constitute another indication for open reduction. However, the indications for open reduction are relative.

The primary purpose for fracture fixation is to restore rigid anatomic alignment of the fracture so that early mobilization can be performed. If the fracture cannot be fixed anatomically owing to severe comminution or inexperience of the surgeon, it is best treated in a closed fashion (Table 7-3).

CLOSED TREATMENT OF FRACTURES

Fractures that are inherently stable or that can be reduced in a closed fashion and made stable should be treated in a closed manner. If the fracture is stable, "buddy taping" to the adjacent digit is all that may be required. Radiographs should be repeated in 7 to 10 days to make sure that the fracture has not angulated or displaced. Fractures that require manipulation often also require external cast immobilization to prevent displacement. The position of immobilization, as described by James [2], is the "intrinsic plus position." Here the wrist is dorsiflexed 30 degrees, the metacarpophalangeal (MCP) joints flexed 70 degrees, and the PIP

Table 7-3. Fractures usually requiring internal fixation

1. Mallet fractures with subluxed joint or 25% percent of articular surface
2. Comminuted mid or proximal phalanx fractures
3. Transverse mid-phalanx fractures
4. Fracture-dislocations of the PIP joints
5. Displaced intraarticular fractures of the DIP, PIP, or MCP joints
6. Juxtaarticular fractures of the DIP and PIP joints that are malrotated
7. Spiral/oblique proximal phalanx fractures
8. Metacarpal head fractures
9. Multiple metacarpal fractures
10. Bennett/Rolando fractures of the first metacarpal
11. Fracture-dislocations of the fifth carpal metacarpal joint
12. Multiply fractured hand

Table 7-4. Average healing time of fractures

Fracture	Healing time (weeks)
Distal phalanx	3
Middle phalanx	4
Metacarpal	4–6

and distal interphalangeal (DIP) joints are held in full extension. The MCP joint is a cam joint, and the collateral ligaments are at maximum stretch at 70 to 90 degrees of flexion. The PIP and DIP joints are hinge joints, and the collateral ligaments are on equal stretch in all positions.

All fractures should be reduced under intermetacarpal or wrist block. Local anesthetic solutions containing epinephrine should never be used in the hand, as local tissue or digital necrosis may occur. Once the digit or hand is anesthetized, the fracture is reduced by distraction, reproduction of the injury, and reduction. Alignment and rotation must be carefully checked both clinically and radiographically.

Fractures of the phalanges are immobilized for 3 weeks and metacarpal fractures for 4 weeks. Full stress should not be placed on the digit or hand for 6 to 8 weeks after fracture. Radiographic healing lags behind clinical healing, and one must not delay movement of the digit based on the radiographic findings. If a digit has been immobilized the recommended period of time, and there is no more tenderness over the fracture site, the fracture can be considered to be clinically healed, and one can proceed with slow, gentle mobilization of the adjacent joints (Table 7-4).

Complications

The primary complication associated with closed treatment is malunion (Fig. 7-1). This complication is, however, preventable. One must carefully examine the digit after reduction to make sure that the rotatory alignment is acceptable. Immediate postreduction and subsequent periodic radiographic evaluations are necessary to

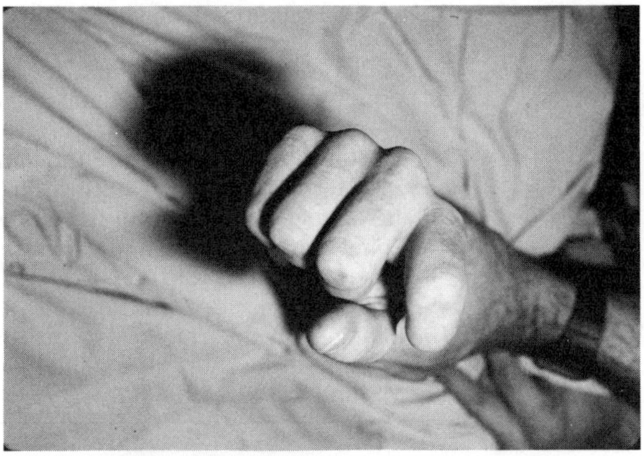

Fig. 7-1. A. Malunited spiral proximal phalanx fracture of the index finger due to inadequate immobilization. This fracture would have been better treated by internal fixation, as spiral proximal phalanx fractures are inherently unstable. B, C. Intraoperative photograph of a metacarpal rotational osteotomy to correct alignment of the malunited proximal phalanx fracture.

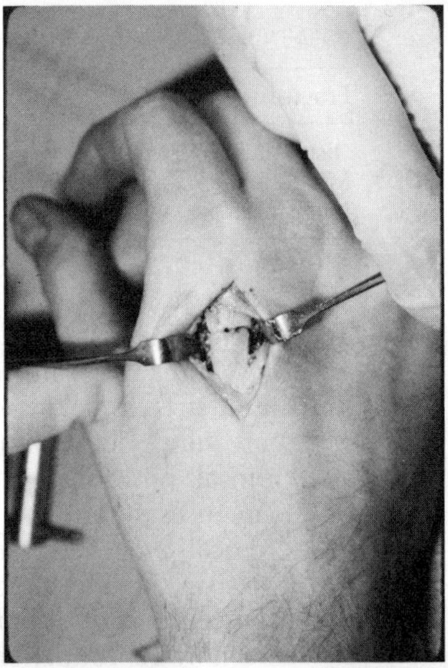

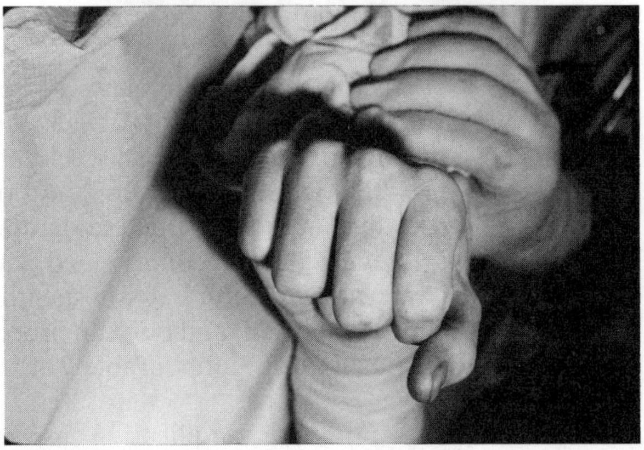

make sure that the reduction has been maintained. Stiffness and joint contractures may be seen with closed treatment. The more severe the mechanism of injury and the older the patient, the higher the risk for stiffness and joint contracture. It is rare to see a joint contracture in a closed fracture in a young individual who has not sustained severe soft-tissue injury. Closed treatment is the gold standard by which we must judge our results of open reduction and internal fixation of fractures.

INTERNAL FIXATION

K-wires, tension band wiring, intraosseous wiring, and AO (ASIF; see below) minifragment screws and plates have all been utilized successfully for the open reduction and internal fixation of fractures. The stability of internal fixation of oblique proximal phalanx fractures has been studied by Black and associates [3]. The strongest fixation was the dorsal plate, followed by the dorsal plate and interfragmentary lag screws. Two interfragmentary lag screws were the next strongest followed by tension band techniques and then crossed K-wires. The intact proximal phalanx was stronger than all internal fixation techniques. Miniplates are rarely used in the proximal phalanges and are more suitable for use in the metacarpals.

The type of internal fixation used is determined by the fracture pattern and the technical expertise of the surgeon. One must remember that the goal is rigid, anatomic internal fixation. This goal can be obtained by any of these techniques.

The complications of open reduction are tendon adhesions secondary to surgical dissection, infection, failure of fixation, and secondary malunion due to loss of fixation. Tendon rupture has been reported with the use of plate and screws in the proximal phalanx.

Surgical Approaches

The second to fifth metacarpal shafts and bases are readily approached by straight dorsal incisions just lateral or medial to the extensor digitorum communis tendon. The incision should not be directly over the tendon in order to reduce the incidence of postoperative adhesions. The dorsal sensory branches of the radial and ulnar nerves should be identified and protected to prevent painful neuroma formation. The tendon is retracted to the side, and the periosteum is split longitudinally (Fig. 7-2). Interosseous muscles may have to be subperiosteally dissected from the bone for exposure. After fixation is applied, the periosteum should be closed with small absorbable sutures, e.g., 5-0 Vicryl. Approaches to the metacarpal head and metacarpal neck necessitate splitting of the extensor apparatus in the direction of its fibers. The metacarpal head can be exposed by subsequent flexion of the digit. The bases of the second and third metacarpals require partial dissection of the extensor carpi radialis longus and brevis insertions from the base of the metacarpal. The fifth metacarpal requires partial removal of the extensor carpi ulnaris tendon insertion. The base of the first metacarpal should be approached through a J-shaped incision. The incision begins on the

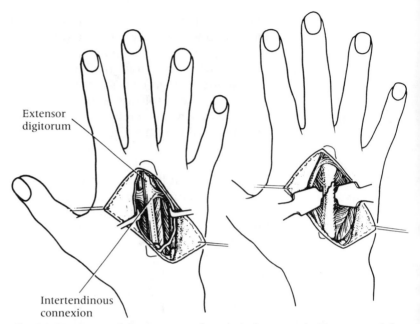

Extensor
digitorum

Intertendinous
connexion

Fig. 7-2. Fractures of the metacarpals: surgical approach. Exposure of the
fracture after retraction of tendons, nerves, and veins. (From U. Heim
and K. M. Pfeiffer. *Small Fragment Set Manual.* Heidelberg:
Springer-Verlag, 1974. With permission.)

volar radial side of the first metacarpal and is carried along the distal
flexion crease of the wrist to the radial side of the flexor carpi radialis
tendon. The thenar muscles are than taken subperiosteally off the
first metacarpal shaft. The attachment of the abductor pollicis longus
to the shaft may be left intact or removed for better exposure. It
should be reattached after the fixation is applied. This exposure
provides excellent access to the metacarpal shaft and the first
carpometacarpal joint (Fig. 7-3). One must avoid injury to the
sensory radial nerve and the lateral antebrachial cutaneous nerve, as
they often overlap in this area. The volar radial artery also pierces the
thenar musculature at the ulnarmost extent of this incision.

The phalanges may be approached through a dorsal extensor
splitting incision as described by Pratt [4]. Fractures that are juxtaarticular or intraarticular, at either the PIP or the MCP joint, require
splitting of the extensor tendon longitudinally. Mid-shaft proximal
phalanx fractures may be approached through a mid-axial incision,
and the lateral bands may be retracted dorsally for exposure. The
dorsal sensory branch of the digital nerve must be identified and
protected. Dorsal fracture-dislocations of the PIP joint are best
approached through a mid-axial incision at either one or both sides
of the joint if additional exposure is required. The transverse lamina
should be split and the collateral ligament dissected off the base of
the mid-phalanx for exposure.

Volar fracture-dislocations, that is, bony boutonnière deformities,

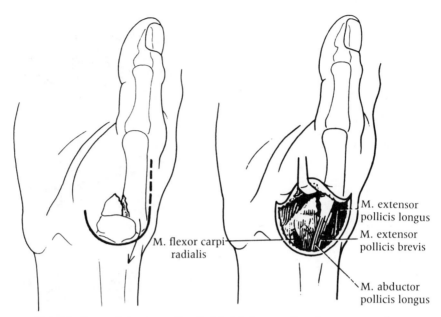

Fig. 7-3. Bennett fracture, the Gedda-Moberg radiopalmar approach.
(From U. Heim and K. M. Pfeiffer. *Small Fragment Set Manual.*
Heidelberg: Springer-Verlag, 1974. With permission.)

should be approached dorsally. An attempt should be made to leave
the central slip intact. If it is not possible, it may be removed;
however, it should be attached back to bone through drill holes.

The mid-phalanx should be approached through a mid-axial
incision. The attachment of the central slip and the terminal slip
make fracture fixation through a dorsal incision difficult if not
impossible. Mid-axial incisions, on one side or bilaterally, give
excellent exposure of the shaft of the mid-phalanx (Fig. 7-4).
Fractures of the neck of the mid-phalanx or intraarticular DIP joint
fractures and mallet fractures that involve more than 25 percent of
the articular surface of the distal phalanx or that are associated with
a volar subluxation of the DIP joint require an extensor splitting
approach. If necessary, removal of the terminal slip with subsequent
reattachment into bone may be performed. The exposure must be
adequate to visualize all fracture fragments in order to obtain
anatomic rigid internal fixation.

Fixation Techniques   *Percutaneous Pinning*
Unstable fractures may be treated by closed reduction and percutaneous K-wire fixation. Percutaneous fixation is best suited for
spiral proximal phalanx fractures, angulated transverse metacarpal
fractures, and fracture-dislocations of the first and fifth carpometacarpal joints. Percutaneous fixation is often more difficult than open
reduction and internal fixation. The use of an image intensifier and
a power K-wire driver as well as a knowledgeable assistant are
mandatory. The fracture must be anatomically reduced prior to the

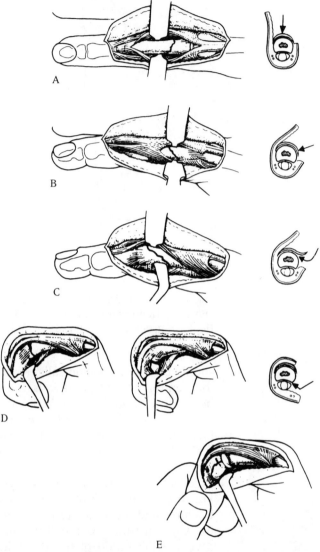

Fig. 7-4. Fractures of the phalanges: approaches and topography of the extensor mechanism. *A.* Dorsal incision of the extensor aponeurosis in basal fractures of the proximal phalanx. *B.* Lateral incision of the interosseous aponeurosis in fractures of the middle of the proximal phalanx. *C.* Lateral approach with elevation of interosseous aponeurosis in distal fractures of the proximal phalanx. *D.* Approach to articular fractures in the PIP joint: opening of the flexor tendon sheath. *E.* Exposure of the PIP joint after division of the collateral ligament. (From U. Heim and K. M. Pfeiffer. *Small Fragment Set Manual.* Heidelberg: Springer-Verlag, 1974. With permission.)

pins being driven. Often the fracture can be displaced by the force of the advancing K-wires and thus pinned in distraction. Fractures cannot be compressed with percutaneous fixation. When pinning phalanges, the lateral bands may be skewered by the K-wires, making early motion difficult. If the K-wires are left protruding through the skin and motion is begun, the skin may become irritated, and subsequent infection may develop.

Multiple attempts at percutaneous pinning may turn a simple closed oblique proximal phalanx fracture into a comminuted open fracture that is impossible to fixate.

If one is proficient at percutaneous pinning, the advantages are obvious. The absence of surgical dissection reduces the number of adhesions that may occur with open reduction. The risk of infection is less, and operative time and anesthesia requirements are decreased.

If one elects to pin the fracture percutaneously, at least two K-wires of 0.035 or 0.045 inch are required to prevent rotation and loss of reduction. Viegas and associates [5] tested the rigidity of fixation of K-wires utilized for closed percutaneous pinning. They recommended four crossed 0.028-inch K-wires for transverse fractures and three oblique 0.035-inch K-wires oriented perpendicular to the fracture plane in oblique fractures to obtain maximal rigidity.

The contraindications to percutaneous K-wire fixation are comminution of the fracture site, lack of adequate radiographic facilities, and lack of experience with this technique on the part of the operating surgeon.

Open Reduction and Internal Fixation with K-Wires

The technically easiest type of fixation, in my experience, is K-wire placement in an open fashion. The fracture is exposed as previously described. It is held in a reduced position and clamped to provide anatomic alignment. The K-wires are driven across the fracture site to obtain rigid fixation. At least two K-wires are necessary to stabilize any fracture, as one K-wire allows rotation. I routinely cut these wires directly on bone and do not attempt to remove them unless they migrate. Motion is begun as soon as possible (Fig. 7-5). During more than 10 years of utilizing this technique, I have not found K-wire migration to be a problem. Those that do migrate subcutaneously are easily removed under local anesthesia. None has caused neurovascular or tendon injury.

Purists would argue that true compression of a fracture cannot be obtained with this technique, and they are correct. Only lag screw techniques can provide compression. However, K-wire fixation is a much more forgiving technique and provides good results. The goals of rigid internal fixation and early motion are easily obtained, and it is probably the easiest technique to master (Fig. 7-6).

For comminuted fractures, multiple 0.028-inch K-wires are utilized. Proximal and mid-phalanx, spiral, oblique, and transverse fractures can all be fixed with crossed or multiple oblique 0.035-inch

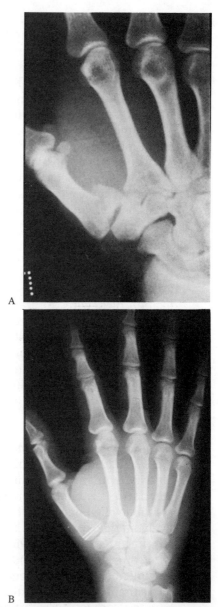

Fig. 7-5. Preoperative (*A*) and postoperative (*B*) radiographs of Bennett's fracture of the first metacarpal. Open reduction and internal fixation were performed with two 0.35-inch K-wires cut on bone.

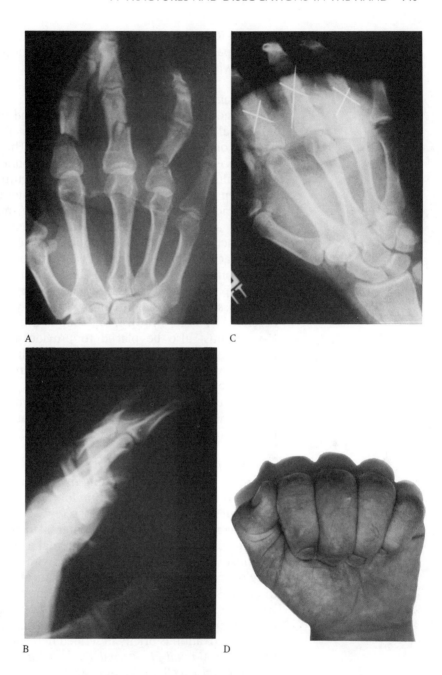

A

C

B

D

Fig. 7-6. A, B. Preoperative radiographs of a multiply fractured hand. Note the three open and volarly angulated proximal phalanx fractures. *C.* Immediate postoperative radiographs. Anatomic rigid fixation was obtained with crossed 0.35-inch K-wires cut on bone. *D.* Early range of motion exercises with K-wires in place resulted in full painless range of motion. K-wires were not removed and have not migrated in 6 years.

K-wires. Crossed 0.045-inch K-wires can be used for transverse metacarpal fractures. Spiral proximal metacarpal fractures are better fixated with lag screws, miniplates, or both.

Intraosseous Wiring/Tension Band Techniques

The tension side of both the metacarpal and proximal phalanges is the dorsal aspect. Eccentric loading due to flexion forces produces gapping on the tension side of the fracture. The use of figure-of-eight wire placed dorsal to the mid-axis of the bone absorbs these forces and results in axial compression at the fracture site.

The tension wire must be utilized with K-wires to prevent rotation at the fracture site. The tension band wire should be small gauge, such as a 26 monofilament wire, utilized in conjunction with 0.035-inch K-wires. This technique can be used only in noncommuted fractures, and the compression side of the fracture must have stable contact. The technique is best suited to transverse and short oblique phalangeal and metacarpal fractures (Fig. 7-7).

Intraosseous wires, with or without K-wire fixation, was well described by Lister in [6]. If one loop of intraosseous wire is used, a K-wire must also be placed to provide additional stability and prevent rotation. The 90-90 intraosseous wires prevent rotation, and K-wire fixation is not necessary. This technique is best utilized for transverse fractures, short oblique fractures, or avulsion fractures of the collateral ligaments. This type of fixation has also been valuable in replantation surgery, as a minimal amount of dissection is required to place the intraosseous wires.

AO/ASIF Techniques

The most technically demanding method of internal fixation in the hand is the AO/ASIF (Association for the Study of Internal Fixation) techniques. This system utilizes screws 2.7, 2.0, and 1.5 mm in diameter and miniplates for rigid internal fixation. It is recommended that the reader attend a course in internal fixation prior to attempting to utilize this system. Once familiar with the system, one should develop expertise fixing transverse fractures of the metacarpals with miniplates and then proceed to spiral proximal phalanx fractures. Although this technique provides the best fixation available, it is unforgiving and not for the novice. The technique of lag screw and miniplate fixation is briefly described here, but the reader is referred to the *AO Manual of Internal Fixation* for complete details of this complex, yet excellent fixation system.

Lag Screw Technique. Use of the lag screw is one of the techniques that can compress a fracture. K-wires provide internal splinting but not compression. Compression facilitates per primum bone healing. The principle of lagging is to overdrill the proximal fragment to create a glide hole that is equal to the external diameter of the screw (Fig. 7-8). When the screw is placed, after tapping, it converts the

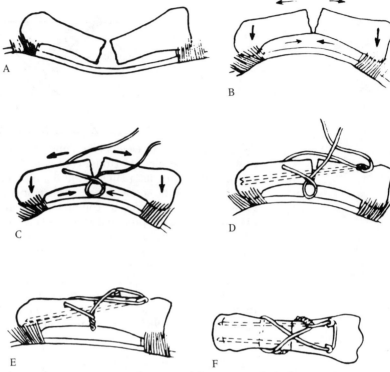

Figure 7-7. A. Transverse fracture of the proximal phalanx with the customary volar angulation. *B.* The fracture is reduced, and the hand is placed in the position of function. When flexion exercises of the digits are initiated, there is compression at the volar apex of the fracture but distraction and gapping dorsally. *C.* A tension band wire is placed through the distal fragment. *D.* Two small longitudinal K-wires are placed through the proximal fragment, across the fracture site, and into the distal fragment. The figure-of-eight tension band is then looped underneath the K-wires. *E.* The two loops in the figure-of-eight tension band are then tightened simultaneously, closing the fracture gap and allowing dynamic compression to occur uniformly across the surface area of the fracture site while a similar amount of tension is absorbed by the tension band wire itself. *F.* Dorsal view of the tension band wire, which is further neutralized against rotational and bending forces by the two longitudinal wires. (From A. E. Freeland, M. E. Jabaley, and J. L. Hughes. *Stable Fixation of the Hand and Wrist.* Berlin: Springer-Verlag, 1986. With permission.)

torsional force into a compressive force at the fracture site (Table 7-5).

There are certain rules that must be followed rigidly when using the lag screw technique. The fragments to be fixed must be at least three times the thread diameter of the cortical screw to be used to decrease the risk of shattering the fragment. The screw must be at least three diameters away from the nearest bone edge in large fragments. A screw placed at a right angle to the fracture plane

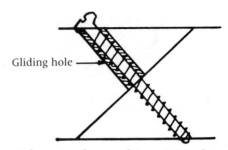

Gliding hole

Fig. 7-8. Sequence of events when applying an interfragmental screw across a fracture site: (1) Drill a core hole the diameter of the screw core across both fragments. (2) Overdrill the proximal fragment with a drill the diameter of the screw threads. This maneuver creates a gliding hole so the two fragments can be compressed when the screw is applied. (3) Countersink the proximal cortex. (4) Measure the depth of the screw with a depth gauge. (5) Tap the distal cortex. The tap must have threads the same diameter and pitch as the screws. (6) Apply the screw. Never use more force to tighten the screw than can be applied with a three-jaw chuck grasp, using the thumb, index, and middle fingers, thereby avoiding stripping. (From A. E. Freeland, M. E. Jabaley, and J. L. Hughes. *Stable Internal Fixation of the Hand and Wrist.* Berlin: Springer-Verlag, 1986. With permission.)

Table 7-5. Steps in lag screw fixation

1. Reduce fracture and hold with clamp.
2. Drill core hole equal to the shaft diameter of the screw.
3. Overdrill the proximal fragment equal to the thread diameter of the screw to create a glide hole.
4. Countersink proximal cortex.
5. Measure depth with gauge.
6. Tap distal cortex equal to the same diameter and pitch as screw.
7. Apply screw to "two finger tightness" to prevent stripping of threads.

provides the best interfragmentary compression but less stability against axial load. A screw placed perpendicular to the long axis of the bone is stable to axial load. Therefore if only one screw can be used for interfragmentary fixation in the diaphysis, the screw should be placed in a plane that bisects a perpendicular to the fracture line and a perpendicular to the long axis of the bone. This method provides the best combination of stability to axial load and good compression (Fig. 7-9). If two screws are used, one can be placed perpendicular to the fracture and the other perpendicular to the long axis of the bone; or both screws can be placed in a direction that bisects the long axis of the bone and fracture axis. Two screws should be used if possible for interfragmentary fixation (Fig. 7-10). Screws alone may be used when the fracture line is twice as long as the diameter of the bone at the level of the fracture. If this is not the case, an additional neutralization plate is necessary. When the screw is placed, one full thread should penetrate the distal cortex.

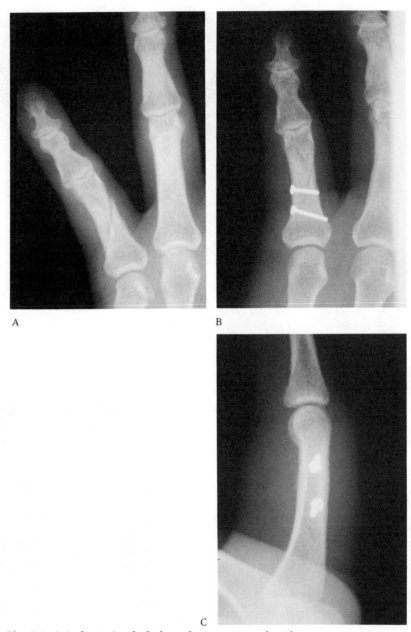

A

B

C

Fig. 7-9. Spiral proximal phalanx fracture treated with two interfragmentary lag screws.

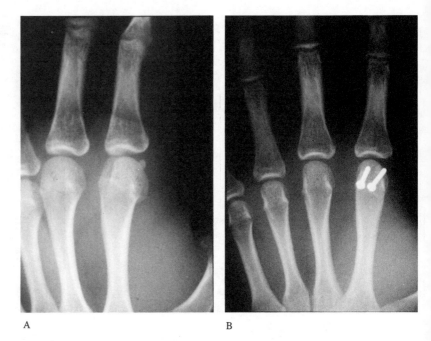

A   B

Fig. 7-10. Intraarticular metacarpal "split" head fracture treated with two interfragmentary lag screws.

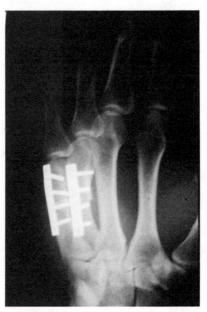

Fig. 7-11. Transverse fourth and fifth metacarpal fractures treated with four-hole miniplates. Four cortices are fixed on either side of the fracture.

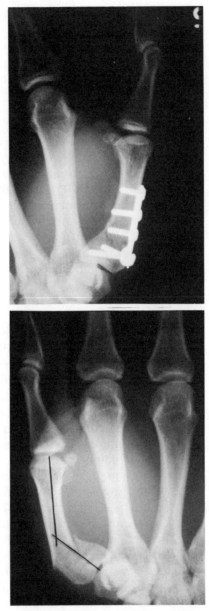

Fig. 7-12. Mini t-plate utilized to fix a juxtaarticular first metacarpal fracture.

Miniplate Fixation. Plates may be used to neutralize, compress, buttress, or bridge a fracture. If a plate is used in the metacarpal, at least four cortices must be fixed or either side of the fracture (Fig. 7-11). In the proximal phalanx, a minimum of three are required on either side of the fracture. Compression is obtained by offsetting drill holes away from the fracture site after two neutral screw holes have been placed on the opposite side of the fracture. As the off-set screws are tightened, they cause the bone to shift toward the fracture site, resulting in compression.

This technique cannot be used for comminuted fractures. For comminuted fractures, the plate can be used to bridge or buttress the fracture site (Fig. 7-12). The reader is referred elsewhere for details of the procedures [7,8]

Conclusion

The surgeon should be familiar with all of the available techniques of internal fixation. The principles of internal fixation can be achieved with all of the previously described techniques. A common mistake is the attempt to make a certain system of internal fixation fit all fracture patterns. Fractures of the hand should be evaluated individually, and the method of fixation used should be based on the fracture pattern and the surgeon's experience. There is no system of internal fixation that is suitable for every conceivable fracture that occurs in the hand. If rigid internal fixation and early mobilization can be accomplished, the goals of internal fixation have been achieved.

FRACTURES IN CHILDREN

Most fractures in the hands of children can be treated by closed reduction and splinting. Owing to lack of cooperation, early motion is often difficult to achieve in children. However, it is also usually not necessary. It is unusual to see stiffness after a fracture in a child.

Fractures in children are classified according to their relation to the epiphysis. The Salter Harris classification is universally accepted to describe fractures in children (Table 7-6). Salter types I and II are most commonly seen. Salter types III and IV are less frequent and usually require open reduction and internal fixation with small K-wires to prevent epiphyseal closure and to realign the joint surface. The Salter V injury results in partial or incomplete closure of the physis and is rare (Fig. 7-13).

The most common fracture in children is the Salter II of the proximal phalanx of the fifth digit, or the "extra octave fracture." It is treated with closed reduction and splinting for 3 weeks. After local anesthesia is obtained, the fracture is reduced by flexing the MCP joint and adducting the digit toward the third metacarpal. Salter I and II open distal phalanx fractures are often mistaken for nail bed injuries. These open fractures should be débrided and reduced. The nail bed should be repaired with 7-0 chromic suture if necessary. Oral antibiotics and splinting of the DIP joint in extension for 3 weeks is the preferred treatment. Occasionally, when seen late, a small fine K-wire is required to hold this fracture in position (Fig. 7-14).

Juxtaarticular fractures with malrotation of the condyles, especially at the PIP joint, are occasionally seen. In my experience, these fractures are difficult to reduce closed and require open reduction and internal fixation with K-wires.

Table 7-6. Salter harris classification of fractures

Type I: The epiphysis is completely separated from the metaphysis without radiographic evidence of a metaphyseal fragment attached to the displaced epiphysis.

Type II: It is the most frequent type of physeal fracture, with the fracture plane traveling transversely through the cartilage plate for a variable distance prior to exiting through the metaphysis on the side opposite the site of fracture initiation.

Type III: An intraarticular fracture of the epiphysis, it occurs with propagation of the fracture crack through the epiphysis to the physis, where it then dissects peripherally to exit from the plate.

Type IV: It is a vertical splitting fracture of the epiphysis that is initiated at the intraarticular surface of the epiphysis, travels longitudinally through the bone, crosses the physis, and exits through the metaphysis.

Type V: A severe crushing injury is applied through the epiphysis to an area of the physis.

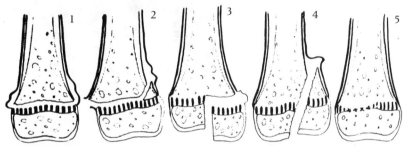

Fig. 7-13. Salter and Harris classification of physeal fractures (see Table 7.5). (From M. Rang. *Children's Fractures.* Philadelphia: Lippincott, 1983. With permission.)

When a small portion of an articular surface can be seen to be displaced on radiography, one must assume that it is a large fragment of bone. The articular cartilage is not visible radiographically, and only a small portion of the subchondral bone can be seen on the radiograph. These fractures usually involve almost the entire articular surface, and they should be treated with open reduction and internal fixation with K-wires.

Repeated attempts at closed reduction may cause severe permanent injury to the physeal plate and should be avoided. Minor degrees of angulation, especially in the plane of the joint motion, can be accepted as they will remodel. *Rotation does not remodel and is unacceptable.* If the digit appears clinically normal after reduction, one can safely assume that the angulation visualized on the radiograph is acceptable. If there is clinical deformity I recommend that it be reduced. The capacity of a child to remodel a fracture declines with age. Therefore the requirements for reduction become more stringent as the child becomes prepubescent, as there is less available time for remodeling the bone.

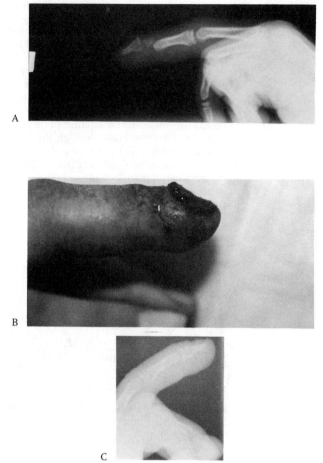

Fig. 7-14. A, B. Open Salter II fracture of distal phalanx in a child. This injury is often mistaken for a nail bed injury and inappropriately treated. *C.* Three months' postoperative radiographs showing reduction of the fraction and an open physeal plate.

DISLOCATIONS

Dislocations may be classified as being open or closed, simple or complex. Simple dislocations are readily reduced in a closed fashion. Complex dislocations cannot be reduced in a closed fashion, usually because of the interposition of soft tissue. At the PIP joint complex dislocations are rare and are usually dorsal lateral dislocations with interposition of the lateral band and collateral ligaments (Fig. 7-15). Complex joint dislocations usually occur in the border digits, thumb, index finger, and fifth finger. The volar plate becomes interposed between the metacarpal head and the base of the proximal phalanx. On radiographs the sesamoid, when present, appears to be in the joint as the sesamoid is contained within the substance of the volar plate (Fig. 7-16).

The DIP joint is frequently dislocated in sports-related injuries. It is easily reduced by direct longitudinal traction. If the wound is open,

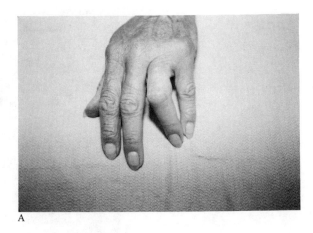

A

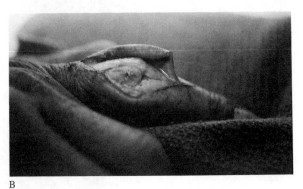

B

Fig. 7-15. A. closed complex dislocation of the PIP joint. Closed reduction was impossible. *B.* Intraoperative photograph demonstrates the lateral band and collateral ligament within the PIP joint, blocking reduction.

it should be débrided prior to reduction. If the reduction is stable, motion can be started as soon as pain permits (Fig. 7-17).

The PIP joint may dislocate in all directions: dorsally, volarly, and dorsolaterally. The dislocation may be open or closed. If open, it should be débrided again prior to reduction. Adequate local anesthesia and flexion of the wrist to relax the flexor tendons followed by longitudinal traction result in rapid reduction. If the dislocation is stable, it may be buddy-taped to the adjacent digit and motion begun as soon as pain permits. If it cannot be reduced closed, most likely the collateral ligament and lateral bands are interposed and open reduction is necessary. Injuries to the PIP joint may result in flexion contractures if not aggressively rehabilitated. These injuries all result in fusiform enlargement of the joint that lasts permanently. One can expect arthralgias for up to 9 months after the injury.

Volar dislocation of the PIP joint is rare and is associated with avulsions of the central slip. After reduction it should pinned in extension with a transarticular K-wire for 6 weeks to allow healing of the central slip (Fig. 7-18).

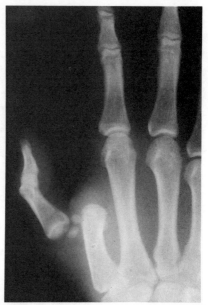

Fig. 7-16. Complex dislocation of the MCP joint of the thumb. The sesamoids, which are located in the volar plate, lie on the dorsal aspect of the first metacarpal, preventing closed reduction.

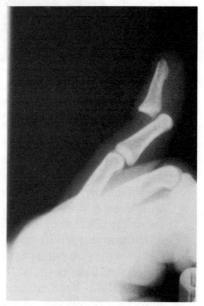

Fig. 7-17. Open dislocation of the DIP joint. Irrigation and débridement should be performed prior to reduction.

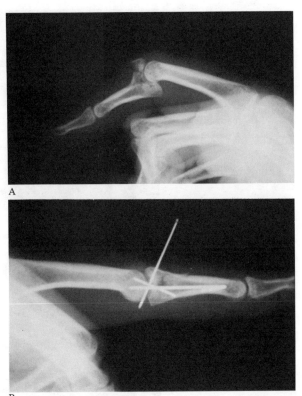

Fig. 7-18. A. Volar fracture dislocation of the PIP joint (bony boutonnière). *B.* Open reduction and internal fixation of the articular surface
is performed. A transarticular K-wire is placed across the PIP joint to
prevent volar subluxation.

Dorsal fracture-dislocations may be treated with early active
motion if there is only a small fragment of the volar surface, that is,
volar plate avulsion. If there is dorsal subluxation associated with a
large comminuted volar fragment of the base of the middle phalanx,
there are various treatment options. Closed reductions and dorsal
extension block splinting may be tried. If the fracture cannot be
reduced, open reduction and internal fixation may be required if the
fragments are large enough. If the fragments are comminuted and the
joint is subluxed dorsally, the options are excision of the comminuted
volar fragments through a volar approach and a volar plate interpositional arthroplasty, as described by Eaton [9]. The other option is the
use of a force coupling device as described by Agee [10]. I have no
experience with this technique, although I have used all of the other
previously described options with varying degrees of success.

Simple MCP joint dislocation may be reduced by distraction and
flexion. These injuries should not be hyperextended after distraction
as this might convert a simple dislocation to a complex dislocation.
Complex MCP joint dislocations require surgical intervention. There
is usually a small dimple of skin on the volar side of the dislocated
joint. The digit is generally hyperextended to approximately 45

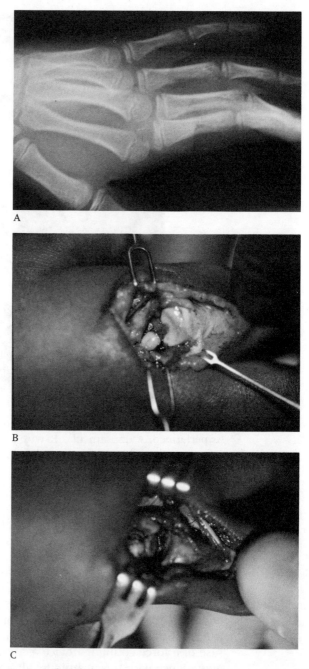

Fig. 7-19. A. Complex dislocation of the index MCP joint in a child. *B.* The dorsal approach described by Becton reveals the volar plate draped over the metacarpal head, preventing reduction. *C.* After the volar plate is split, the joint is easily reduced. The longitudinal incision in the extensor tendon is repaired, and early motion is begun.

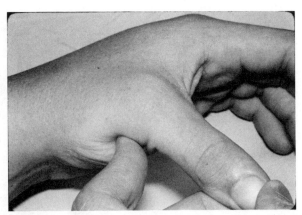

Fig. 7-20. Stress test reveals gross instability of the ulnar collateral-ligament of the MCP joint of the thumb, a gamekeeper's thumb.

degrees, in contrast to the 90 degrees in a simple dislocated joint.

I recommend the dorsal approach as described by Becton [11]. Here the extensor hood is split to expose the head of the metacarpal, which is usually covered by the volar plate. The volar plate is then split, resulting in reduction of the joint. Early active motion is begun (Fig. 7-19). A volar approach can be used, but the most superficial structure encountered is usually the digital nerve, especially in the index finger. This approach, in my opinion, is more hazardous and technically difficult.

Gamekeeper's thumb, or avulsion of the ulnar collateral ligament, usually requires open repair of the ligament. The ulnar collateral ligament may be found to be overlying the adductor aponeurosis, preventing spontaneous healing; this situation is referred to as a Stener lesion. Reattachment of this ligament to bone is necessary to restore stability (Fig. 7-20).

Avulsion fractures of the proximal phalanx of the thumb — "bony gamekeeper's fracture" — may be treated in a closed fashion unless they involve a significant portion of the articular surface, i.e., more than 15 to 20 percent. Open reduction and internal fixation should be performed to prevent secondary degenerative joint disease if more than 20 percent of the articular surface is involved (Fig. 7-21).

Dislocations of the first carpometacarpal joint of the thumb are rare. They are usually easily reduced by longitudinal traction. However, if they are unstable, percutaneous K-wire fixation for 6 weeks is required (Fig. 7-22).

CONCLUSIONS   Fractures and dislocations in the hand are common in an industrialized society. Aggressive, intelligent treatment is required to obtain optimal functional return. Judgments regarding the method and type of treatment should be based on the fracture pattern, associated injuries, and the technical expertise and skill of the operating surgeon.

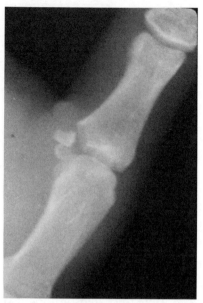

Fig. 7-21. Bony gamekeeper's fracture involving 25 percent of the articular surface. This fracture should be reduced anatomically and pinned with two 0.28-inch K-wires to prevent degenerative osteoarthritis.

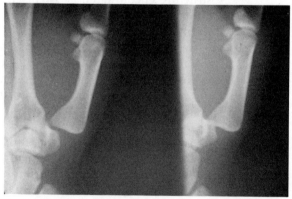

Fig. 7-22. Closed simple dislocation of the first carpometacarpal joint. It can usually be reduced closed. However, if it is unstable and redislocates, percutaneous fixation for 6 weeks is required.

REFERENCES

1. Sloan, J. P., et al. Antibiotics in open fractures of the distal phalanx? *J. Hand Surg. [Br.]* 12:123, 1987.
2. James, J. I. P. Fractures of the proximal and middle phalanges of the fingers. *Acta. Orthop. Scand.* 32: 401–412, 1962.
3. Black D. M., et al. The stability of internal fixation in the proximal phalanx. *J. Hand Surg. [Am.]* 11:672, 1986.
4. Pratt, D. R. Exposing fractures of the proximal phalanx of the finger longitudinally through the dorsal extensor apparatus. *Clin. Orthop.* 15:22–26, 1959.
5. Viegas, S. F., et al. Comparative mechanical properties of various

Kirschner wire configurations in transverse and oblique phalangeal fractures. *J. Hand Surg.* [*Am.*] 13:246, 1988.

6. Lister, G. Intraosseous wiring of the digital skeleton. *J. Hand Surg.* [*Am.*] 3:427, 1978.
7. Freeland, A. E., Jabaley, M. E., and Hughes, J. L. *Stable Fixation of the Hand and Wrist.* Berlin: Springer-Verlag, 1986.
8. Heim, V., and Pfeiffer, K. M. *Small Fragment Set Manual — Technique Recommended by the ASIF Group.* Berlin: Springer-Verlag, 1974.
9. Eaton, R. G., and Mallerich, M. M. Volar plate arthroplasty for the proximal interphalangeal joint: A ten year review. *J. Hand Surg.* 5:260, 1980.
10. Agee, J. M. Unstable fracture dislocations of the proximal interphalangeal joint of the fingers: A preliminary report of a new technique. *J. Hand Surg.* 3:386, 1978.
11. Becton, J. L., Christian J. D., Jr., Goodwin, N. H., and Jackson, T. G. A simplified technique for treating the complex dislocation of the index metacarpal phalangeal joint *J. Bone Joint Surg.* 57A: 698–700, 1975.

SUGGESTED READING

Dabezies, E. J., and Schutte, J. P. Fixation of metacarpal and phalangeal fractures with miniature plates and screws. *J. Hand Surg.* [*Am.*] 11:283, 1986.

Green, D. P. *Operative Hand Surgery,* 2nd ed. New York: Churchill Livingstone, 1988.

Green, D. P., and Anderson, J. R. Closed reduction and percutaneous pin fixation of fractured phalanges. *J. Bone Joint Surg.* [*Am.*] 55:1651, 1973.

Gustilo, R. B., Gruninger, R. P., and Tsukayama, D. T. *Orthopaedic Infection.* Philadelphia: Saunders, 1989.

Melone C. P. Rigid fixation of phalangeal and metacarpal fractures. *Orthop. Clin. North Am.* 17:421, 1986.

Rockwood, C. A., and Green, D. P. *Fractures in Adults,* Vols. 1 and 2. Philadelphia: Lippincott, 1984.

Commentary on Chapter 7

Joseph E. Imbriglia

This chapter provides an excellent summary of the diagnosis and care of hand fractures and dislocations. There are certain points that warrant emphasis.

1. The fracture that creates the most long-term disability is the displaced fracture of the proximal phalanx. These fractures are inherently unstable when they displace and may lead to malunions, nonunions, and concomitant loss of motion at the PIP joint, whose motion is critical for satisfactory finger function. Malunions have resulted from inappropriate closed treatment of these fractures, and nonunions are seen after inappropriate and inadequate internal fixation. We have seen patients who have had open reduction and internal fixation with miniplates that have resulted in severe extensor and flexor tendon scarring and loss of PIP joint motion. We prefer close reduction and percutaneous, longitudinal pinning of displaced, transverse fractures of the proximal phalanx. These fractures most commonly have an apex volar deformity. If the fracture is left angulated, there will be scarring of the superficialis tendon to the fracture, resulting in a PIP flexion contracture and loss of PIP motion. The long, spiral, oblique fractures of the proximal phalanx are treated by open reduction and AO screw fixation. Plates are not necessary in most cases. Cross-pinning of transverse fractures of the proximal phalanx is not a good technique. The cross pins inevitably spear the lateral bands and may actually distract the fracture.

2. In regard to open fractures, Dr. Aulicino stated: "Type III wounds should be left open, and internal fixation is usually not indicated for these injuries." It has been our experience with type III open wounds that some fixation is absolutely necessary. Because of the severe soft-tissue injury accompanying these fractures, the fractures have no intrinsic stability. External or internal fixation may be used depending on the site of the fracture. After providing appropriate fixation, these wounds are left open and are secondarily closed once the surgeon believes the wound is clean.

3. When immobilizing the hand after either closed or open reduction of the fracture, the MCP joints should be places in at least

70 degrees of flexion if possible, thereby preventing loss of flexion at the MCP joints as the fracture heals. Dr. Aulicino stated that the PIP and DIP joints are hinge joints and that the collateral ligaments are stretched in all positions. It is important, however, that the PIP joints be immobilized in the extended position to prevent flexion contractures of these joints. Under no circumstances should the PIP joints be immobilized in a flexed position following a fracture of the proximal phalanx. In fact, the only time the PIP joint is immobilized in flexion is when treating a dorsal fracture-dislocation of this joint.

4. When surgically approaching the fractures of the proximal phalanx or PIP joint, it is best to dissect underneath the extensor mechanism and not split the extensor tendon to obtain exposure. In almost all cases, enough exposure can be gained by retracting the extensor mechanism to perform the necessary operation. We believe that splitting the extensor mechanism and then repairing it results in increased scar formation, with secondary loss of motion.

The amount of disability that results from inappropriately treated fractures of the fingers is tremendous, particularly in the workman. The surgeon must remember that the goal is not simply getting the bones to heal but getting the bones to heal with minimal damage to the soft tissues. It is the soft-tissue scarring that most often results in prolonged disability to these patients. Fixation with K-wires provides strong enough fixation for the fracture to heal but does not require the extensive soft-tissue dissections that are often necessary to put on plates. Appropriate, sensible, surgical care yields satisfactory results with most of these fractures.

8 PRINCIPLES OF ACUTE FLEXOR TENDON REPAIR

Richard J. Greco

Sterling Bunnell once wrote, "One of the most baffling problems in surgery is to restore normal function to a finger in which the tendons have been injured" [1]. Much has been learned about the repair and approach to the treatment of acute flexor tendon injuries, yet these injuries continue to challenge the most accomplished surgeon. Their surgical repair requires an exact knowledge of the anatomy, sound clinical judgment, strict atraumatic technique, and, most importantly, a well planned and well supervised postoperative therapy program.

ANATOMY

A detailed anatomic review of the upper extremity is included in Chapter 4. This section concentrates on the muscles and tendons of the flexor system.

Volar Compartment

The flexor system comprises muscle bellies originating in the proximal two-thirds of the volar compartment of the forearm and tendinous extensions that insert into the wrist or digits. There are two tendons for each finger and one for the thumb. In the fingers the flexor digitorum superficialis (FDS) inserts into the middle phalanx and creates flexion at the proximal interphalangeal (PIP) joint. The flexor digitorum profundus (FDP) inserts into the distal phalanx and flexes the distal interphalangeal (DIP) joint of the respective finger. There is only one long flexor tendon to the thumb, the flexor pollicis longus, and it inserts into the distal phalanx and causes flexion of the interphalangeal joint of the thumb.

The anatomy of the forearm is best understood if viewed in a layer approach. The most superficial layer contains the palmaris longus, flexor carpi radialis, flexor carpi ulnaris, and the pronator teres (Fig. 8-1). These muscle units, which do not cross the wrist, are involved in wrist flexion and forearm pronation.

The second layer contains the flexor digitorum superficialis. It arises from two heads and separates in four separate tendons. The ring and long finger arise from the more superficial muscle belly, and the tendons are more superficial than the tendons of the index and

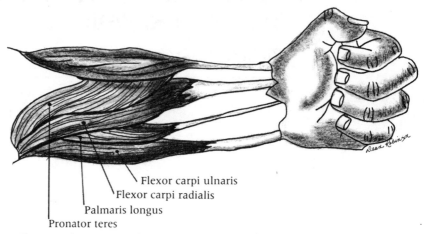

Flexor carpi ulnaris
Flexor carpi radialis
Palmaris longus
Pronator teres

Fig. 8-1. Flexor musculature, superficial group.

little finger in the carpal canal (Fig. 8-2). After exiting the carpal canal, the tendons diverge to their respective digits volar to the FDP tendon. The tendon flattens and splits into two slips that encompass the FDP tendon, pass dorsal to it, and reunite to form a bed for the FDP tendon until it inserts in the proximal one-half of the middle phalanx (Fig.8-3). This area of division is commonly called the "chiasma of Camper." The median nerve courses along the undersurface of the FDS and in its muscle sheath. As the muscle becomes tendinous, the median nerve courses radial and then superficial to the FDS tendons and remains deep to the superficial layer of muscles. The ulnar artery and nerve are found immediately underneath the flexor carpi ulnaris, and the radial artery courses radial to, but at the same level as, the flexor carpi ulnaris in the distal forearm.

The third layer of the forearm consists of the flexor digitorum profundus and the flexor pollicis longus. The conjoined FDP muscle mass separates into four tendons that course dorsal to the FDS tendon and penetrate it at the chiasma of Camper; it then inserts at the base of the distal phalanx. The flexor pollicis longus is located in the radial aspect of the carpal canal, travels through the thenar muscles in a fibroosseous canal, and inserts in the distal phalanx of the thumb (Fig.8-4).

The fourth and deepest layer of the volar forearm contains the pronator quadratus and is not usually important in acute tendon repairs.

Flexor Retinaculum
The flexor retinaculum comprises a system of pulleys and a tendon sheath that begins at the neck of the metacarpal and ends with the insertion of the profundus tendon in the distal phalanx (Fig. 8-5). This system of pulleys is responsible for holding the tendons close to the bone and allowing for the transformation of muscle contraction and excursion into a maximum range of motion for the digital joints they serve. The flexor retinaculum contains both zone 1

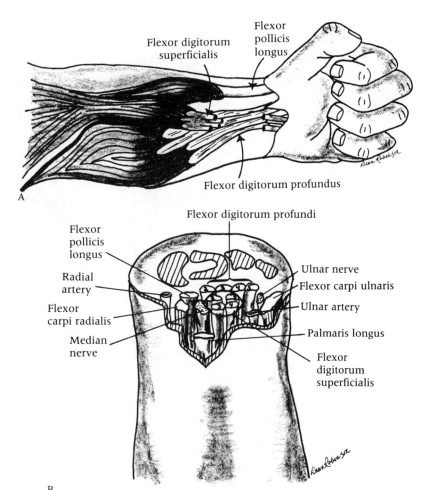

Fig. 8-2. A. Flexor musculature, middle and deep groups. *B.* Cross-sectional anatomy of the wrist.

and zone 2 of Verdan. Zone 2 has been commonly called the "no man's land" of Bunnell and the critical zone of Boyes because of the technical challenge it provides the tendon surgeon.

There are five annular (A) pulleys and three cruciate (C) pulleys in each digit (see Fig. 8-5). The two most important pulleys are named the A2 pulley (base of the proximal phalanx) and the A4 pulley (base of the middle phalanx). They constitute the minimum requirement for efficient function. The flexor retinaculum of the thumb has two annular and one oblique pulley (Fig. 8-4).

Vascular Anatomy of the Flexor Tendon

Tendons are long bundles of collagenous fibers. They have blood supply from their muscles of origin, surrounding paratenon and vincula, and the vessels of the periosteum into which they insert. The intrinsic vascular system is dorsally based, and therefore sutures should be placed in the volar two-thirds of the tendon (Fig. 8-6).

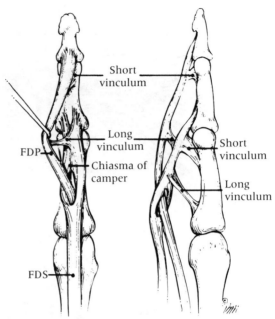

Fig. 8-3. The flexor digitorum profundus (FDP) passes through the tails of the flexor digitorum superficiales (FDS) on the way to its insertion into the distal phalanx. (From L. H. Schneider and J. M. Hunter. Flexor tendons — late reconstruction. In D. Green, ed. Operative Hand Surgery, 2nd ed. New York: Churchill Livingstone, 1988. With permission.)

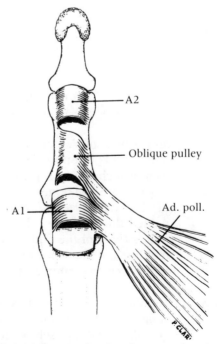

Fig. 8-4. Flexor retinaculum in the thumb. It consist of two annular and an oblique pulley over the proximal phalanx. (From J. R. Doyle and W. F. Blythe. Anatomy of the flexor tendon sheath and pulley of the thumb. *J. Hand Surg.* 2:149, 1977. With permission.)

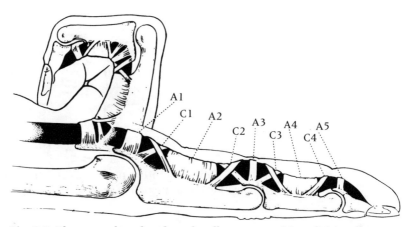

Fig. 8-5. Flexor tendon sheath and pulley system. A2 and A4 pulleys are critical to save or reconstruct to prevent bowstringing during active finger flexion. (From H. E. Kleinert, et al. Current state of flexor tendon surgery. *Ann. Chir. Main.* 3(1):7, 1984. With permission.)

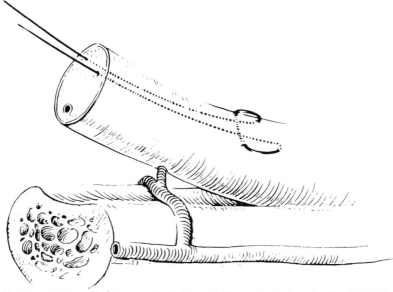

Fig. 8-6. Suture placement should avoid the intrinsic longitudinal blood supply located in the dorsal one-third of the tendon. (From H. E. Kleinert, et al. Complications of tendon surgery in the hand. In S. Sandzen, ed. *Current Management of Complications in Orthopaedic Surgery: The Hand and Wrist.* Baltimore: Williams & Wilkins, 1985. With permission.)

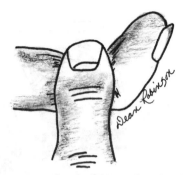

Fig. 8-7. Flexor digitorum profundus (FDP) function is assessed by isolated flexion at the DIP joint.

EVALUATION

The basic evaluation of the upper extremity is reviewed in Chapter 4; therefore this discussion is limited to the examination of the upper extremity in reference to flexor tendon function. One must remember to examine the entire patient prior to concentrating on the examination of the upper extremity. One can learn far more from examining the extremity distal to the site of injury than by probing the wound. It is again emphasized that one should do a thorough neurologic and vascular examination and document these findings. Tetanus and antibiotic prophylaxis should be considered.

There are four basic components to the examination of flexor tendon function.

1. *Active motion tests.* In the awake, cooperative patient special maneuvers can be used to separate and test the functions of the FDP and FDS independently. It is the most informative part of the flexor examination. It is useful to examine each digit of the uninjured hand first to be sure the patient fully understands the activities to be tested. By blocking and allowing only DIP flexion one can test sequentially the FDP functions of each digit (Fig. 8-7). Next, one restrains the FDP of all other digits by holding the digits in extension and asking the patient to flex the unrestrained digit. Full flexion at the PIP joint demonstrates an intact FDS tendon. Baker et al. [2] have shown that 34 percent of all little fingers have an insufficient FDS tendon. These maneuvers are done against light resistance; and if pain is elicited, one should be suspicious of a partial laceration of the involved tendon.
2. *Observation at rest.* One observes the cascade of the digits with the patient relaxed or under anesthesia. There should be a normal progression of increasing flexion as one proceeds from the index to the little finger. One finger in the extended position with an otherwise normal cascade is suspicious of a flexor tendon injury.
3. *Squeeze test.* If the injury is distal to the forearm, one can cause flexion of intact flexor tendons by placing pressure on the volar forearm proximal to the level of injury. Intact musculotendon

units cause finger flexion. Partial lacerations give false-negative results.
4. *Tenodesis effect.* Gentle flexion and extension at the wrist should make all the fingers flex and extend in a normal cascade fashion. Again, fingers with disrupted flexor tendons remain in an extended position.

It is important to assess the amount of accompanying bony and soft-tissue injury, the degree of contamination, and the length of time since the injury occurred. A radiograph of the involved area is important for defining the degree of bone pathology and for locating any radiopaque foreign bodies.

CLASSIFICATION OF FLEXOR INJURIES

When experienced hand surgeons reviewed the functional results of their repairs of acute flexor tendon injuries they noted a significant association of functional recovery with the location in the tendon system where the injury had occurred. Verdan [3] separated the flexor tendon system into five zones based on the tendons, flexor retinaculum, and carpal ligament anatomy. This classification has allowed direct comparison of varied techniques of repair, postoperative management, and their subsequent functional outcome at comparable levels from multiple institutions. It has also allowed us to individualize the approach to the acute tendon injury based on the expected outcomes from the chosen techniques in that particular zone.

I have found the modification of Verdan's zone system, as accepted by the International Federation of Societies for Surgery of the Hand, useful when evaluating flexor tendon injuries (Fig. 8-8). The following zones are used for examining the fingers.

Zone 5:   Musculotendinous junctures to the proximal edge of the carpal canal.

Zone 4:   Underlies the transverse carpal ligament; the anatomic limits are the hook of the hamate and tuberosity of the scaphoid proximally and the pisiform and trapezium distally. The volar wrist crease is a surface marker for the division of zones 4 and 5.

Zone 3:   Between the restraint of the carpal ligament and that created by the flexor retinaculum.

Zone 2:   Bunnell's "no man's land," which anatomically starts at the entrance of the flexor retinaculum at the level of the neck of the metacarpal and ends with the insertion of the FDS into the mid-portion of the middle phalanx. Both tendons are contained by a tight fibroosseous tunnel and are in intimate contact in this region. The distal palmar crease is a surface marker for the start of zone 2.

Zone 1:   Distal to the FDS insertion and terminating in the FDP insertion. (Only the FDP tendon is found in this zone.)

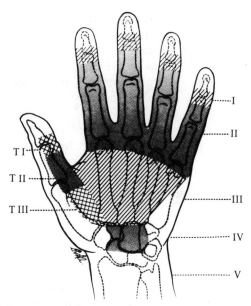

Fig. 8-8. Verdan's zones of flexor tendon injury are based on the level of transected tendon, not the skin laceration. (From H. E. Kleinert and C. E. Verdon. Report of the committee on tendon injuries. *J. Hand Surg.* 8:794–798, 1983. With permission.)

The following zones are useful when describing injuries to the thumb (zones 4 and 5 are the same). It is important to note that there is only one tendon that traverses this fibroosseous tunnel.

Zone T3:   Area of the thenar muscles
Zone T2:   From the neck of the metacarpal to the neck of the proximal phalanx and coinciding with the flexor retinaculum of the thumb
Zone T1:   End of the retinaculum to the insertion of the flexor pollicis longus

Note that it is the location of the tendon injury with the wrist and digits in extension and not the surface laceration that determines the appropriate zone discussed. The relation of the skin and tendon injuries depends on the position of the fingers and extremity at the time of injury.

ACUTE PRECAUTIONS

After the timing of the operative intervention is established, a soft, bulky dressing and a dorsal protective splint are appropriate (see Chapter 19). The traumatized area should be kept elevated to reduce swelling and the patient prepared for the operating room. If there is significant bleeding, a pressure dressing is placed and the patient taken promptly to the operating room. *Blind clamping of structures in the emergency room is fraught with dangerous consequences.* If the bleeding is not controlled by the pressure dressing, a tourniquet or

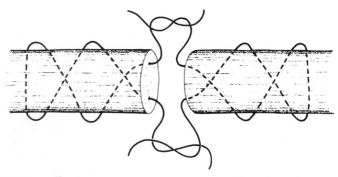

Fig. 8-9. Bunnell crisscross suture. (From L. H. Schneider. *Flexor Tendon Injuries. Monographs in Hand Surgery.* Boston: Little, Brown, 1985. With permission.)

inflated blood pressure cuff can be used and immediate exploration in the operating room undertaken. One must closely observe the amount of time extremity is ischemic.

SUTURE MATERIAL AND TECHNIQUE

Much controversy exists as to the ideal tendon suture and the appropriate method to secure the tendon stumps. Stainless steel suture is still used by many, but it is not as flexible as man-made materials and therefore not ideal for zone 2 repairs. Braided sutures and monofilament nylon and Prolene are flexible but may stretch with tension. All of these 4-0 sutures have adequate tensile strength. I have used 4-0 nylon and Prolene with good success.

The suture technique is also controversial; and when a particular variation of the technique is necessary it is described in that zone. The Bunnell suture was a significant advance in tendon surgery (Fig. 8-9). With prolonged experience it was noted that with tension the repair tended to gap, leading to increased adhesions in this area. The Kessler suture, and then its modification (Fig. 8-10), were tested in animal models, and it was shown that the Bunnell suture had more of a "strangling" effect on the tendon than the "grasping" Kessler suture; moreover, there was a threefold difference in strength on the fifth postoperative day in favor of the Kessler suture.

I prefer to use the Tajima modification of the Kessler suture (Fig. 8-11). It allows placement of the suture as the tendon stumps are dissected, a subsequent atraumatic way of handling the stumps, and a secure juncture. The disadvantage of this technique is the bulk and risk of two knots unraveling.

A shallow, inverting, continuous epitendinous suture is used for all zone 2 repairs and in any are where the coaptation of the tendon causes everted edges. It is important to emphasize that it must be an inverting suture repair (Fig. 8-12). It is not necessary for zone 5 injuries.

When repairing distal profundus tendon injuries with a inadequate distal stump, a periosteal flap is raised proximal to the distal stump

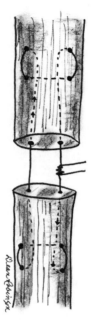

Fig. 8-10. Modified Kessler suture.

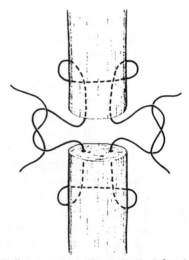

Fig. 8-11. Modified Tajima suture. (From L. H. Schneider. *Flexor Tendon Injuries. Monographs in Hand Surgery.* Boston: Little, Brown, 1985. With permission.)

and distal to the volar plate. A cortical defect is created in the volar cortex using a bone awl or a bur and then a small curet. A modified Bunnell crisscross suture is placed with two crosses at the end of the profundus tendon. A pull-out suture is placed after the first transverse pass. Two straight Keith needles in a motorized pin driver are inserted through the distal phalanx and nail. Care must be taken to

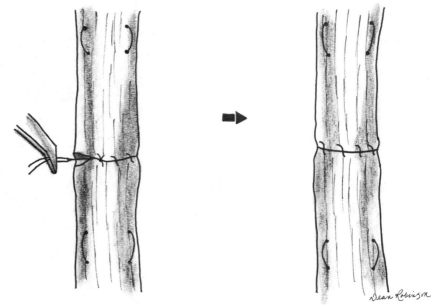

Fig. 8-12. Inverting epitendinous suture.

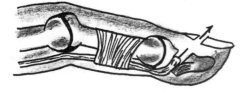

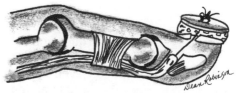

Fig. 8-13. Bunnell distal juncture for tendon grafts and reinsertion of FDP into the distal phalanx.

place them through the middle of the nail and not through the proximal nail bed. The needles on the suture are removed, and the suture is fed into the eyes of the Keith needles. The Keith needle is then pulled through the distal phalanx and secured using the standard button technique (Fig. 8-13). Gauze padding is placed between the nail and the button before the sutures are tied over the button. Additional 4-0 sutures are used to secure the distal stump remnant and the periosteum to the reinserted tendon.

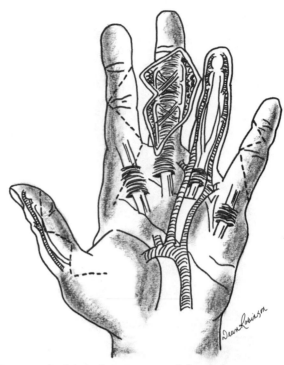

Fig. 8-14. Brunner incisions for exposure of the digits.

OPERATIVE APPROACH

Tendon repair is not the first priority in the multiple injury patient, the massive crush injury, or the contaminated injury that cannot be converted to a clean wound by surgical débridement. The surgeon's responsibility is to clean and débride the wound, stabilize fractures, obtain adequate skin coverage, and obtain a healed wound without infection. *Absolute contraindications* to a zone 2 repair include human bite lacerations, inadequate skin coverage, and evidence of cellulitis.

All tendon repairs should be done in an operating room with adequate lighting, instruments, and anesthesia, and under tourniquet control. An axillary block is ideal, with general anesthesia equivalent — if not contraindicated. Prophylactic antibiotics are given for at least 24 hours postoperatively and longer if the wound is contaminated. The wound is carefully cleaned and débrided. High pressure irrigation by a 35-ml syringe and a 19-gauge needle helps decrease wound infection rates.

Discussion of the operative approach is broken down by the zones previously described. In general, skin incisions should be carefully planned, attempting to utilize the laceration and avoiding straight volar incisions that cross flexion creases. Bruner incisions for exposure of the injury are useful (Fig. 8-14). However, if the injury is transverse and in the digital crease, a Bruner incision may produce two flaps with tip angles of 45 degrees that may have an inadequate blood supply for survival. In these situations, the incision should start from the wound in the mid-lateral line, turning to pass to the other side of the digit after a sufficiently wide tip has been created for flap survival. After dissection of the tendons and their sheaths, as needed, the neurovascular structures are evaluated if they are in the zone of injury. The fractures and joint injuries are stabilized before the tendons are repaired. The neurovascular repairs are best done last unless the hand or finger is compromised.

Careful "atraumatic technique" is essential, and only the cut ends of the tendon should be handled. Minimal débridement of the tendon stumps is done, only when necessary, with a fresh sharp blade on a tongue blade background.

Primary repair is direct end-to-end repair of the tendons within the first 24 hours. End-to-end repair after this time is considered to be a delayed primary repair. When appropriately performed, there is no adverse effect on the end result when a delayed primary repair is elected and performed during the first 4 weeks. After 4 weeks, unless the tendon unit is being held at length by an intact vincula or bone fragment, the shortening of the muscle-tendon unit is detrimental to the ability to perform a primary repair, and tendon grafts or two-stage reconstruction may become necessary. I believe that primary repair is often easier technically and the length of disability is less because there is no delay. However, when there is no qualified hand surgeon available, closure of the wound, oral antibiotics, and appropriate splinting are preferred over repair by unqualified surgeons not familiar with the demands of tendon surgery.

Zone 5

Zone 5 has the optimal chance for recovery of tendon function, although the concomitant nerve injuries often leave a significant postoperative functional deficit.

One-half modified Kessler sutures are placed in the proximal and distal tendon stumps as they are dissected free (Fig. 8-10). This method allows handling the tendons in an atraumatic way and begins the repair process. A 3-0 nylon or Prolene suture is used for repair at the tendinous levels. After all tendon sutures are placed, the median and ulnar nerves and the radial and ulnar arteries are evaluated and prepared for repair. If the vessels are not injured, the tourniquet is released, bleeding is controlled, the corresponding tendons are secured, and finally the nerve repairs are performed. If the repair is at the level of the muscle bellies, a 3-0 PDS or Vicryl suture is utilized in a figure-of-eight fashion for the repair. No epitendinous suture is required in zone 5.

The repair is performed in a logical and orderly fashion. After identification of all tendons, nerves, and vessels to be repaired, the repair begins from the deepest layer to the most superficial. If the vessels require repair, the tendons underneath the vessels are approximated first, the vessels are repaired with the assistance of the microscope, and the tourniquet is then released. After the patency of the vessel is ensured, hemostasis is obtained, the nerves are repaired, and the remaining tendons are approximated. If the injury is in the distal one-third of the forearm, the transverse carpal ligament is released so the tendon repairs can pass without difficulty.

Repair of the flexor carpi radialis and ulnaris completes the repair. No attempts at palmaris repair is recommended. Chase [4] did not repair the flexor carpi ulnaris if the ulnar nerve was to be repaired. He believed that the increase scarring formed is detrimental. At the completion of the closure, 3-0 nylon sutures are placed in the nails for postoperative controlled motion therapy (or hooks are glued on postoperatively). A dorsal splint with the wrist at neutral and the fingers in the position of safety is utilized (see Chapter 19). If the repairs are in the distal one-third of the forearm, the wrist is splinted in 35 degrees of flexion.

Zone 4

Nine tendons and the median nerve are located behind the transverse carpal ligament in zone 4. A vertical zigzag incision is used for exposure. There are two schools of thought regarding whether to leave the distal aspect of the ligament intact or to release the entire carpal ligament. Impingement of this pulley on the repaired tendons should be tested for and guarded against. Flexor bowstringing has been reported when the entire ligament is transected.

What one repairs in this zone depends on the number of structures injured. If all nine tendons are transected, only the flexor pollicis longus, profundus tendons, and median nerve are repaired. The superficialis tendons are excised from the area. If all other structures are intact, and only one or two superficialis tendons are injured, they can be repaired primarily. A 3-0 modified Kessler suture is adequate for repair at this level.

The median nerve is repaired after the tendon junctures are secure (see Chapter 10 for techniques). An "awake stimulation" for identification of the motor branch proximally and distally makes scientific sense but has not been proved clinically yet. The carpal ligament is left open and the skin closed. A dorsal splint with the wrist in 35 degrees of flexion is utilized.

Zone 3

Primary or delayed primary repair of both the flexor digiti superficialis and profundus tendons is the treatment of choice for clean, sharp injuries. If the tendon stumps are ragged or the repair seems to jeopardize tendon excursion, the flexor digitorum profundus is repaired and the flexor digitorum superficialis is resected widely so that the flexor digitorum profundus is not compromised. Concomitant neurovascular injury is common and must be repaired.

A zigzag approach is utilized in the palm. Care during dissection is necessary to avoid further neurovascular injuries. The proximal stump of the profundus tendon is held by the lumbrical origin and prevents more proximal slippage of the ends. The palmar fascia is excised and a modified Kessler suture is utilized for repair. A 4-0 nylon or Prolene suture is used; and if good coaptation of the junctures is achieved, the 6-0 epitendinous suture is not necessary. Postoperative controlled motion therapy is utilized with a dorsally based splint (Fig. 8-15).

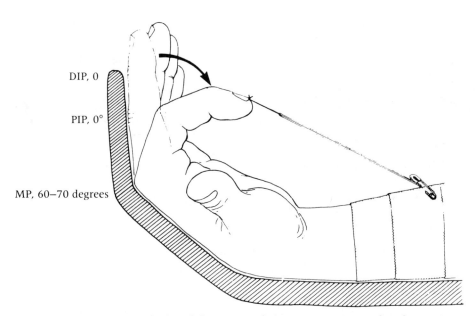

DIP, 0

PIP, 0°

MP, 60–70 degrees

Fig. 8-15. Protected mobilization with active extension and early passive gliding of the tendon repair.

Zone 2

Zone 2, coined as "no man's land" by Bunnell, describes the area where the superficialis and profundus tendons are held closely together in the fibroosseous tunnel. This region presents the most difficulty for the surgeon to restore active flexion to the finger. Repair during the first 3 weeks have resulted in comparable results; however, repair during the first 10 days is recommended. If severe aggravating factors such as skin loss, crushing joint injuries, or fractures with precarious stabilization are encountered, secondary reconstruction should be utilized.

A zigzag Bruner incision is used for exposure when possible. Careful dissection of the neurovascular bundles is performed. It is important to expose 1 to 2 cm of tendon sheath both proximally and distally. The sheath is opened with transverse or L-shaped incisions in the cruciate portions of the pulley system. Care is taken to preserve the A2 and A4 pulleys as an absolute minimum (Fig. 8-16).

One flexes the distal finger to determine where the sheath should be opened for repair. If 1 cm of tendon can be expressed distal to the major pulley, the repair can be performed proximal to this pulley. If less than 0.5 cm of tendon is expressed, it is necessary to perform the repair distal to the pulley. A flap of the sheath is elevated, leaving an adequate margin of sheath for closure along the vertical aspect of the opening (Fig. 8-17).

The proximal stumps are milked distally with the wrist and proximal finger flexed. The two tendon ends are kept together so as to not interrupt their vascular connections. A fine Keith needle is placed through the sheath and tendons proximally to keep the

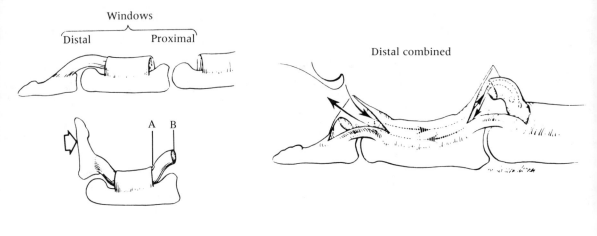

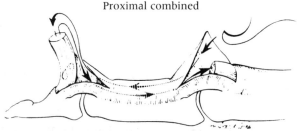

Fig. 8-16. Windows in the flexor sheath were described by Lister to provide access and spare major pulleys. (From G. D. Lister. *Hand* 15(2):123, 1983. With permission.)

proximal stumps from retracting. "Atraumatic" technique is necessary, and only the cut ends should be handled. A fine-tooth forceps is sufficient because the tendon is secured proximally with the Keith needle or a 25-gauge needle. One-half of a Kessler suture is placed in the volar one-half of the profundus tendon (to spare the intrinsic tendon blood supply). The corresponding distal profundus core suture is placed, and these sutures are then set aside until after the superficialis repair.

If the proximal stumps cannot be milked distally, control can be obtained at the level of the distal palmar crease and proximal to the A1 pulley. A Hunter silicone prosthesis or a fine red rubber catheter can be passed from the distal sheath opening to the palm through the fibroosseous tunnel. The tendons are then attached to the catheter and guided distally to the repair site. An alternative technique includes placing the sutures in the proximal and distal stumps of the tendons through transverse incisions in the sheath more proximally and subsequently retrieving the sutures with a Swanson suture passer through an area in the sheath where both tendons can be retrieved without tension.

The superficialis repair depends on which portion of the tendon is injured. When the injury is distal to the decussation, two separate horizontal mattress sutures of 4-0 nylon are used in the medial and

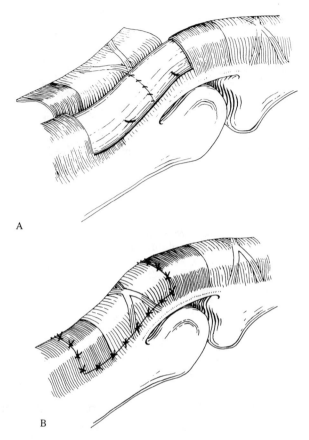

A

B

Fig. 8-17. A. Tendon repair can be performed with the sheath reflected. (From L. H. Schneider. *Flexor Tendon Injuries Monographs in Hand Surgery.* Boston: Little, Brown, 1985. With permission.) *B.* The sheath is repaired.

lateral tails of the tendon. If the transection is proximal to the decussation, a modified Kessler suture of 4-0 nylon or Prolene is used. Care is taken to tie the suture so that the knot lies in the tendon substance and the tendon is not excessively bunched up. The sutures are kept long until after the 6-0 Prolene or nylon continuous, inverting, epitendinous suture is placed. The latter is used to form a smooth juncture. The profundus tendon is then approximated with the previously placed sutures, and an epitendinous suture is placed.

When the superficialis tendon cannot be repaired, the proximal end is pulled into the wound and severed, allowing it to retract proximally. The distal aspect is not removed because a highly vascular bed in which adhesions would be formed would be created, and the hyperextension deformity in lax individuals is prevented.

If the injury is located near the A1 pulley, the pulley is resected, converting a zone 2 injury to a zone 3 injury. Passive motion can be utilized to determine if the junctures will freely pass in the fibroosseous tunnel. Again there are two schools of thought as to whether the sheath should be closed or resected. The arguments for

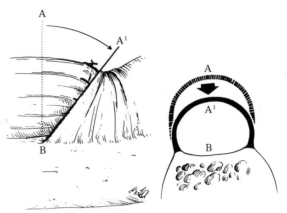

Fig. 8-18. Unrepaired tendon sheath can snag the repair and decrease tendon gliding. (From H. E. Kleinert, S. Schepel, and D. Gillt. *Surg. Clin. North Am.* 61:267, 1981. With permission.)

closing the sheath are that fewer adhesions form, better peritendon nutrition is provided, and the open end of the sheath may cause the tendon repair to snag (Fig. 8-18). The sheath is closed with fine 6-0 or 7-0 Prolene sutures. On many occasions the sheath cannot be closed, and it is then resected adequately (approximately 1.5 cm) to allow free passage of the tendon repairs. One must preserve the A2 and A4 pulleys.

After the tendons have been repaired, the injured neurovascular structures are repaired, the tourniquet is released, hemostasis is obtained, the skin is closed, and 3-0 nylon sutures are placed in the nails for postoperative therapy. A dorsal plaster splint is then fashioned with the wrist in 45 degrees of flexion and the MCP joints at 45 degrees of flexion. The splint must allow full extension of PIP and DIP motion. Rubberbands should be placed to keep the fingers in flexion and allow active extension to occur against their resistance.

Zone 1

Zone 1 is distal to the superficialis insertion, and only the profundus is injured. Although a functional hand is possible without repair, strength is less and there is loss of active DIP flexion. Young, healthy people should be offered early repair. About 35 percent of individuals have an insufficient superficialis to the little finger and require flexor digitorum profundus repair for a functional finger.

There are three basic types of zone 1 injury:

1. Distal vincula intact: This situation is rare, and little dissection is necessary. The proximal tendon stump is held from retracting by the short vincula.
2. Long vinculum intact: The profundus is held from retraction at the level of the decussation.
3. No vincula intact: The profundus has retracted into the palm where it is held by the attachments of the lumbricals. This presentation is most common and requires the most dissection

and potential scarring while attempting to thread the tendon stump through the chiasma of Camper and the fibroosseous tunnel.

A zigzag Bruner incision is carried out from the middle of the distal phalanx and ending at the PIP crease. The flexor sheath and neurovascular bundles are then dissected, and the location of the proximal tendon stump is identified. If it is located at the decussation of the flexor digitorum superficialis, a small transverse incision is made in the sheath, a one-half modified Kessler suture of 4-0 nylon or Prolene is placed in the profundus end, and a suture passer is moved retrogradely from the distal sheath opening. If a suture passer is not available, one can use a No. 28 wire suture bent in half as a passer, and the suture and tendon stump are then threaded up the flexor retinaculum. Care is taken not to injure the superficialis tendon. Again, a fine Keith needle or a 25-gauge needle can be used to secure the tendon more proximally and lead to a repair without tension.

If there is an adequate distal profundus stump, an end-to-end repair is performed, with an additional one-half modified Kessler suture being placed in the distal stump. After the juncture is secured, a 6-0 continuous nylon or Prolene epitendinous suture is placed if the juncture does not pass smoothly through the sheath. It is often impossible to perform posteriorly and is often unnecessary. Advancement and reinsertion of the profundus into the distal phalanx is advocated by many if less than 1 cm of distal stump remains. Because one advances more than one expects in most situations, which leads to a flexion deformity at the DIP joint, advancement is used only when inadequate distal stump is available for repair.

If the profundus is located in the palm, one to two attempts at retrieving the tendon stump through a small transverse incision in the retinaculum at the level of the PIP is attempted with a fine clamp while the palm is massaged to push the tendon end distally. If this method is unsuccessful, the skin incision is carried more proximally to the base of the finger. Another transverse incision is made in the sheath, and the tendon is retrieved. One retrieves the tendon with the suture passer after placing one-half of the modified Kessler suture in the tendon stump or by guiding a Hunter's silicone rod down the sheath from the distal opening, securing the tendon end to it, and threading them both up the flexor retinaculum. Under no circumstance should the uninjured flexor digitorum superficialis tendon be purposely injured to obtain a flexor digitorum profundus repair. Occasionally, one must expose the tendon at the distal palmar crease at the level of the A1 pulley and subsequently thread the tendon up the retinaculum as described previously. The flexor retinaculum is then repaired with 6-0 or 7-0 Prolene sutures.

After the tendon has been repaired, the injured neurovascular structures are repaired, the tourniquet is released, hemostasis is obtained, the skin is closed, and a 3-0 nylon suture is placed in the nail for postoperative therapy. A dorsal plaster splint is then fashioned with the wrist in 45 degrees of flexion and MCP joints at 45 degrees of flexion. The splint must allow full extension of PIP and DIP motion. Rubberbands should be placed to keep the fingers in flexion and allow active extension to occur against their resistance.

If there is an inadequate distal stump for tendon repair, one must advance and reinsert the profundus tendon with the pull-out wire and button technique as described in the Suture Material and Technique section, above. One must be careful not to overadvance the tendon and cause a relative weakening of the other profundi.

Avulsion Injuries of the Profundus Tendon

Avulsion of the profundus tendon is a fairly common injury and usually occurs at its bony insertion and not in the tendon substance. This injury is most common in young athletes and involves the ring finger in many cases. The insertion in this finger is anatomically weaker than in other fingers. Patients present with a history of a sudden extension injury to an actively flexing finger. They have been told that they have a "jammed finger"; and only careful examination can detect the inability to flex the DIP joint. Radiographs of the involved finger may detect avulsed segments of distal phalanx. Unfortunately, a delay in diagnosis may severely jeopardize the final result. Leddy and Packer [5] have classified these injuries in three main types.

Type I: The profundus ruptures and retracts into the palm. No intact vincula are present. The inability to flex the DIP joint and a tender mass in the palm are helpful for the diagnosis.

Type II: The ruptured profundus retracts to the level of the DIP joint. No DIP motion, decreased PIP motion, and swelling and tenderness are noted over the PIP joint. Lateral radiographs may reveal a bony fragment at the level of the PIP joint. The long vincula is still intact in these injuries.

Type III: A large fragment of the distal phalanx is avulsed from the distal phalanx and caught up at the A4 pulley. Swelling and tenderness over the middle phalanx and inability to flex the DIP joint are helpful in the diagnosis. A lateral radiograph of the finger should reveal a large fragment of bone just proximal to the DIP joint.

Treatment

Treatment of the avulsed profundus tendon depends on the location of the proximal tendon stump, the size of the bony fragment avulsed from the distal phalanx, and the length of time since the injury occurred.

Type I. These tendons should be reinserted within 7 to 10 days before they become necrotic and contracted. The modified Bunnell technique is used as described above. The proximal tendon stump is located through an incision parallel to the distal palmar crease proximal to the A1 pulley. A distal Bruner zigzag incision is utilized over the DIP joint, and the tendon is threaded up the flexor retinaculum as described under zone 1 repairs.

Type II. These tendons should be reinserted using the modified Bunnell technique also. Because the vincula is intact, up to 3 months can go by before repair, and a satisfactory result can be expected. The exposure necessary is from the distal phalanx to the proximal stump at the level of the middle phalanx. A Bruner zigzag skin incision and a small transverse incision in the sheath are usually necessary to obtain control of the proximal tendon stump. It is threaded to the distal phalanx as described for zone 1 repairs.

Type III. The large fragment can be secured with open reduction and internal fixation of the bony fragment with K-wires. The exposure is needed only over the distal aspect of the digit. The fragment is usually easily retrieved.

It is important not to accept a tendon repair that is too tight. If the tendon is advanced too far and the finger cannot come into full extension, the rest of the profundi have weakened activity, and flexion deformity is likely to occur at that DIP joint. This problem is referred to as a syndrome of quadriga.

Thumb. Zones 1, 3, 4, and 5 are treated in the same manner as described for zones 1, 3, 4, and 5 for the fingers. Zone 2 is different from that of the fingers because there is only one tendon present and the flexor retinaculum is different (see Fig. 8-4). Either the A1 or the oblique pulley must be preserved for an adequate functional result. If the vincula are intact, retrieval of the tendon stump should be easy. If the vincula is disrupted, a small catheter is passed through the sheath into the distal forearm where it can be easily palpated. A small transverse incision is made, and the flexor pollicis longus is attached to the catheter and subsequently threaded to the distal stump with the wrist in the flexed position. A transfixion needle can be used proximally, and an atraumatic zone II repair is done with a 4-0 modified Kessler suture and a 6-0 epitendinous suture. The sheath is closed with 6-0 or 7-0 Prolene sutures. Postoperatively, rubberband traction is utilized as in the other digits; however, the point of proximal fixation of the rubberband should be 10 cm proximal to the wrist and over the ulna.

One should avoid the temptation to open the transverse carpal ligament to search for the proximal end. It is usually in the forearm, and the intact carpal ligament allows the surgeon to splint the patient with the wrist in flexion and gives better long-term mechanical advantage to the repaired tendon.

**PARTIAL
LACERATIONS**

All tendon lacerations should be explored, even if there is near-normal function of the digit. The most common complications of missed partial lacerations are rupture of the tendon, triggering within the tendon sheath, and entrapment of the tendon flap in the opening of the sheath. If the injury is less than 60 percent of the tendon, the flap should be débrided to prevent triggering or entrapment. The temptation to repair all injuries should be resisted because more adhesions will form and the strength of a repaired tendon with less than a 60 percent injury is less than one not repaired.

For tendon injuries outside the flexor retinaculum, débridement of the tendon flaps is performed as necessary for lesions of 60 percent or less, and an early protected motion program is used for 4 weeks with elastic traction on the fingernails. For injuries larger than 60 percent, a modified Kessler suture is utilized to increase the potential for healing and decrease the possibility of complications.

Partial injuries in the flexor retinaculum are dealt with in a similar manner. For lacerations of less than 30 percent, the flap is débrided, the sheath closed, and an early protective motion program used. For lacerations between 30 and 60 percent, small 6-0 epitendinous tacking sutures would be used to avoid triggering and entrapment if approximation was easy. If repair would cause distortion of the tendon, débridement of flaps and closure of the sheath are performed. Again an early protected motion program is used for 4 weeks. For lacerations of more than 60 percent, the repair utilizes a 4-0 modified Kessler suture and a 6-0 epitendinous suture. The sheath is closed, and a postoperative protected passive motion program is begun with elastic traction.

REFERENCES

1. Bunnell, S. *Surgery of the Hand.* Philadelphia: Lippincott, 1944.
2. Baker, D. S., Gaul, J. S., Williams, V. K., and Graves, M. The little finger superficiales: Clinical investigation of its anatomic and functional shortcomings. *J. Hand Surg.* 6:374, 1981.
3. Verdan, C. E., Primary and secondary repair of flexor and extensor injuries. In J. E. Flynn (Ed.). *Hand Surgery* (3rd ed.) Baltimore: Williams and Wilkins, 1966.
4. Chase, R. A., *Atlas of Hand Surgery,* Saunders, 1973.
5. Leddy, J. P., and Packer, J. W., Avulsion of the profundus tendon insertion in athletes. *J. Hand Surg.* 2:66, 1977.

Commentary on Chapter 8

Lawrence H. Schneider

Direct flexor tendon repair has always been advocated when the flexor tendon was divided at the various levels of injury outside the difficult zone 2. However, up to the 1970s the direct repair of flexor tendon injuries was rarely undertaken for the zone 2 flexor tendon injury. We were taught to close the skin and prepare the patient for a palm to fingertip free flexor tendon graft, which was done 3 weeks or more later, thereby avoiding surgery within the flexor retinaculum, the so-called no man's land. Today it is safe to say that direct early repair is the preferred treatment for flexor tendon injuries at all levels.

What has changed our thinking? First, removal of the rigid time constraints within which it was thought that this surgery had to be done. The results obtained by the master tendon repairers such as Verdan in Switzerland and Kleinert in the United States, greatly advanced the cause of the early direct repair. Newer knowledge about the way flexor tendons heal, better suture material, and finer instruments and techniques along with the availability of trained surgeons have made it an available technique. It is now agreed that it is a simpler technique with which to return patients to function than the difficult free tendon graft, even though it is still not a simple operative procedure. The surgeon must pay strict attention to the details of the operative procedure, as outlined by Dr. Greco. It is also stressed that wound conditions must be adequate before early direct repair is feasible. Postoperative therapy is at least as important as the surgery itself, and provision must be made for postoperative supervision preferably with the services of trained therapists.

Adhesion formation is still the foremost enemy to the recovery of function after flexor tendon repair. It has been shown that each time a needle penetrates the delicate tendon surface or a forceps tip injures the tendon surface an adhesion forms at that site. There must be no careless probing or handling of the tissues with forceps, scissors, or knife. The reader must keep this point in mind and train one's self to resist purposeless handling of the tendons and surrounding structures when working on these delicate tissues. Attention to the details of the operative care and postoperative program will reward patient and surgeon alike.

9 PRINCIPLES OF ACUTE EXTENSOR TENDON INJURIES

Richard J. Greco

Extension of the finger is a complex motion, more intricate than flexion. Paradoxically, injury to the extensor tendon system is often given less attention than it is due. If the injury is treated early and appropriately, a good result can be anticipated; however, delayed, late treatment does not carry the same favorable prognosis.

ANATOMY

A detailed anatomic review of the upper extremity is included in Chapter 4. This section concentrates on the muscles, tendons, and extensor mechanism of the extensor system.

Dorsal Forearm Compartment

The extensor system is comprised of muscle bellies originating in the proximal two-thirds of the dorsal compartment of the forearm and their tendinous extensions that insert into the wrist or digits, the "extrinsic system," the components of which are innervated by the radial nerve. It also includes the "intrinsic system," which is innervated by the ulnar and median nerves. The extrinsic system originates in the forearm and gains entrance to the hand through a series of fibroosseous canals overlying the wrist; it is covered by the extensor retinaculum.

The "extrinsic" extensor tendons can be divided into the "superficial" and "deep" muscle groups. The superficial group includes the wrist extensors extensor carpi radialis brevis and longus (ECRB, ECRL) and extensor carpi ulnaris (ECU), the common finger extensors (extensor digiti), and the extensor digiti minimi. These tendons arise from the distal humerus and the lateral epicondyle of the humerus. The deep muscle group includes the extensor pollicis longus (EPL) and brevis (EPB), the abductor pollicis longus (APL), the extensor indicis (EI), and the supinator muscles. The supinator arises from the humerus; and the EPL, EPB, EI, and APL originate from the radius, ulna, and interosseous membrane. (Figs. 9-1 and 9-2).

The radial nerve gives off branches to the branchioradialis and ECRL at the level of the lateral epicondyle before dividing into the posterior interosseous (motor) and superficial (sensory) branches.

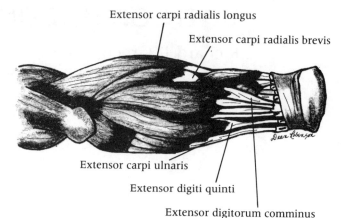

Fig. 9-1. Extensor musculature, superficial group.

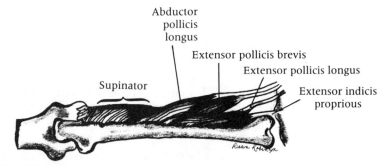

Fig. 9-2. Extensor musculature, deep group.

The superficial branch of the radial nerve then runs under the cover of the branchioradialis, penetrating it in the distal forearm to pass to the dorsal wrist and hand.

The wrist extensors extend the wrist, allow the hand to be positioned for finger flexion, and stabilize the wrist for effective power grip. They insert into the bases of the metacarpal bones — the ECRL to the second, the ECRB to the third, and the ECU to the fifth. The ECRL has the greatest muscle mass (strength), the ECRB has the most efficient moment arm for wrist extension, and the ECU has the greatest leverage arm for ulnar deviation of the wrist.

The extensor digitorum travels under the extensor retinaculum and divides into four tendons for finger extension. These tendons insert into the middle and distal phalanges through the dorsal extensor aponeurosis, as described below. The tendons are connected by distal intertendinous connections (*juncturae tendinum*), and all arise from a common muscle origin. Together they produce simultaneous extension of the index, middle, ring, and little fingers.

The extensor digiti minimi and the extensor indicis effect complete independent extension of the small and index fingers, respectively. The independent tendons are uniformly found ulnar to the digitorum tendons at the metacarpophalangeal (MCP) joint, and they insert into the extensor hood. The extensor indicis is the most distal and ulnar of the deep muscle group (Fig. 9-2).

The abductor pollicis longus is the most radial of the deep group and comes to the surface between the extensor digiti and the ECRB. It subsequently crosses over the ECRB and the ECRL before inserting into the base of the thumb metacarpal. Contraction of the abductor pollicis longus causes extension of the thumb metacarpal and radial abduction of the thumb.

The extensor pollicis brevis is ulnar to the abductor pollicis longus and accompanies it under the extensor retinaculum until it inserts into the dorsal portion of the proximal phalanx of the thumb. The function of the extensor pollicis brevis is to extend the proximal phalanx of the thumb.

The extensor pollicis longus originates ulnar to the abductor pollicis longus and the extensor pollicis brevis in the forearm. It travels obliquely across the carpus ulnar to the dorsal tubercle of the radius. It inserts into the base of the distal phalanx and causes independent extension across both the MCP and interphalangeal joints of the thumb. Multiple slips of the extensor pollicis brevis, abductor pollicis longus, and extensor pollicis brevis tendons are often found.

Extensor Retinaculum Ligament
The skin over the dorsum of the hand is pliable and redundant, and it lacks the fibrous septal connections to the palmar fascia that characterize the palmar skin. The skin redundancy is taken up during fist formation. A superficial areolar layer containing the dorsal veins, lymphatics, and sensory nerves allows further gliding of the skin over the deep fascia and underlying tendons. There is a potential space and gliding interface between the superficial and deep fascias.

The deep fascia of the extensor surface of the forearm is thick over the wrist joint and forms the extensor retinaculum. Vertical septa from this dorsal carpal ligament connect to the radius and ulna, creating six fibroosseous canals (Fig. 9-3). These fascial constraints contain the extensor tendons and their synovial sheaths. The retinaculum functions to prevent bowstringing of the tendons across the wrist. The first compartment contains the abductor pollicis and longus and extensor pollicis brevis, the second the ERCB and ECRL, the third the extensor pollicis longus, the fourth the extensor digiti and extensor indicis, the fifth the extensor digiti minimi, and the sixth the extensor carpi ulnaris.

Extensor Dorsal Aponeurosis Mechanism

The "extrinsic" extensor tendons fuse with the aponeurotic expansion of the intrinsic muscles over their corresponding MCP joints. The "dorsal apparatus," together with transverse and oblique fibers, anchor and centralize the extensor tendon over the long axis of the MCP joint. The sagittal bands are a continuation of the dorsal intertendinous fascia and course obliquely on each side of the MCP

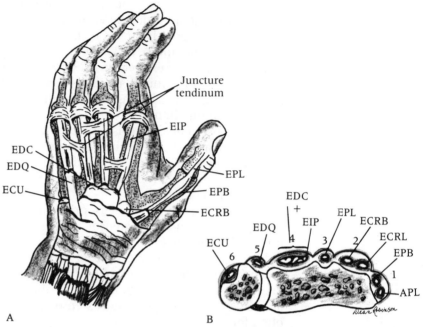

Fig. 9-3. A. The extensor retinaculum consists of six fibroosseous canals and helps prevent bowstringing. *B.* Cross-sectional area of the retinaculum at the level of the wrist.

joint capsule to insert into the volar plate and proximal phalanx (Fig. 9-4). The contraction of the extrinsic extensor tendons causes extension of the proximal phalanx at the MCP joint through these bands. Their geometric orientation prevents active hyperextension of the MCP joint by becoming progressively more transverse in orientation until the axis of force is parallel to the fibers (Fig. 9-5). The obliquity of these fibers permits the extensor tendon to glide distally with flexion and proximally with extension.

The extensor tendon then splits into three relatively noncompliant bands: one central slip and two lateral slips (Fig. 9-4). The central slip is comprised of a major portion of the extrinsic extensor tendon and slips from the intrinsic tendons; it inserts into the dorsal tubercle at the base of the middle phalanx. Its primary function is to extend the proximal interphalangeal (PIP) joint.

The lateral slips merge with the interosseous (intrinsic) muscle tendons just distal to the MCP joint to form the conjoined lateral bands (Fig. 9-4). A few millimeters more distally on the radial side, the tendon of the lumbrical muscle joins the lateral bands. The lateral bands course palmar to the axis of flexion and extension at the MCP joint, dorsal to the axis at the PIP joint, and fuse again in the midline dorsally to insert into the base of the distal phalanx. Therefore the lateral bands and the intrinsic muscles cause flexion at the MCP joint and extension of the PIP and distal interphalangeal (DIP) joints.

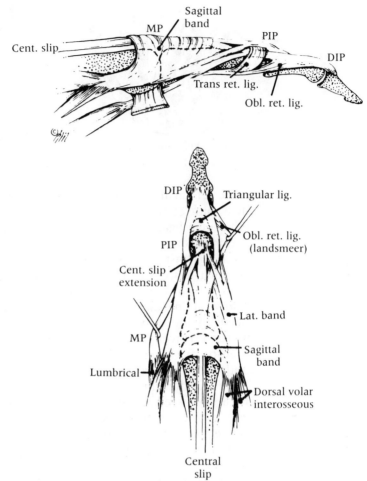

Fig. 9-4. "Extensor hood" mechanism. (From J. R. Doyle. Extensor tendons — acute injuries. In D. Green, ed. *Operative Hand Surgery,* 2nd ed. New York: Churchill Livingstone, 1988. With permission.)

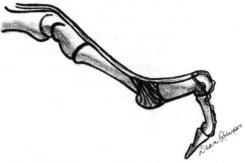

Fig. 9-5. When the MCP joint is hyperextended, the sagittal bands become horizontal and the extensor tendon loses distal motion.

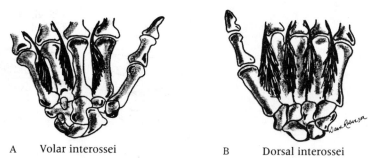

A   Volar interossei   B   Dorsal interossei

Fig. 9-6. A. Three palmar interossei. *B.* Four dorsal interossei.

The retinacular system is an analog of the sagittal bands of the MCP joint at the PIP joint. Consisting of oblique and transverse retinacular ligaments, it connects the lateral bands to the flexor tendon sheath. The dorsal transverse fibers distal to the central slip insertion constitute the triangular ligament (Fig. 9-4) and restrain the volar descent of the lateral bands during flexion. The palmar fibers restrain the dorsal ascent of the bands during extension. The oblique retinacular ligament of Landsmeer connects the flexor sheath of the proximal phalanx to the terminal extensor tendon insertion. Traveling palmar to the PIP joint, it contributes little to the extensor mechanism in the normal finger but contributes significantly to deformities of the imbalanced finger.

The four dorsal interossei muscles are the abductors of the fingers and are centered around the axis of the middle finger. The first is on the radial side of the index finger, the second on the radial side of the middle finger, the third on the ulnar side of the middle finger, and the fourth on the ulnar side of the ring finger. Each of the dorsal interossei, except the third, has two separate muscle bellies (Fig. 9-6A). The superficial muscle belly inserts via a medial tendon underneath the lateral bands onto the proximal phalanx, and its only function is abduction and flexion of the proximal phalanx at the MCP joint. The deep muscle bellies continue as the lateral tendon and fuse with the lateral slips of the extensor tendon to form the lateral bands. Through the lateral bands, the deep bellies cause flexion and abduction of the proximal phalanx and subsequent extension of the PIP and DIP joints.

The three volar interossei muscles are adductors of the fingers around the axis of the middle finger. They insert on the adductor side of the lateral bands of the index, ring, and little fingers (Fig.9-6B). They cause flexion and adduction of the proximal phalanx and extend the PIP and DIP joints. Usually, all of the interossei muscles are innervated by the ulnar nerve. The lumbrical muscles arise from the profundus tendons in the palm, pass palmar to the transverse metacarpal ligament, and join the radial lateral bands at the middle of the proximal phalanx. They cause flexion at the MCP joint and extension at the PIP and DIP joints. When they contract, they pull the lateral bands proximally and the profundus tendons distally, causing a decreased flexion force on the distal phalanx and a more effective extension to the interphalangeal joints. The radial two lumbricales are innervated by the median nerve and the ulnar two by the ulnar nerve.

EVALUATION

The basic evaluation of the arm is outlined in Chapter 4. Therefore this discussion is limited to examination of the arm in reference to extensor tendon function. One can learn far more from examining the extremity distal to the site of injury than one can by probing the wound.

There are three basic components to the examination of extensor tendon function.

1. Observation at rest: The examiner observes the lineup of the digits with the patient relaxed or under anesthesia. There should be a normal progression of increasing flexion as one proceeds from the index to the little finger. The joint of the finger involved with an extensor tendon injury may have slightly increased flexion when compared to the other fingers at rest. Injury to the extensor tendon proximal to the central slip insertion will lead to a flexion deformity of the PIP joint. If the DIP joint is in an exaggerated flexed position, injury to the distal extensor tendon should be considered.

2. Tenodesis effect: With the arm fully relaxed, gentle passive flexion and extension at the wrist should make all the fingers flex and extend in a normal cascade fashion. Fingers with disrupted extensor tendons remain in a relatively more flexed posture compared to the other fingers. When evaluating extensor tendon injuries, it is important to assess the degree of accompanying bony and soft tissue injury. Anteroposterior and especially lateral radiographs of the involved area are important to define the degree of injury. Many of the tendon "ruptures" are associated with a dorsal avulsion fracture, especially of the base of the middle and distal phalanges.

3. Active motion tests: In the awake, cooperative patient special maneuvers are used to evaluate the functions of the individual extensor muscle units independently, constituting the most informative part of the extensor examination. It is useful to perform the complete examination on the uninjured arm first so that one is sure the patient fully understands the activities to be tested. The extensor examinations, as described below, are performed against light resistance. Observation and palpation of the extensor tendon being tested is useful and is possible because of the relatively thin dorsal skin.

Wrist Extensors

The examiner has the patient extend the wrist against resistance in radial deviation (ECRL), in ulnar deviation (extensor carpi ulnaris), and in the midline (ECRB), palpating for the intact tendons at their

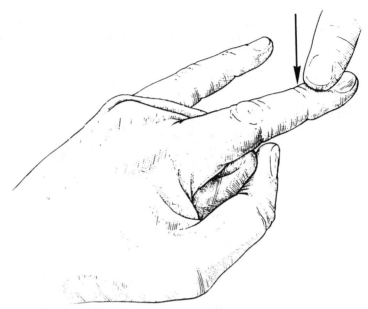

Fig. 9-7. Testing of the indicis proprius tendon. (From R. Tubiana. *Examination of the Hand and Upper Limb*. Philadelphia: Saunders, 1984. With permission.)

insertions into the following metacarpal bases: ECRL, second; ECRB, third; and extensor carpi ulnaris, fifth.

Finger Extensors

The examiner should first dorsiflex the patient's wrist to eliminate the automatic MCP extension, which occurs by a tenodesis effect when the wrist is in flexion. The patient is then asked to extend the proximal phalanges and any evidence of a loss of extension is observed. This test for the extensor digiti is repeated again against light resistance on the dorsal proximal phalanx. An additional useful test, described by Chamay [1], involves placing the patient's hand palm down and flat against the table and sequentially having the patient lift each finger from the table. This motion can be performed only by the extrinsic extensors, not the intrinsic muscles.

The independent tendons of the index (extensor indicis) and little (extensor digiti minimi) fingers are tested by completely flexing the middle and ring finger's MCP joints to eliminate the action of their extensor digiti contribution. The patient is then asked to extend the index and little fingers against light resistance (Fig. 9-7).

Extensor Hood Mechanism

MCP Joint

During flexion and extension of the MCP joint, one should observe any loss of the ability to actively extend the proximal phalanx and any subluxation of the tendon to either side of the midline. Subluxation of the extensor tendon is caused by a longitudinal disruption of the dorsal apparatus over the MCP joint opposite to the side of subluxation.

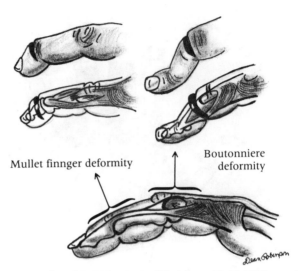

Mullet finnger deformity

Boutonniere
deformity

Fig. 9-8. Extensor hood injuries. (Modified from H. E. Kleinert. *Technics in Surgery: Hand Injuries.* Somerville, NJ: Ethicon, 1989. With permission.)

PIP Joint

To test the integrity of the central slips, the patient's fingers are placed with the PIP joints flexed at 90 degrees over the side of a table; active extension of the middle phalanx is then tested. If the central slip is intact, the middle phalanx extends with a flail DIP joint. If the central slip is transected, extension is performed by pull-through of the lateral bands, thereby causing hyperextension of the DIP joint and an absent or weak extension force on the middle phalanx at the PIP joint. If complete dorsal apparatus incompetence is present, the unrestrained action of the flexor digitorum sublimus causes flexion of the middle phalanx, the flexor profundus loses relative length, and the origin of the lumbrical is retracted. The retraction of the lumbrical muscle causes tension on the lateral bands and subsequent extension of the distal phalanx. This deformity is commonly referred to as the ''buttonhole'' or ''boutonnière'' deformity (Fig. 9-8).

DIP Joint

To test the integrity of the distal extensor tendon, the patient is asked to actively extend the DIP joint while stabilizing the middle phalanx. The inability to extend the distal phalanx at the DIP joint indicates an injury to the terminal extensor tendon, commonly referred to as a ''mallet finger'' (Fig. 9-8).

Thumb Extensors

The extensor pollicis longus is tested by active extension of the interphalangeal joint of the thumb against light resistance. The extensor pollicis brevis is tested by active extension of the thumb

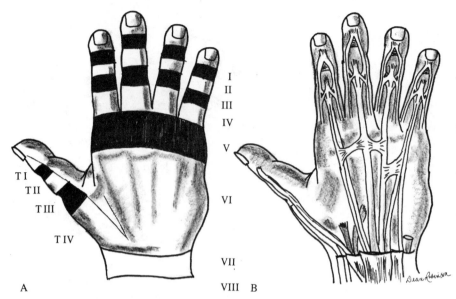

Fig. 9-9. Verdan's extensor tendon's zones of injury.

proximal phalanx with the interphalangeal joint in slight flexion. The patient is asked to move the thumb in radial abduction, that is, to extend the thumb metacarpal, and the tension of the abductor pollicis longus is felt on the extensor border of the anatomic snuffbox.

CLASSIFICATION OF EXTENSOR INJURIES

Experienced hand surgeons have noted a correlation between the functional recovery they were able to achieve and the location of the acute extensor tendon injures. Verdan [2] subsequently classified the extensor tendon system into eight zones for treatment and comparison of results. The odd-numbered zones overlie the joints of the wrist and fingers, and the even-numbered zones are the intervening segments between these joints. Classification of extensor tendon injuries has allowed hand surgeons from numerous institutions to compare different methods of management at specific zones of injury. I have used the modification of Verdan's zone system as accepted by the International Federation of Societies for Surgery of the Hand when evaluating extensor tendon injuries (Fig. 9-9).

Zone 1: area over the distal phalanx and over the DIP joint
Zone 2: dorsum of the middle phalanx
Zone 3: area over the PIP joint
Zone 4: dorsum of the proximal phalanx
Zone 5: area over the MCP joint
Zone 6: dorsum of the hand
Zone 7: area over the wrist (in fibroosseous canal)
Zone 8: distal forearm

The system for the thumb is as follows.

Zone T1:   area over the interphalangeal joint
Zone T2:   dorsum of the proximal phalanx
Zone T3:   area over the MCP joint
Zone T4:   dorsum of the first metacarpal
Zone   7:   area over the wrist (in fibroosseous canal)
Zone   8:   distal forearm

ACUTE PRECAUTIONS

After a decision is made concerning the timing of the operative intervention, a volar protective splint is appropriate (see Chapter 19). The hand should be kept elevated to reduce swelling. Significant bleeding on the dorsum of the forearm or hand is rare and usually venous. Typically, it can be controlled by a pressure dressing and elevation. If it cannot be controlled by the pressure dressing, a tourniquet or inflated blood pressure cuff can be used for short periods until operative exploration can be performed emergently. *Blind clamping of "bleeders" in the emergency room is fraught with injury to important neurovascular structures.*

The examiner should have a high degree of suspicion with lacerations over the MCP joint because they are frequently secondary to a "closed fist injury" and must be treated as a human bite. They typically occur when the "knuckle" area strikes a tooth during a fight. The patient, because of ignorance or embarrassment, may consciously or unconsciously attempt to misinform the examiner as to the nature of the injury. The important point is that the wound may appear benign initially, but it is usually inoculated with a potent mixture of bacteria. (See the recommended management in Chapter 12.)

OPERATIVE APPROACH

Tendon repair is often not the first priority in patients with multiple trauma, massive crush, or contaminated injuries that cannot be converted to a clean wound by surgical débridement. The surgeon's responsibility is to clean and débride the wound, stabilize fractures, obtain adequate skin coverage, and obtain a healed wound without infection. Absolute contraindications to immediate tendon reconstruction include human bite lacerations, inadequate skin coverage, and evidence of cellulitis.

Most tendon repairs should be done in a facility with adequate lighting, instruments, anesthesia, and under tourniquet control. An axillary block or general anesthesia is usually necessary because of tourniquet pain. Injuries of the distal finger can often be treated with a digital block and a digital tourniquet. The wound is carefully cleaned and débrided. High pressure irrigation by a 35-ml syringe and a 19-gauge needle is used to decrease the risk of wound infection. Prophylactic antibiotics are given for at least 24 hours postoperatively and longer if the wound is contaminated. Because of the close proximity of the interphalangeal joints to the extensor tendons, the possibility of an open contaminated joint should be explored and if necessary the joint irrigated with antibiotic solution. After appropriate irrigation, the joint capsules should be repaired separately.

The operative approach is discussed according to the zones previously described. In general, skin incisions should be carefully planned, attempting to utilize the laceration and avoiding straight dorsal incisions that cross the joint creases. The fractures and joint injuries are stabilized before the tendons are repaired.

"Atraumatic technique" is essential, and only the cut ends of the tendon should be handled. The tendon stumps should be minimally débrided and then only when necessary. A new, sharp scalpel blade is used against a wooden tongue blade surface. The extensor tendons have less excursion than flexor tendons, and preservation of length is far more critical in their repair. On the other hand, a loosely approximated tendon repair may lead to a lengthened extensor tendon and an extension lag. This lag cannot be recovered nonoperatively.

As a general rule, the management of extensor tendon injuries between joints is the same as the treatment of injuries over the more distal joint zone.

Zone 1

Injuries in zone 1 produce an inability to actively extend the DIP joint and are called "mallet fingers." The mechanism of injury varies.

1. Open laceration of the terminal tendon in zones 1 or 2.
2. Closed rupture of the terminal tendon, usually secondary to an acute forced flexion of an extended digit.
3. Closed rupture associated with an avulsion fracture of the dorsal lip of the distal phalanx.
4. Epiphyseal plate separation of the distal phalanx after a fingertip crush injury in a child. The tendon insertion is intact, and a mallet deformity can occur.

When dealing with the typical closed mallet deformity, one must realize that the terminal extensor tendon is thin and difficult to suture and the tendon ends do not retract far. The best functional results have been obtained by immobilization of the DIP joint in extension for 6 to 8 weeks with an additional 2 to 4 weeks of nighttime splinting. A polyethylene Stack splint is convenient (Fig. 9-10), but a volar finger splint immobilizing only the DIP joint is adequate. The only significant poor prognostic factor in long-term results is the presence of an associated fracture. If an extensor lag reappears, continued immobilization is necessary. It is emphasized that the *splinting must be uninterrupted and continuous.*

Closed mallet injuries associated with a dorsal avulsion fracture and a volar subluxation of the remaining portion of the distal phalanx may also be treated satisfactorily with Stack splinting.

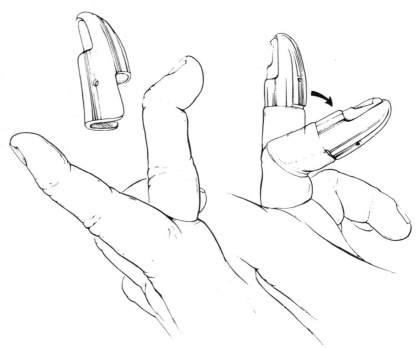

Fig. 9-10. Stack splint. (From J. R. Doyle. Extensor tendons — acute injuries. In D. Green, ed. *Operative Hand Surgery,* 2nd ed. New York: Churchill Livingstone, 1988. With permission.)

The best results are obtained if splinting is initiated within 10 days of the injury; however, splinting is useful even 6 months after the injury. In special groups of patients where external splinting is nearly impossible because of job restraints (surgeons), internal splinting of the DIP joint in full extension with an obliquely placed, buried K-wire (0.035 mm) is a reasonable alternative, although it carries increased risks of pulp scarring and osteomyelitis.

Many authors recommend open reduction and internal fixation of dorsal articular fractures if the fragment is more than one-third of the articular surface. The fragments are fragile, and the operation is difficult to perform successfully. Webbe and Schneider [3] have shown that nonoperative management with DIP splinting produces equivalent results, and that the percent of the articular surface involvement is not important. They suggested that the patients must be warned that even after bone remodeling a bump persists on the dorsum of the joint regardless of the method of treatment.

Open lacerations of the extensor tendon are best treated by horizontal mattress suture repair using fine nylon (6-0) when the tendon is accessible. If the tendon does not separate easily from the overlying skin, simple figure-of-eight sutures (4-0 or 5-0 nylon), which simultaneously approximates the skin and tendon substance, are inserted. Care must be taken to not injure the nail bed, as the germinal matrix extends 5 mm farther proximally than the nail fold. If there is significant tendon loss, stabilization of the DIP joint in full extension with appropriate skin coverage is provided acutely, and reconstruction is delayed.

Zone 2

Injuries on the dorsum of the middle phalanx are common, and a subsequent flexion deformity of the DIP joint occurs. Clean transections of the extensor tendon can be repaired with horizontal mattress sutures of 5-0 nylon, and the DIP joint is splinted with a K-wire or Stack splint for 4 to 6 weeks. If the periosteum is injured, it should be repaired separately; however, significant adhesions may still form.

Zone 3

The area over the PIP joint is one of the most complex regions of the extensor tendon system because at this level there are three main portions of the extensor mechanism: a central slip and two lateral bands. Injuries can be caused by open laceration of the tendon, closed avulsion of the dorsal articular surface of the middle phalanx by an acute forceful flexion of the PIP joint, and fracture-dislocation of the PIP joint.

If this injury is neglected or misdiagnosed, the lateral bands progressively displace palmarly. The head of the proximal phalanx protrudes through the extensor hood, and the force of the lateral bands now creates hyperextension of the DIP joint, and boutonnière deformity is established. This pattern is usually not seen in the acute injury because the tearing and subsequent volar displacement of the lateral bands occurs secondarily.

The extensor tendon lengths are such that extension of the DIP and PIP joints occurs simultaneously. If the tendon length is altered at any level, extension becomes altered and the finger collapses into a segmental zigzag deformity. With these collapsing deformities, the overall length of the finger is shorter than normal and the excessive pull delivered to one joint implies a loss of pull at the other joints (Fig. 9-11).

The key to treatment of extensor tendon injuries in this zone is immobilization of the PIP joint in extension for 4 to 6 weeks, leaving the DIP joint free to allow distal and dorsal motion of the lateral bands. With acute open injuries, after appropriate irrigation of the PIP joint, the joint capsule should be closed separately. The central tendon is repaired or reattached to the base of the middle phalanx. If necessary, the lateral bands and the triangular ligament are repaired to keep the lateral bands in appropriate position. For 1 week the wrist is splinted in 35 degrees of extension, the MCP in 10 degrees of flexion, and the PIP in full extension; the DIP is allowed full motion. This phase is followed by immobilization of only the PIP joint in full extension for an additional 5 to 6 weeks. A "safety pin splint" is useful for this immobilization. Splinting of the PIP joint in extension is used for closed ruptures of the central slip that

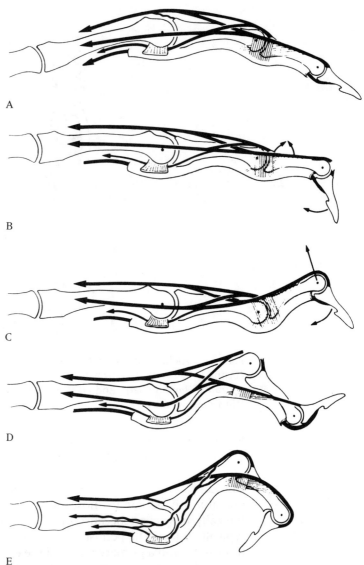

Fig. 9-11. Digital kinetic chain and its deformity. *A.* Normal balance of the chain. *B.* Mallet deformity. *C.* Swan neck deformity. *D.* Boutonnière deformity. *E.* Claw deformity. (From R. Tubiana. *Examination of the Hand and Upper Limb.* Philadelphia: Saunders, 1984. With permission.)

are less than 12 weeks old. Operative intervention is indicated for injuries with a nonreducible dorsal fragment of the middle phalanx, proximal phalanx fractures, and fracture-dislocations of the PIP joint. In these situations, direct suture repair with mattress sutures (5-0 nylon) is indicated. PIP extension splinting is mandatory postoperatively.

When there has been a loss of central tendon substance or an inadequate shredded tendon exists, both lateral bands can be split

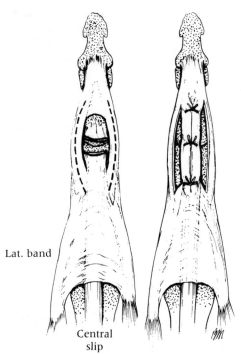

Lat. band

Central
slip

Fig. 9-12. Aiche, Barsky, and Weiner repair for central slip deficiency. (From J. R. Doyle. Extensor tendons — acute injuries. In D. Green, ed. *Operative Hand Surgery,* 2nd ed. New York: Churchill Livingstone, 1988. With permission.)

longitudinally, as described by Aiche and coworkers [4], and reapproximated in the midline with 5-0 nylon sutures (Fig. 9-12).

Zone 4

Clinical findings for injuries over the dorsum of the proximal phalanx are similar to those of zone 3 injuries. The findings are typically less severe because the PIP joint and the lateral bands are typically intact. The periosteum should be closed as a separate layer if possible, and a primary repair of the extensor tendon is performed. Immobilization should be performed as described for zone 3 injuries. Secondary extensor tenolysis procedures are often required.

Zone 5

One must be suspicious that an injury over the MCP joint has been caused by a closed fist injury. If it has, refer to Chapter 12 for the appropriate management.

Two basic types of injury occur at the MCP joint. Transverse transection of the extensor tendon causes an inability to extend the proximal phalanx. The joint capsule and extensor tendon should be repaired primarily using fine nonabsorbable suture as necessary. A longitudinal tear of the sagittal band leads to subluxation of the central extensor tendon toward the uninjured side. A precise repair with centralization of the extensor tendon with 5-0 nylon sutures is performed. If this procedure is not possible, the transverse fibers of the hood can be anchored to the MCP capsule, or a tendon sling can be fashioned. Postoperatively, after repair of the extensor tendons in zone 5, the wrist is splinted in 35 degrees of extension, the MCP joint in 30 degrees of flexion, and the interphalangeal joints in extension for 3 to 4 weeks. Dynamic extension splinting may be indicated for carefully selected and motivated patients.

It is important to repair the extensor digitorum contribution to the index and little fingers, even if the extensor indicis and extensor digiti minimi tendons are intact.

Zone 6

Extensor tendon injuries to the dorsum of the hand may be associated with significant soft tissue injuries. Partial or total laceration of the extensor tendon requires simple mattress suture of the involved tendons with 4-0 nonabsorbable sutures. The proximal end may have retracted and may require extension of the wound and proximal massage of the muscle to retrieve the tendon end. It is possible to prevent retraction of the proximal tendon end by placing a 25-gauge needle through the skin and tendon at the level of the extensor retinaculum. If significant tendon loss has occurred, side-to-side tendon transfer or primary tendon transfers are acceptable. These procedures should be performed by a knowledgeable hand surgeon.

Postoperatively, patients are immobilized for 4 weeks with the wrist extended 35 degrees and the proximal phalanges flexed at either 70 degrees or 15 degrees at the MCP joints. Alternatively, dynamic extension splinting may be considered in selected, motivated patients. The wrist is splinted in 35 degrees of extension; the MCPs are positioned in a resting position of 0 degrees and are allowed 30 degrees of active flexion. Such splinting creates the necessary 5 mm of extensor digiti carpi tendon excursion for improved long-term motion.

Zone 7

Extensor tendon injuries within the fibroosseous canals are often difficult to manage because any impingement of the repair or postoperative adhesions underneath the extensor retinaculum may lead to impairment of finger flexion. After performing an end-to-end repair with 4-0 nylon with a modified Kessler technique (see Chapter 8) or mattress suture technique, the repair is tested for impingement under the extensor retinaculum passively. If the repaired tendon does not slide through easily, part of the extensor retinaculum may be excised or the tendon totally transposed outside the canal (if necessary) to obtain unimpeded motion. The small amount of postoperative bowstringing does not functionally impair the patient.

All of the extensor tendon injuries in zone 7 should be repaired. Postoperatively, the wrist is immobilized in 35 degrees of extension and the MCP in 15 degrees of flexion for 4 to 6 weeks. Passive range of motion is begun at 4 weeks.

Zone 8

Repair of extensor tendons in the distal forearm is relatively simple using modified Kessler or mattress sutures of 4-0 or 3-0 nonadsorbable material. If the muscle–tendon junctures are injured, repair is somewhat more difficult, and it is important to include the fibrous septae of the muscle in the sutures to strengthen the repair. All the tendons should be repaired. Splinting of the wrist in 35 degrees of extension for 4 to 6 weeks postoperatively is imperative to allow adequate healing.

REFERENCES

1. Chamay, J. C. Extensor tendon lesions of the dorsum of the hand and wrist. In E. C. Verdan (Ed.) *Tendon Surgery of the Thumb.* New York: Churchill Livingstone, 1979.
2. Verdan, C. E. Primary and secondary repair of flexor and extensor injuries. In J. E. Flynn (Ed.) *Hand Surgery* (3rd ed.) Baltimore: Williams and Wilkins, 1966.
3. Webbe, M.A. and Schneider L. H. Mallet fractures. *J. Bone Joint Surg.* 69:892–896, 1987.
4. Aiche, A., Barsky, A. J., and Weiner, D. L. Prevention of Boutinniere deformity. *Plast. Reconstr. Surg.* 46:164–167, 1979.

SUGGESTED READING

Hunter, J., Schneider, L., and Mackin, E. J. (eds.), *Tendon Surgery in the Hand.* St. Louis: Mosby, 1987.
Verdan, C. (ed.), *Tendon Surgery of the Hand.* New York: Churchill Livingstone, 1979.
Zancolli, E. *Structural and Dynamic Bases of Hand Surgery,* 2nd ed. Philadelphia: Lippincott, 1979.

Commentary on Chapter 9

Robert A. Chase

Extensor tendon injuries are often assigned a low level of priority without attention to the level of injury, type of injury, or the injury to adjacent bone or joint. If the outcome after such an injury is a severe boutonnière injury, a dropped tip with a severe snapping recurvatum deformity of the PIP joint, or if the extensor tendon adheres to bone over the metacarpal or proximal phalynx preventing metacarpal phalangeal or PIP joint flexion, the result of this "low priority" injury is disabling. With proper attention, care, and understanding, these problems can be avoided. Extensor tendon injuries may be repaired without serious threat to primary neurovascular structures. Thus many of these injuries may be cared for by surgery using local anesthesia and without tourniquet ischemia. If there ever was a place for hand surgeons who are thoroughly addicted to the use of a tourniquet to consider carefully the illogic of general anesthesia or brachial plexus block simply to allow use of a tourniquet, this is it. Have we forgotten the techniques of real-time hemostasis just because use of a tourniquet for a bloodless field is possible in the limb? There are too many recorded complications from general or brachial block anesthesia given for dorsal hand or digital surgery that could have been done using no tourniquet and local anesthesia. Big anesthesia for small surgery is unwarranted.

Emphasis should be placed on the fact noted by Dr. Greco that transection of the extensor central slip in zone 3 may not be followed immediately by an inability to extend the PIP joint. The lateral bands, still in anatomic position, may effectively, though less powerfully, extend the joint. Unless repair or a rigorous splinting regimen is followed, development of an inability to fully extend the PIP joint with progression to a full-blown boutonnière deformity may develop over weeks or even months.

Routine use of antibiotics for every extensor injury is mindless and robotic. Moreover, I remain unconvinced that high pressure "water pick" style irrigation is appropriate in an area characterized by loose areolar subcutaneous and subtendinous fascia into which materials including microorganisms may be driven by such pressure.

Mallet fingers resulting from central insertion tendon injuries in zone 1 may be successfully treated by rigorous splinting of the DIP joint in hyperextension. An individually fashioned and fitted extension splint using one of the heat-malleable plastics may be more reliable than a Stack splint. Such a splint may be carried proximal to the PIP joint only to block it from full extension to ensure that no proximal pull on the injured extensor occurs. Furthermore, with an individually tailored splint, it is possible to leave the tactile tip exposed to make several weeks of splinting more tolerable. I have yet to be convinced that splinting alone suffices when intra-articular fractures of the distal phalanx and unstable palmar subluxation under the influence of the flexor digitorum profundus pertains. It remains a place for reduction and internal fixation.

One generalization concerning the anatomy and biomechanics of tendons, whether flexor or extensor, should be emphasized. A tendon muscle unit influences every joint between its proximal and distal attachments. Furthermore, the antagonist of that unit at any one joint may, through its action, augment the influence of the muscle tendon unit at the other joints. Thus it is not correct to say that the function of the extensor pollicis brevis is to extend the MCP joint of the thumb. It also secondarily abducts the first metacarpal at the metacarpal trapezial joint and acts to radially deviate the wrist. So, if an antagonist of the extensor pollicis brevis at the wrist pulls the wrist into ulnar deviation, the influence of the extensor pollicis brevis is augmented as a first metacarpal abductor and MCP extensor. These relations of tendons need to be kept in mind when planning surgery, splinting, and rehabilitation.

10 PRINCIPLES OF ACUTE NERVE REPAIR

John H. Moore Jr.

It may be admitted that experience is the best teacher, but the man who relies on his own experience gets a very limited education.

— ANONYMOUS

The hand serves as a primary tactile window to the external environment. It is a receptor for temperature, pain, texture, and recognition. In addition, the hand allows us to manipulate the environment through complex, coordinated motor activities of the upper extremity. Therefore nerve injuries of the upper extremity can alter not only the perception of our environment but also our ability to control it.

Ideally, upper extremity nerve injuries should be treated acutely. Tissue planes are then fresh and unscarred, yielding improved identification of vital structures. Not infrequently immediate repair is not possible, however, because of wound contamination. Precise clinical and anatomic knowledge is imperative for identification of the level and extent of injury and allows more precise coaptation of the nerve with minimal intraneural scarring. Poor planning or execution can result in long-term, devastating functional impairment.

ANATOMY
Microscopic Anatomy

A *neuron* is a nerve cell. Axons of the neuron transmit efferent conduction, and dendrites accept afferent conduction from another neuron at junctions called *synapses*. Individual axons of peripheral nerves are surrounded by connective tissue called *endoneurium*. They are then arranged in groups called *fascicles* (funiculi). The connective tissue that surrounds this grouping is called the *perineurium*. Peripheral nerves contain groups of fascicles, which are surrounded by circumferential connective tissue, the *epineurium*. This layer often contains blood vessels (Fig. 10-1).

The vascular supply of a peripheral nerve is segmental. Arteriae nervorum vascularize a nerve segment. Longitudinal epineural and perineural plexuses traverse the nerve with rich interconnections between the segments.

Controversy exists as to the amount of fascicular branching that occurs in a peripheral nerve. Sunderland [1] has identified multiple branches over short segments. In contrast, Jabaley [2] has noted that

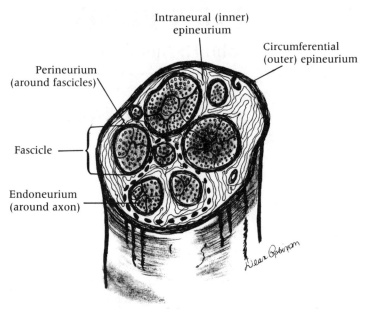

Intraneural (inner)
epineurium

Circumferential
(outer) epineurium

Perineurium
(around fascicles)

Fascicle

Endoneurium
(around axon)

Fig. 10-1. Microscopic anatomy of the nerve. (From P. L. Hodges, T. E. Spicer, and J. B. Tebbetts. Hand II — nerves and tendon transfers. *Selected Readings in Plastic Surgery* 3(34):5, 1986. With permission.)

branching does occur but not as frequently as previously described (Fig. 10-2). Sensory and motor signals are not all-or-none phenomena but, rather, the end result of a vast interplay of signals that are modified at many levels before their input is received by the end-organ, making complete recovery almost impossible.

Macroscopic Anatomy

Digital Nerves

The common digital nerves arise from the median and ulnar nerves and are purely sensory (Fig. 10-3). They course underneath the palmar fascia and give rise to the individual digital nerves of the fingers.

The median nerve gives rise to four branches that supply innervation to the thumb, index and middle fingers, and radial aspect of the ring finger. The ulnar nerve gives rise to two branches that supply innervation to the little finger and the ulnar aspect of the ring finger.

Digital nerves lie in the palmar aspect of the hand (Fig. 10-4). In the digit the nerve is intimately associated with the digital artery and is bordered by Cleland's ligament dorsally and the digital artery and Grayson's ligament palmarly. At the level of the distal interphalangeal (DIP) joint, the digital nerve terminates into three branches: nail bed, tip, and pulp.

The dorsal sensory branch arises from the digital nerve proper at the level of the proximal phalanx and innervates the dorsal skin to the proximal and middle phalanges. There are communications with dorsal sensory branches of the radial and ulnar nerves at these levels.

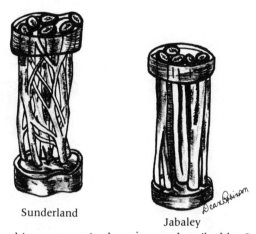

Sunderland

Jabaley

Fig. 10-2. Branching patterns in the nerve as described by Sunderland and Jabaley. (Modified from G. K. Frykman, A. Wolfe, and T. Coyle. An algorithm for management of peripheral nerve injuries. *Orthop. Clin. North Am.* 12:239, 1981. With permission.)

Palmar

Dorsal

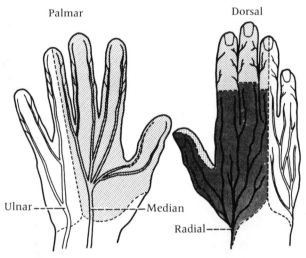

Ulnar

Median

Radial

Fig. 10-3. Distribution of major nerve sensory innervation of the hand. (From American Society of the Hand. *The Hand: Examination and Diagnosis*, 2nd ed. New York: Churchill Livingstone, 1983. With permission.)

Median Nerve. The median nerve is the principal motor and sensory unit of the upper extremity (Fig. 10-5). It originates from the lateral and medial cords of the branchial plexus and is paired with the branchial artery in the upper arm. There are no motor or sensory branches in the arm, and the median nerve enters the forearm between the two heads of the pronator teres muscle(Fig. 10-6).

The median nerve courses on the inferior surface of the flexor digitorum superficialis muscle belly and gives off direct motor branches to the pronator teres, flexor carpi radialis, palmaris longus,

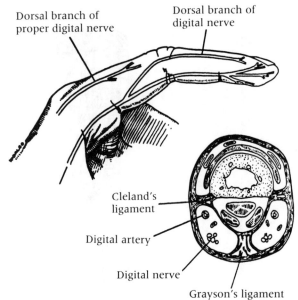

Dorsal branch of
proper digital nerve

Dorsal branch of
digital nerve

Cleland's
ligament

Digital artery

Digital nerve

Grayson's ligament

Fig. 10-4. Digital nerve anatomy. (From W. W. Shaw and D. A. Hidalgo. *Microsurgery in Trauma.* Mt. Kisco, NY: Futura, 1987. With permission.)

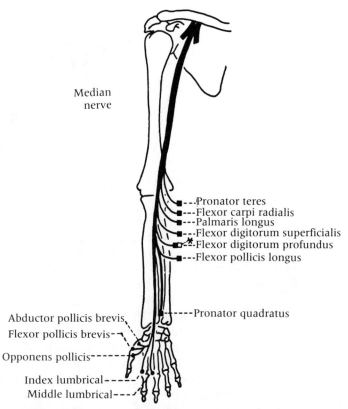

Median
nerve

Pronator teres
Flexor carpi radialis
Palmaris longus
Flexor digitorum superficialis
Flexor digitorum profundus
Flexor pollicis longus

Pronator quadratus

Abductor pollicis brevis
Flexor pollicis brevis
Opponens pollicis
Index lumbrical
Middle lumbrical

Fig. 10-5. Motor innervation of the forearm and arm by the median nerve. (From American Society of the Hand. *The Hand: Examination and Diagnosis,* 2nd ed. New York: Churchill Livingstone, 1983. With permission.)

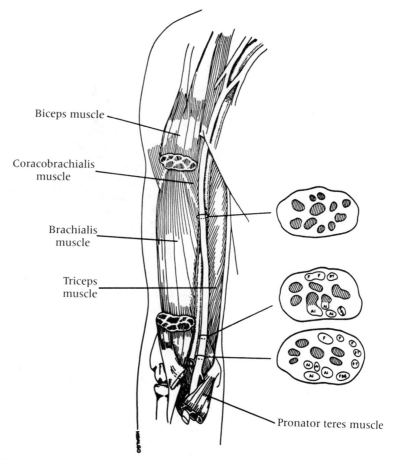

Fig. 10-6. Median nerve, upper arm. (From W. W. Shaw and D. A. Hidalgo. *Microsurgery in Trauma.* Mt. Kisco, NY: Futura, 1987. With permission.)

and flexor digitorum superficialis. The *anterior interosseous branch* forms at the level of the elbow and runs on the interosseous membrane. It innervates the flexor digitorum profundus to the index and long finger, the flexor pollicis longus, and the pronator quadratus (Fig. 10-7).

In the distal forearm the median nerve travels under the tendon of the palmaris longus and the transverse carpal ligament. In the hand, the nerve provides motor innervation to the muscles of the thenar eminence and the index and middle finger lumbricales. The *palmar cutaneous sensory branch* begins in the distal forearm and supplies sensation to the palmar and thenar eminence (Fig. 10-8).

Intraneural anatomy is varied and complex in the arm (See Fig. 10-6–10-8). At the level of the elbow, the fascicle to the pronator teres and flexor carpi radialis occupy the volar and ulnar aspects of the median nerve. The anterior interosseous branch and the branch to the flexor digiti superficialis is more dorsal. In the mid-forearm,

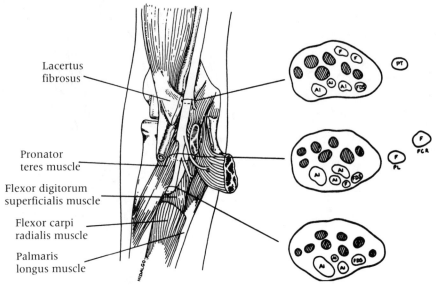

Fig. 10-7. Median nerve, elbow. (From W. W. Shaw and D. A. Hidalgo. *Microsurgery in Trauma.* Mt. Kisco, NY: Futura, 1987. With permission.)

the palmar cutaneous branch is more radial, with most of the fascicles being sensory. The thenar motor branches occupy the radial position in the median nerve at the wrist.

Ulnar Nerve. The ulnar nerve originates from the medial cord of the branchial plexus and travels along the medial aspect of the arm. The medial antebranchial cutaneous nerve arises at the mid-arm level and supplies sensation to the medial arm and forearm. The ulnar nerve enters the forearm between the two heads of the flexor carpi ulnaris (FCU) and gives off its first motor branches, which supply the FCU (Fig. 10-9).

The ulnar nerve continues through the forearm in a plane between the FCU and the flexor digiti profundus (FDP) muscle units. Motor branches are supplied to the FCU and the FDP muscles of the ring and little fingers as the ulnar nerve is en route to the hand.

At the wrist, a dorsal ulnar sensory branch arises before the ulnar nerve traverses Guyon's canal (Fig. 10-10). The nerve then separates into superficial sensory digital nerves and a deep motor branch to the hypothenar muscles, ring and little finger lumbricales, all palmar and dorsal interossei, the adductor pollicis, and the deep head of the flexor pollicis brevis.

Intraneural neuroanatomy shows mixing of fibers in the arms. At the level of the elbow, fascicles to the flexors are located posteriorly and dorsal cutaneous fibers ulnarly. In the mid-forearm, the motor fibers are in a central position and gradually travel to a dorsoulnar position at the wrist (see Fig. 10-9 and 10-10).

There is frequently a communication between the median and ulnar nerve in the forearm called the Martin-Gruber anastomosis.

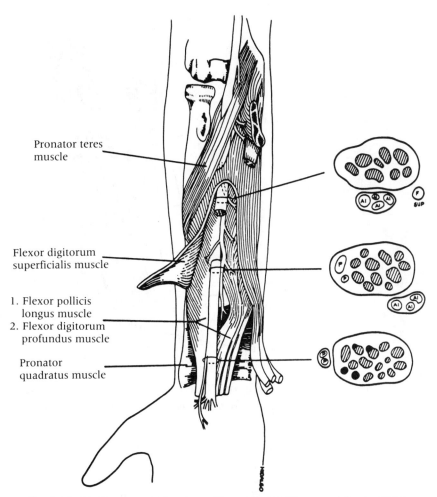

Pronator teres
muscle

Flexor digitorum
superficialis muscle

1. Flexor pollicis
   longus muscle
2. Flexor digitorum
   profundus muscle

Pronator
quadratus muscle

Fig. 10-8. Median nerve, forearm. (From W. W. Shaw and D. A. Hidalgo. *Microsurgery in Trauma.* Mt. Kisco, NY: Futura, 1987. With permission.)

The median nerve sends motor fibers for the radial intrinsics (adductor pollicis and first interosseous) through the ulnar nerve to the hand. A high laceration of the ulnar nerve above this crossover would create paralysis of all the intrinsics typically innervated by the ulnar nerve and a sparing of these radial intrinisic muscles.

Radial Nerve
The radial nerve originates from the posterior cord of the branchial plexus, beginning medial to the triceps, and travels posteriorly thorugh the muscle and behind the shaft of the humerus. The nerve then courses anteromedially between the branchialis and branchioradialis over the lateral epicondyle (Fig. 10-11). In the arm it innervates the teres major, triceps, brachioradialis, aconeus, and extensor carpi radialis longus (ECRL).

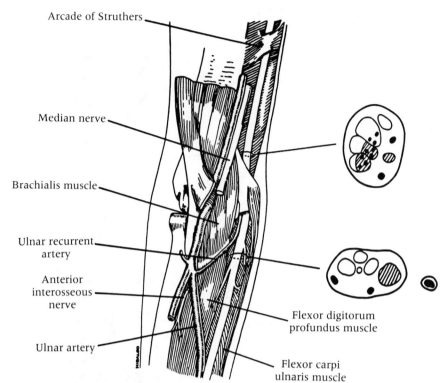

Fig. 10-9. Ulnar nerve, elbow. (From W. W. Shaw and D. A. Hidalgo. *Microsurgery in Trauma.* Mt. Kisco, NY: Futura, 1987. With permission.)

Just distal to the lateral epicondyle, the main nerve divides into two branches. The superficial branch innervates the ECRL and the extensor carpi radialis brevis (ECRB) and provides radial sensation to the hand. The deep branch, the posterior interosseous nerve, runs through the two heads of the supinator underneath the arcade of Forshe and innervates the supinator, the extensor digitorum communis, extensor digiti minimi, extensor carpi ulnaris, extensor pollicis longus, abductor pollicis longus, extensor pollicis brevis, and extensor indicis proprius.

In general, the sensory fascicles are more superficial and the motor fascicles are deep in the radial nerve (see Fig. 10-11). The motor branches take off on the ulnar side of the radial nerve, with the motor branch to the long head of the triceps being the only exception — branching off the radial side of the nerve.

Branchial Plexus

Next to the brain and spinal cord, the branchial plexus is one of the most complex nervous structures in the body. The intricate anatomic relation is beyond the scope of this handbook, but a brief overview is presented. The branchial plexus arises from the rootlets of C5 to C8 and T1 with occasional contributions from C4 and T2 (Fig. 10-12).

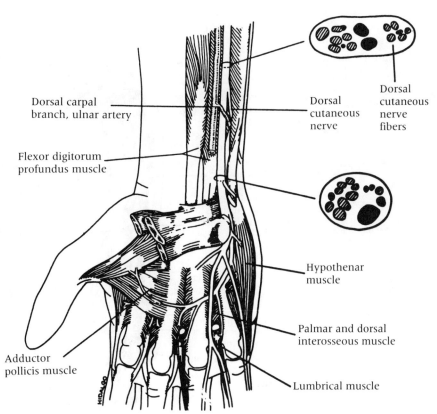

Dorsal carpal branch, ulnar artery

Flexor digitorum profundus muscle

Dorsal cutaneous nerve

Dorsal cutaneous nerve fibers

Hypothenar muscle

Palmar and dorsal interosseous muscle

Adductor pollicis muscle

Lumbrical muscle

Fig. 10-10. Ulnar nerve at the wrist. (From W. W. Shaw and D. A. Hidalgo. *Microsurgery in Trauma.* Mt. Kisco, NY: Futura, 1987. With permission.)

The upper, middle, and lower trunks arise from the branching of the spinal cord roots at the level of the clavicle and in close association with the subclavian vessels. The trunks then intermingle to form the posterior, lateral, and medial cords at a point just distal to the clavicle. The major peripheral nerves derive from these cords.

The posterior cord gives rise to the axillary and radial nerves. The lateral cord gives rise to the musculocutaneous nerve and contributes to the median nerve. The medial cord contributes to the median nerve and forms the ulnar nerve. Thus the median, ulnar, and musculocutaneous nerves are more susceptible to a penetrating injury because of their superficial position, and the axillary and radial nerves are commonly injured during shoulder dislocation.

The axillary nerve provides motor innervation to the deltoid muscle and sensation to the posterior aspect of the shoulder. The musculocutaneous nerve innervates the coracobranchialis, biceps branchi, and branchialis muscles, and it supplies sensation to the proximal radial portion of the forearm.

Mixed motor and sensory neurons are common in these larger

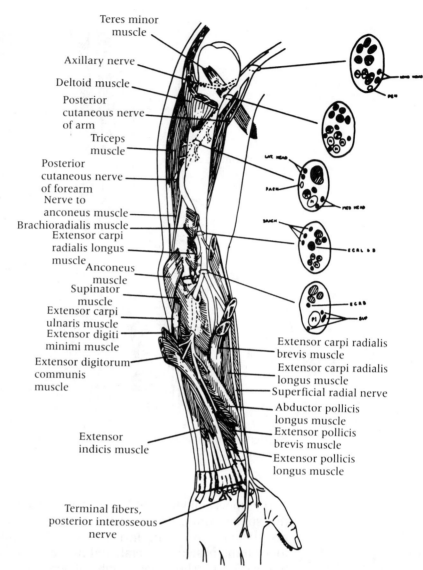

Teres minor muscle
Axillary nerve
Deltoid muscle
Posterior cutaneous nerve of arm
Triceps muscle
Posterior cutaneous nerve of forearm
Nerve to anconeus muscle
Brachioradialis muscle
Extensor carpi radialis longus muscle
Anconeus muscle
Supinator muscle
Extensor carpi ulnaris muscle
Extensor digiti minimi muscle
Extensor digitorum communis muscle
Extensor indicis muscle
Extensor carpi radialis brevis muscle
Extensor carpi radialis longus muscle
Superficial radial nerve
Abductor pollicis longus muscle
Extensor pollicis brevis muscle
Extensor pollicis longus muscle
Terminal fibers, posterior interosseous nerve

Fig. 10-11. Radial nerve, overview. (From W. W. Shaw and D. A. Hidalgo. *Microsurgery in Trauma.* Mt. Kisco, NY: Futura, 1987. With permission.)

fascicles. There are 8 to 11 fascicles in the trunks, and 13 to 18 in the cords. Many anatomic variants are present.

Summary
Most extensors of the hand are radially innervated, and most extrinsic flexors of the hand are medially innervated. Most intrinsic muscles of the hand (except the abductor pollicis longus, superficial head of the flexor pollicis brevis, opponens, and index and middle lumbricales) are ulnar innervated.

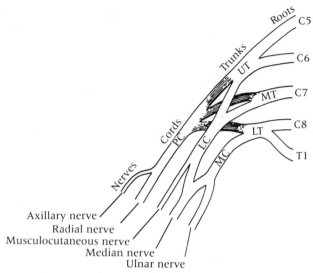

Fig. 10-12. Anatomic representation of the branchial plexus.(From W. W. Shaw and D. A. Hidalgo. *Microsurgery in Trauma.* Mt. Kisco, NY: Futura, 1987. With permission.)

EVALUATION

All injuries of the upper extremity, whether blunt or penetrating, require an adequate neurologic evaluation. As with any examination, an accurate history is essential and guides the examiner's physical evaluation.

Traction/avulsion injuries are frequently much more neurologically complex than lacerations. The neurons are frequently contused along a large segment of the nerve. Motor vehicle accidents are frequently a mixed injury: laceration and traction. Industrial accidents depend on the mechanism of injury. Understanding the exact mechanism of injury and the way the offending equipment works is essential for recreating the type of forces to which the extremity was exposed. Friends and coworkers can frequently describe the accident and how the machinery works. Most importantly, this interview allows the physician to establish a rapport with the patient and increases patient cooperation during the physical examination, which is integral to ascertaining a reliable diagnosis.

Frequently, these patients may have associated injuries, most commonly of the cervical spine, vascular system, chest, or abdomen. The patient must be totally evaluated by a traumatologist before the upper extremity injury is addressed operatively.

One should begin the physical examination on the uninjured extremity, which allows the patient to understand more clearly what is expected of him or her and is reassuring about what the examination entails. It also helps establish a sensory examination baseline for comparison.

The complete physical examination of the upper extremity is

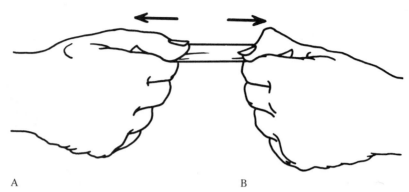

Fig. 10-13. Froment's sign is positive in hand B. (From American Society of the Hand. *The Hand: Examination and Diagnosis.* 2nd ed. New York: Churchill Livingstone, 1983. With permission.)

discussed in Chapter 4. Here we concentrate on the neurologic examination. It is most useful to begin with a distal sensory examination of the digits. *Light touch* is tested with an examiner's fingertip or a cotton-tipped applicator. Any discrepancy from normal (tingling sensations, numbness, or "feels funny") is recorded. Next, a *moving two-point discrimination test* is performed for all digits. The simplest method is to use a bent paper clip, although there are commercially available units. The upper limit of normal is approximately 7 to 8 mm. The radial and ulnar aspects of each digit are evaluated separately, and the palm and first web space must be included in this sensory evaluation.

In general, if the moving two-point discrimination test is abnormal or the patient says there is abnormal sensation, one should suspect a more proximal injury to the nerve supplying that sensory distribution. The static two-point discrimination or vibratory studies are not particularly useful in the emergency room situation.

A gross motor examination is then performed to detect denervated muscles distal to the site of the nerve injury. Peripheral motor examination may be helpful for determining the level of the injury; however, it can be hampered by patient pain or musculotendinous injuries.

Ulnar nerve motor function can be assessed in two ways: (1) Innervation of the interossei can be tested by asking the patient to abduct and adduct the extended fingers around the middle finger axis. Also, *Froment's sign* (interphalangeal joint flexion of the thumb when forcibly holding a piece of paper between the thumb and radial side of the index finger) signifies loss of the adductor pollicis function (Fig. 10-13). (2)Flexor digiti profundus function of the little finger is also supplied by the ulnar nerve and can be tested directly.

Median nerve motor function can be tested most easily by testing flexor digiti superficialis and profundus functions separately (see Fig. 4-21) The flexor pollicis longus can be tested by asking the

Table 10-1. Nerve injuries according to two classification systems

Seddon system	Sunderland system	Structure disrupted	Prognosis
Neurapraxia	1st Degree	Minimal, axon	Complete recovery in days/months
Axonotmesis	2nd Degree	Complete, axon (wallerian degeneration)	Complete return in months
Neurotmesis	3rd Degree	Axon, endoneurium	Mild/moderate reduction of function
Neurotmesis	4th Degree	Axon, endoneurium, perineurium	Moderate reduction of function
Neurotmesis	5th Degree	Axon, endoneurium, perineurium, epineurium (all structures)	Marked reduction of functional return

Source: P. L. Hadges, T. E. Spicer, and J. B. Tebbetts. Hand II — nerves and tendon transfers. *Selected Readings in Plastic Surgery,* 3(34): 5, 1986. With permission.

patient to bend the thumb interphalangeal joint. With resisted wrist flexion, the function of the flexor carpi radialis and pronator teres can be assessed.

The *radial nerve* can be evaluated by having the patient extend the wrist (ECRL, ECRB) and the digits (extensors indicis proprius, digitorum communis, digitorum minimus). One must remember that the intrinsics (ulnar innervated) cause extension of the PIP and DIP joints, but with MCP joints flexed.

Examination of the wound should be the concluding portion of the evaluation. The wound should not be probed; and if the injury already demands operative treatment (see Chapter 4), the examination may be postponed until the patient is in the operating room and adequate anesthesia is administered.

CLASSIFICATION

Classically, nerve injuries have been categorized by the degree of axonal injury, as described by Seddon [3] and Sunderland [4] (Table 10-1). Acutely, these injuries may all display the same physical findings: total loss of axonal function of the involved nerve segment. The recovery and prognosis, however, are different.

Unless the severed ends of a nerve are seen in the wound, classification is usually delayed until after exploration of the injured nerve and observation of the total extent of nerve injury. With closed injuries, electromyographic and nerve conduction studies can help to classify the degree of injury (Table 10-2). These classifications are useful when discussing the prognosis of the functional recovery to be expected for the patient.

Table 10-2. Results of electrical studies in normal nerves, complete nerve disruption, incomplete nerve lesions, and neurapraxia

| | Electromyogram | | Nerve conduction study | |
Condition	*Fibrillations, and positive, sharp waves*	Voluntary motor unit potentials	Sensory and motor latency	Amplitude
Normal	Absent	Present	Normal	Normal
Complete lesion	Present	Absent	Absent	Absent
Incomplete lesion	Present	Decrease in number	Normal or slightly prolonged	Reduced
Neurapraxia	Absent	Absent	Absent across block; normal above and below block	Normal above

Source: G. K. Frykman, A. Wolf, and T. Coyle, An algorithm for management of peripheral nerve injuries. *Orthop. Clin. North Am.* 12:239, 1981. With permission.

MANAGEMENT

Once the extremity has been evaluated, the decision regarding the need for acute surgery is made. If significant bleeding is present, pressure should be held on the wound. If this measure does not resolve the bleeding, the patient should be taken urgently to the operating room for exploration. No probing or clamping should be performed in the emergency room.

If a delayed operative intervention is elected, the patient should be placed in an appropriate splint (see Chapter 20). This maneuver prevents additional trauma, as from motion of unstable fractures, and makes the patient more comfortable.

It is important to inform the patient and family of the extent of injury, overall prognosis, and length of rehabilitation that will be required. There are many factors that have been shown statistically to influence the outcome of nerve injuries, including age, location, concomitant soft tissue injury, distance from innervated muscles, and timing of repair.

In general, young patients have better neurologic return of function than older patients; sharp transections fare better than avulsed segments; distal injuries fare better than proximal injuries; muscle reinnervation is better in a patient with a transection close to the motor unit than in a patient injured a distance proximal to the innervated muscle; and significant concomitant soft-tissue injury diminishes the likelihood of a good neurologic return.

The timing of the nerve repair can also influence the final results. If the patient is stable and there is no significant soft-tissue injury, an early or acute repair is technically easier and leads to a better outcome, in my experience. Fascicular sprouting and scarring in the distal endoneurial tubules make secondary closure more difficult.

Primary and delayed (10–14 days) primary repairs yield similar results with peripheral nerve repair. Branchial plexus injuries appear to have better functional results if explored and repaired within 6 months from the time of injury.

OPERATIVE REPAIR

One can compare the repair of a major nerve transection to the repair of a cleft lip: The act is one of the most important events in that patient's life. His or her function (appearance with a cleft) depends on the preparation and coaptation of the transected nerve ends. Although the repair is hidden in the depths of the extremity, its results will be evident. Therefore all repairs should be performed by a surgeon experienced in hand/microsurgery who has a thorough understanding of the anatomy of the upper extremity. The use of magnification and tourniquet ischemia are helpful adjuncts for a good repair.

Once the extremity has been cleaned, it is exsanguinated by elevation or a compressive wrap, and an arm tourniquet is inflated to approximately 100 mm Hg above the systolic blood pressure (approximately 250–300 mm Hg). If the nerve ends are not present on wound exploration, proximal and distal extension of the exposure may be necessary. The dissection should be gentle and meticulous, and one should proceed from the noninjured zone to the injured zone. During exposure of the nerve, one should be careful not to disturb the vascular supply and small branches associated with the nerve. It is not necessary or desirable to circumferentially isolate the nerve over long distances. Circumferential exposure is needed only at the site of repair.

Nerves have a multitude of sensory and motor fascicles. Precise coaption is necessary to ensure that the motor fascicles are joined to corresponding motor, and not sensory, fascicles. The location of longitudinal vessels on the severed ends and knowledge of intraneural anatomy are useful guides for orientating the severed nerve ends.

Intraoperative nerve stimulation may prove beneficial; however, at this time it is not commonplace. In general, a hand surgeon can line up the severed fascicles with a reasonable degree of certainty based on the intraneural anatomy and with the help of the operating microscope. It may be impossible, however, if there is a significant nerve gap.

The principles for management of a peripheral nerve injury are no different from those used for management of other soft-tissue injuries: All devitalized tissues must be débrided back to viable tissues, and the surgeon must have the ability to provide viable soft-tissue coverage for the nerve repair.

Mild stretching and moderate mobilization of the transected nerve ends are acceptable; however, if the nerve gap is more than 2.5 cm, a primary repair creates more than 50 g of tension and more intraneural scarring is likely to occur secondary to decreased blood flow. Excess mobilization of the injured nerve ends (6–8 cm) also leads to increased intraneural scarring secondary to diminished blood flow.

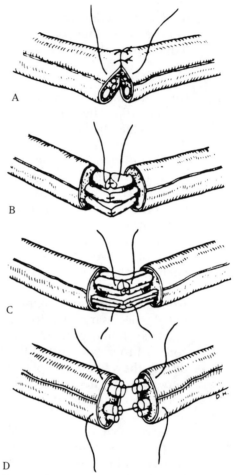

Fig. 10-14. Nerve repairs. *A.* Epineurial repair. *B.* Fascicular repair. *C.* Group fascicular repair. *D.* Epiperineural repair. (From W.W. Shaw and D.A. Hidalgo. *Microsurgery in Trauma.* Mt. Kisco, NY: Futura, 1987. With permission.)

Poor functional results are associated with intraneural scarring, and therefore nerve grafting is recommended in these situations.

Epineural Repair

Epineural repair is the standard nerve repair to which other techniques are compared (Fig. 10-14). Following débridement, the proximal and distal nerve endings are aligned as previously detailed. The epineurium is coapted under magnification with interrupted 8–0 to 11–0 sutures. This technique is technically easy and relatively quick, creates little intraneural trauma, and many times can be done under loupe magnification. The main disadvantage is the lack of precise coaptation of appropriate fascicles and the risk that portions of the epineurium would lie between the planes of the fascicles. In general, this repair is best suited for pure motor or sensory nerves or when there are only a few fascicles present.

Fascicular (Perineural) Repair

Fascicular or perineural repair allows coaptation of individual fascicles and therefore allows more precise coaptation of motor and sensory fibers. It is usually accomplished with 10-0 or 11-0) sutures under an operating microscope after microdissection of the transected nerve endings. The main disadvantages are increased intraneural scarring secondary to dissection and suture material and increased operative time.

The superiority of one technique over the other is still a matter of debate. Jabaley [2] has suggested that the fascicular technique is applicable where the microscopic intraneural anatomy is well defined and precise realignment is possible. However, the type of repair utilized depends on the nature of the wound, the status of the transected nerve, and the surgeon's expertise.

Nerve Grafting

When the nerve gap exceeds 2.5 cm after reasonable mobilization of the transected nerve endings, nerve grafting may be necessary. Débridement is performed under the operating microscope back to "normal-appearing" nerve, and the fascicles are gently dissected out (see Fig. 10-14). A donor nerve of adequate length is harvested. In general, the radial and ulnar nerves require four or five grafts, and the median nerve requires five or six grafts. These grafts are cut longer than the defect, and a fascicular repair is performed. The functional result of nerve grafting is better than that of nerve repair under significant tension.

In general, the sural nerve is the most common donor nerve utilized because it is desirable to leave the smallest functional deficit possible from the donor site, although any sensory nerve can be used. On occasion, nerve can be harvested from unsalvageable amputated portions of the extremity if they are not locally traumatized.

Microsurgical vascularized nerve grafts may have a place in secondary reconstruction for proximal extremity defects in poorly vascularized beds, but they are not utilized in the acute setting.

Branchial Plexus Injury

The general acute care of a branchial plexus injury is outlined here. Because of the complex anatomy and the severe risk of uninformed exploration to the extremity's function, these injuries should be cared for by a surgeon familiar with this area. Thorough débridement of all devitalized tissue is performed, and vascularized soft-tissue coverage is provided. Severed nerve endings should be tagged; silicone rods can be helpful in this setting, as they are easy to locate at a secondary procedure.

The standard preoperative reconstructive workup includes a thorough clinical examination, a cervical myelogram, a computed tomography scan, and an electromyographic study across the plexus to pinpoint the plexus injury as accurately as possible and to rule out any cervical rootlet avulsions. Reexploration and repair of the branchial plexus is a long, tedious operation requiring multiple nerve grafts from normal nerve to normal nerve. For details the reader is referred to the work of Milessi [5] and Terzis [6].

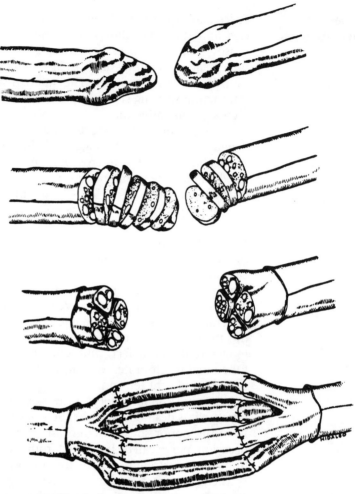

Fig. 10-15. Scar must be removed from nerve ends. Repair may require grafts. (From W. W. Shaw and D. A. Hidalgo. *Microsurgery in Trauma.* Mt. Kisco, NY: Futura, 1987. With permission.)

PARTIAL TRANSECTIONS

In many instances the nerve has a partial transection or hematoma. Partial transections are an indication for limited intrafascicular dissection and repair or grafting with a fascicular technique. The surgeon must be cognizant of potentially increasing the amount of intraneural scarring that will form. Therefore intraneural hematoma in an intact nerve is not an indication for intrafascicular exploration. Serial examinations and electromyographic evaluations can guide the surgeon toward subsequent reexploration when necessary.

POSTOPERATIVE CARE

After treatment of a peripheral nerve injury, the surgeon and patient must realize that full functional recovery may not be obtained for 3 to 5 years. Thus repeated examinations and patience are indicated. Highet's scheme of motor and sensory recovery is the most useful system for evaluating the end results (Table 10-3).

Table 10-3. Highet's method of end result evaluation

Motor Recovery

M0   No contraction
M1   Return of perceptible contraction in the proximal muscles.
M2   Return of perceptible contraction in both proximal and distal muscles.
M3   Return of function in both proximal and distal muscles of such a de-
       gree that all important muscles are sufficiently powerful to act
       against resistance.
M4   Return of function as in stage 3; in addition, all synergic and indepen-
       dent movements are possible.
M5   Complete recovery.

Sensory Recovery

S0   Absence of sensibility in the autonomous area.
S1   Recovery of deep cutaneous pain sensibility within the autonomous
       area of the nerve.
S2   Return of some degree of superficial cutaneous pain and tactile sensi-
       bility within the autonomous area of the nerve.
S3   Return of superficial cutaneous pain and tactile sensibility throughout
       the autonomous area, with disappearance of any previous overre-
       sponse.
S3+ Return of sensibility as in stage 3; in addition, there is some recovery
       of two-point discrimination within the autonomous area.
S4   Complete recovery.

Proximal muscles are defined as extrinsic, and distal muscles as intrinsic, in
the hand.
Source: Shaw Wilgus, E. F. Nerve repair and grafting. In D. P. Green, ed.
Operative Hand Surgery, 2nd ed. New York: Churchill Livingstone, 1988. With
permission.

Postoperatively, the wound should be protected for approximately
3 weeks. Supervised range of motion is then initiated, and splints are
fabricated to prevent associated secondary contractures. At 2 to 3
months after the injury, strengthening exercises and sensory reeducation is begun.

Tinel's sign is monitored on regular intervals. It should move
progressively at a rate of 1 inch per month. Two-point perception
and vibration are tested. When vibration at 256 cycles per second is
noted, sensory reeducation is begun.

If there is not an advancing Tinel's sign by 3 to 6 months,
electromyography should be performed. If no improvement is seen
at 6 months, serious consideration should be given to exploration of
the repaired nerve.

COMPLICATIONS   Complications of any injury include bleeding, infection, and wound
dehiscence. Most complications of nerve repair are found many
weeks after the repair. Inadequate progression of Tinel's sign may be
secondary to poor coaptation, coaptation of incorrect structures,
scarring, and local ischemia. Reexploration and nerve grafts in a well
vascularized bed are then required.

With the disruption of axons, sprouting from the severed ends occurs. If the nerve has been coapted appropriately, one hopes that it will be organized into nerve reinnervation. If the growth is disorganized, a neuroma may form. Primary nerve repair is the best method of preventing, and therefore treating, potential sensory neuromas.

Small, benign-appearing lacerations in the region of the palmar cutaneous sensory branch of the median nerve (see Fig. 10-8) or the dorsal sensory branch of the radial nerve (see Fig. 10-11) should be tested closely for possible nerve injury. The sensory neuromas that form with untreated, and occasionally treated, injuries can become problematic because of their associated pain and hypersensitivity. Often these symptoms can interfere with hand function and therapy, and they occasionally lead to reflex sympathetic dystrophy and total disability of the involved extremity. Injection of neuromas with steroids, desensitization therapy, and operative resection and relocation of neuromas can be helpful.

SUMMARY

Peripheral nerve surgery usually occurs in conjunction with injuries to the bones, tendons, vessels, and soft tissue, and frequently nerve repair is the final stage of the surgical procedure. The extra time spent for meticulous débridement and coaptation of the nerve endings is rewarded many times over during the patient'r recuperation. Knowledge of the anatomy and patience during the dissection are key elements. Similarly, hand therapy and splinting techniques must be involved early in the postoperative course to maximize function. The rehabilitation of nerve injuries is a team effort.

REFERENCES

1. Sunderland, S. The intra nerve topography of the radial, median and ulnar nerves. *Brain* 68:243, 1945.
2. Jabaley, M. E., Wallace, W. H., and Heckler, F. R. Internal topography of major nerves of the forearm and hand: A current View. *J. Hand Surg.* 5:1, 1980.
3. Seddon, H. J. Three types of nerve injury. *Brain* 66:237, 1947.
4. Sunderland, S. A classification of pheripheal nerve injuries producing loss of function. *Brain* 74:491, 1951.
5. Milessi, H. Surgical management of branchial plexus injuries. *J. Hand Surg.* 2:367, 1977.
6. Terzis, J. K. *Microreconstruction of Nerve Injuries.* Philadelphia: Saunders, 1987.

SUGGESTED READING

American Society of the Hand. *The Hand: Examination and Diagnosis,* 2nd ed. New York: Churchill Livingstone, 1983.
Green, D. (ed.), *Operative Hand Surgery.* New York: Churchill Livingstone, 1982.
Mackinnon, S. E., and Dellon, A. L. *Surgery of the Peripheral Nerve.* New York: Thieme, 1988.
Omer, G. E., and Spinner, M. *Management of Peripheral Nerve Problems.* Philadelphia: Saunders, 1980.
Shaw, W. W., and Hidalgo, D. A., *Microsurgery in Trauma.* Mount Kisco, NY: Futura, 1987.
Spinner, M. *Injuries to the Major Branches of the Peripheral Nerves of the Forearm.* Philadelphia: Saunders, 1978.

Commentary on Chapter 10

E. Douglas Newton

Management of injury to the peripheral nerve begins with clinical suspicion of injury to the nerve and physical examination appropriate to that suspicion. If we are talking about the upper extremity, as we seem to be here, then examination begins in the neck and proceeds distally. One should be careful to include the truncal musculature of the upper extremity in the exam as this may reveal or differentiate brachial plexus injury. Also, Horner's syndrome may be present in lower brachial plexus avulsion.

The neurologic exam should be done early and often. Sensorium and cooperativeness of the patient should be noted in the record of the exam. Drawings of areas of hypesthesia are most helpful to subsequent examiners in determining baseline levels, and discreet skin markings are useful in this regard as well.

Dr. Moore does not find the tuning fork useful in the emergency situation; Dr. Dellon uses the wrong end; for my part, I can't seem to find a tuning fork when I need it. The concept, however, of using a standard, nonthreatening form of stimulation (avoid pricks!) is good and can make our examinations more consistent and therefore more valid. The two tables below provide a clear cut specific testing site for various nerves (Tables 10C-1 and 10C-2)

The divided nerve is not a true emergency demanding immediate operative intervention, but the acutely compressed nerve is. In situations where there is an acutely compressed nerve (e.g., crush injuries, ischemia; skeletal instability, and thermal electrical burns) acute knee nerve decompression may be indicated. Nerve decompression may require faciotomy ascarotomy or division of anatomical constrictive structures, such as the carpal tunnel, tarsal tunnel, Guyon's cannal, and others.

On the other hand, a closed injury with neural deficit may be an indication to delay operative intervention (when there is no other indication to generate) to determine the degree of injury by observation for return of function; or it may be an indication to await the full evolution of the extent of injury along the nerve segment. In either case, timing of the intervention is of the essence: the observer must be acutely aware that end organs do not wait forever for their lost central connections and time must intervene between the ana-

Table 10-C1. Muscle function related to specific peripheral nerve: Localization of injury site

Lack of	Suggests injury to	At
Thumb extension, or MP finger extension, or ulnar wrist extension if also	Radial nerve	Proximal forearm, at superficial head of supinator
Extensor carpi radialis brevis or brachio-radialis if also	Radial nerve	Antecubital fossa, proximal to posterior interosseous nerve
Triceps	Radial nerve	Proximal humerus
First dorsal interosseous if also	Ulnar nerve	Palm
Abductor digiti minimi if also	Ulnar nerve	Guyon's canal
Flexor profundus to little finger if also	Ulnar nerve	Proximal forearm
Ulnar wrist flexor	Ulnar nerve	Cubital tunnel
Abductor pollicis brevis if also	Median nerve	Carpal tunnel
Flexor sublimis if also	Median nerve	Midforearm
Flexor policis longus, index profundus, or pronator quadratus if also	Median nerve	Proximal forearm (anterior interosseous nerve)
Pronator teres, flexor carpi radialis	Median nerve	Antecubital fossa

Source: A. L. Dellon, Peripheral Nerve Injury. In N. G. Georgiade, et al. (Eds.) *Essentials of Plastic, Maxillofacial, and Reconstructive Surgery.* Baltimore: Williams and Wilkins, 1980. With permission.

tomical repair and the arrival of the axonal sprout at the end organ. I find it useful at the first post-injury office visit to set a date by which time we should operate and to describe to the patient what we are looking for in terms of growth of axons and reinnervation. At the same time we discuss potential for return of function, necessity of preventing contractures, and sensory and motor reeducation. All the points must be reinforced and discussed many times, I have found.

Operative technique should cleave to the cardinal virtues of plastic surgery: meticulous attention to detail, careful hemostasis, gentle handling of tissues, reverence for blood supply, avoidance of large amounts of foreign material, *ad nauseam.* The operator must keep in mind that the purpose is not to provide a watertight closure of epineurium as he or she would a blood vessel, but simply to allow the nerve ends to lie gently abutting one another, "to be satisfied," as told to John D. Franklin by Bernard McO'Brien.

Remember that the nerve endings are unsatisfied and all we have to do is put them together and stand back.

Table 10-C2. Sensory area to test for unambiguous diagnosis of peripheral nerve injury

Injured nerve	Test area
Digital	Lateral-volar area of distal interphalangeal joint
Median	Index finger pulp
Ulnar, distal ⅓ forearm	Little finger pulp
Ulnar, proximal to midforearm	Entire little finger
Dorsal branch, ulnar	Dorsal ulnar aspect of hand
Radial	Dorsal metacarpophalangeal of index or thumb (rarely, no autonomous zone)
Posterior interosseous	None, innervates dorsal wrist capsule
Lateral antebrachial	None, extensive overlap with radial
Medial antebrachial	Medial posterior area, proximal forearm
Musculocutaneous	Radial volar forearm, proximally
Deep peroneal	Web space, big and second toe
Superficial peroneal	Dorsum of foot, proximally
Common peroneal	Entire dorsum of foot
Sural	Lateral aspect of pxoximal foot
Medial plantar	Big or second toe pulp
Lateral plantar	Little toe pulp
Saphenous	Medial aspect, distal leg
Lateral femoral	Anterolateral thigh, proximally
Femoral	Anterior thigh distally
Posterior tibial	Pulp of all toes
Calcaneal	Heel

Source: A. L. Dellon, Peripheral nerve injury. In N. G. Georgiade, et al. (Eds.) *Essentials of Plastic, Maxillofacial, and Reconstructive Surgery.* Baltimore: Williams and Wilkins, 1980. With permission.

11 SOFT-TISSUE COVERAGE OF THE UPPER EXTREMITY

Paul D. Fischer

The human upper extremity provides both tactile feedback from the environment and a mechanism by which an individual can manipulate his or her surroundings. These roles require constant exposure to potentially hazardous circumstances, and therefore injuries to the arm and hand are some of the most common conditions dealt with by the emergency physician and reconstructive surgeon.

When reconstructing soft-tissue deficits of the upper limb one must recognize the different tissue requirements of each of the arm and hand surfaces. A "reconstructive ladder" can be employed (Fig. 11-1) but often should be modified to provide for the unique functional characteristics of the area involved. Palm skin, for example, is thick and glabrous without sebaceous glands, and it is adherent to the underlying fascial architecture, whereas the skin of the dorsum of the hand is elastic and loose. Volar arm skin is thinner and has less hair than dorsal arm skin. All joints in the upper extremity require covering with supple tissue that allows motion. Finally, the need for sensation varies markedly in different areas of the hand and arm.

To perform the best reconstruction of soft-tissue loss in the upper extremity, therefore, the characteristics of color match, sensibility, durability, and ability to preserve joint function must be kept in mind. In addition, rarely is there a surface-tissue loss in the upper extremity without some other vascular, muscular, or nervous injury; and one must always be thinking ahead to possible secondary reconstruction needs so as not to limit the potential recovery of the patient by performing a poorly thought out initial repair.

EVALUATION

Evaluation of the injured upper extremity begins with the history and physical examination. The *time* since the injury should be noted, the first 6 hours after the trauma being the "golden period" when bacterial contamination is low, and the chances of wound infection after closure are least. In reality, many injured patients are not seen at the treating institution until well after their injury has occurred, and it is not unreasonable to close a "tidy wound" even after 24 hours if concomitant antibiotics are used.

237

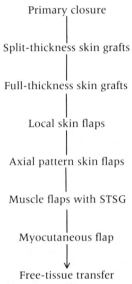

Soft-tissue coverage

reconstructive ladder

Primary closure

Split-thickness skin grafts

Full-thickness skin grafts

Local skin flaps

Axial pattern skin flaps

Muscle flaps with STSG

Myocutaneous flap

Free-tissue transfer

Fig. 11-1. The simplest option to perform the needed task should be used.

Where the injury occurred should be noted to assess the relative bacterial exposure of the wound. Was the patient working in a manure pile or a sterile laboratory? What are the most likely organisms contaminating the wound (Table 11-1)?

The *mechanism of injury* should be explored, specifically noting any crushing modalities, which would increase the potential amount of devitalized tissue. What was the posture of the patient's hand or arm at the time of the accident? Was there bleeding suggestive of major arterial injury? Did sensory or motor changes occur immediately or develop gradually?

If the patient was referred from another institution, one should know *how the wound was handled* there. *Tetanus immunization status* should be checked. Was the wound irrigated, and were antibiotics administered? Finally, one should not overlook other injuries by just focusing on the extremity problem.

Examination

Refer to Chapter 4 for a complete examination of the upper extremity during emergent situations. Here we focus on specific aspects of the examination that directly relate to soft-tissue coverage and reconstruction.

An initial key decision is whether the injury requires the services of an operating room for repair, and this decision is usually based on the results of a thorough neurovascular and functional hand examination. There is rarely need to "probe" a wound in the relatively

Table 11-1. Most likely organisms contaminating a wound

Accident location	Major bacterial cultures
Farm wounds[a]	Mixed gram-positive and gram-negative
Home/industrial wounds[a]	Gram-positive
Bites	
Human	*S. aureus*
	Eikenella corrodens[b] — unique to human bites
Animal	*Pasteurella multicida*[b]

[a] Prophylactic antibiotics are *not* recommended for farm wounds. These wounds should be thoroughly débrided and treated depending on culture results. Prophylactic antibiotics *are* recommended for home/industrial wounds, as a single organism is often cultured. Prophylactic antibiotics do not avert subsequent infection without thorough wound débridement.
[b] Sensitive only to penicillin or tetracycline.

unsterile emergency room if the examination reveals a surface deficit too large to repair outside of an operating room. Similarly, if a vascular or neurologic problem that requires further investigation is demonstrated, one should not risk increasing the chance of infection and further damage by relatively "blind" probing in the emergency room. This approach also spares the patient unnecessary discomfort.

Not all hand and arm injuries need to be handled in the operating room, however, as there are many relatively minor situations that are appropriately treated in the emergency room. *These injuries must be handled according to the following guidelines of good wound care.* A poorly handled "minor" injury can rapidly become a major operative problem.

Begin by noting the posture of the extremity, its motor and sensory function, and the appearance and size of the wound. Is there soft-tissue loss or merely skin contraction simulating a coverage problem? Are there exposed tendons, nerves, blood vessels, or bones? Is there an underlying fracture? Radiographs are usually obtained on all but the most trivial extremity injuries to check for fractures and foreign bodies. Note that only approximately 10 percent of glass in today's society is visible with radiography. Remember to check the entire radiograph systematically so as to not miss concomitant injuries.

Any constricting garment or jewelry should be removed. The treatment is then completed in the emergency room if appropriate, or the extremity is splinted and elevated to await further repair in the operating room.

Wound Classification

One should attempt to classify the wound regarding its potential for contamination and ischemic loss. The system proposed by Rank and Wakefield [1] is both useful and simple, grouping the wounds into "tidy" and "untidy" categories.

Injuries that are produced by tearing, crushing, exploding, or combustion have devitalized tissue and associated edema, vascular thrombosis, and significant contamination; and they are classified as untidy. These wounds are best treated by irrigation and débride-ment, splinting, and reexploration within 25 to 48 hours, with further débridement as needed and delayed closure. *All human bites and burns are considered untidy wounds.*

Injuries produced by sharp, relatively clean objects with little crush component are classified as tidy. They can usually be closed after the initial thorough cleaning and débridement.

Another classification system divides closure of extremity wounds into primary, delayed primary, or secondary closure categories. *Primary closure*, or closure performed as the initial treatment, is appropriate for clean, minimally contaminated wounds after thor-ough débridement. *Delayed primary closure*, or closure accomplished 2 to 7 days after initial treatment, is appropriate for contaminated wounds or wounds with a significant crush component that requires a second or third trip to the operating room for evaluation and continued débridement before final reconstruction. *Secondary closure*, or closure after healing by a secondary intention, is appropriate for grossly contaminated wounds (e.g., human bites). Exposure of vital underlying structures (e.g., major nerves) necessitates some flexibil-ity when applying this classification system.

Skin substitutes can be used to cover areas not yet ready for closure or that are likely to spontaneously reepithelialize. Porcine skin and Biobrane are often used for burns. Duoderm (a hydrophilic colloid dressing) can be useful for thin partial-thickness losses.

Do not forget to splint the extremity appropriately (see Chapter 19) between operative treatments to avoid contractures.

INITIAL TREATMENT

Irrigation and débridement after appropriate anesthesia is given are the most important parts of wound care of the upper extremity. In the operating room I prefer to use 2 to 4 liters of isotonic saline containing 50,000 units of bacitracin or 1 g of a first-generation cephalosporin per liter powered through a pulse lavage system (e.g., Surgilav). In the emergency room at least 200 ml of saline delivered through an 18-gauge angiocatheter from a 30-ml syringe also generates the minimally acceptable 7 pounds per square inch pressure needed for wound irrigation.

Visualization is an important part of wound care and is most easily accomplished in both the emergency and operating rooms using an upper arm blood pressure cuff inflated to a pressure 150 mm Hg greater than the patient's systolic pressure. Exsanguination prior to cuff inflation can be accomplished with a Martin (Esmarch) elastic wrap or Ace wrap or by elevating the extremity above the level of the heart for 2 to 3 minutes. Remember that a patient's tolerance to a constricting pressure of 280 to 300 mm Hg in the upper arm without arm anesthesia is limited, usually 30 to 45 minutes. *If tourniquet control is needed for longer than this time in the emergency room, you are treating the wound in the wrong place.* There is no shame in backing out of an intended emergency room repair if the wound is found to be more formidable than initially thought.

For injuries limited to the finger, a finger tourniquet constructed of a Penrose drain can be used, wrapped around the base of the finger. It is held in place by a clamp, or rubber glove finger rolled from fingertip to base can be used. (Fig. 11-2).

RECONSTRUCTIVE OPTIONS

Assuming that the remaining uninjured tissue around a wound is insufficient in amount or character for closure, one must decide on a reconstructive method that brings in new tissue to the deficient area.

Skin Grafts

A skin graft is one of the most common and simple methods of providing coverage for upper extremity tissue loss. Such grafts can be divided into two groups: (1) split-thickness skin grafts (STSGs), where skin is harvested leaving some dermis on the donor site and some in the graft; and (2) full-thickness skin grafts (FTSGs) where the entire dermis is included with the harvested skin (Fig. 11-3).

Because they are thinner, STSGs have the advantage of better take on marginal beds compared to FTSGs, although they also ultimately contract more. As a general rule (but certainly not a binding one), STSGs are used on dorsal hand deficits and arm deficits, whereas FTSGs are preferred for palmar losses and sometimes losses across joints.

To understand this choice one must remember that the amount of dermis retained in the graft is one of the determinants of wound contracture. Thus in situations where there is a skin loss crossing a joint, for example (provided there is a vascular bed to support a free graft), one could choose an FTSG (or flap, see below) to limit contracture and allow as full range of motion as possible. In addition, the amount of included dermis also determines the thickness of coverage, and therefore an FTSG is preferred to replace the thicker palmar skin.

Tendon without paratenon and bone without periosteum cannot support an STSG or FTSG. Although not ideal, as seen from microsurgical free flap transfer experiences, blood vessels reperfuse grafted skin and thus can be covered by skin grafts.

Split-Thickness Skin Grafts
Donor sites for STSGs are unlimited. Any area with intact skin is able to donate its superficial surface. The temptation to use other areas in the prepped field of the arm and hand should be avoided. Although the color match may be better and it is convenient, the donor scar is often too conspicuous to be recommended. Most often standard areas on the thighs or buttocks are employed.

The STSGs can be obtained in a variety of ways using a large scalpel blade, Weck or Goulian knife, or any of the various power dermatomes (e.g., Padgett, Zimmer, Brown) available on the market. The thickness of the graft should be between 0.012 and 0.015 inch

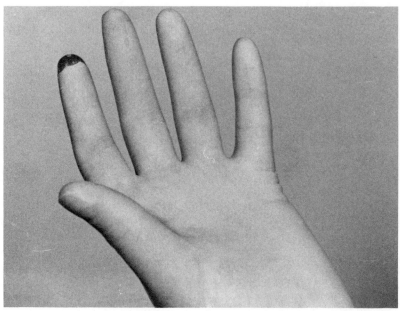

A

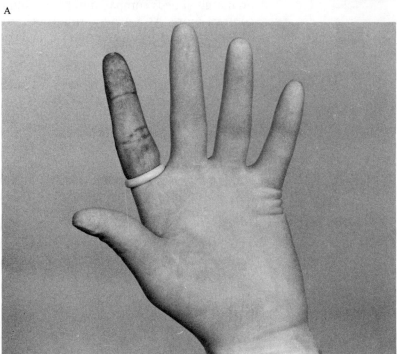

B

Fig. 11-2. A., B. A sterile rubber glove (one-half size too small) is placed over the prepped hand. The glove tip of the involved digit is cut off and rolled down to exsanguinate the area and provide a bloodless finger.

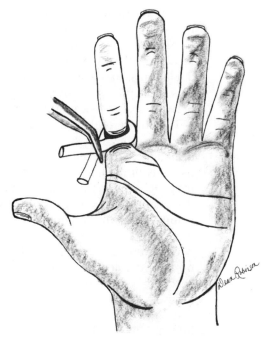

Fig. 11-2. (continued) C. An alternative method is to place a Penrose drain with a clamp on both ends to provide a relatively safe tourniquet effect.

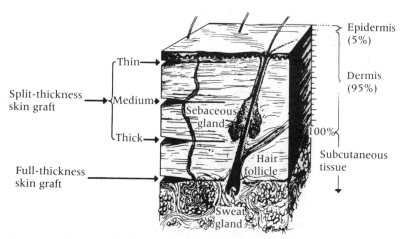

Fig. 11-3. Skin graft thickness. The true depth depends on the thickness of the epidermis and dermis in the region from which the skin is harvested. It varies in different regions of the body. (From W.C. Grabb, and J.W. Smith, eds. *Plastic Surgery*, 3rd ed. Boston: Little Brown, 1979. With permission.)

in adults. In infants, small children, and certain elderly adults a thickness of 0.008 inches is more appropriate as their dermis is thinner. Harvesting the standard adult STSG in these individuals can result in removal of the full thickness of skin at the donor site.

Plantar skin has skin characteristics similar to those of palmar skin. It is particularly useful in black patients where the color difference between palmar skin and skin from other areas is noticeable.

The choice of meshing an STSG depends on the clinical situation. The advantages of such a procedure are increased egress ports for drainage and increased ability to cover larger areas when donor tissue is limited, as for major burns where the hand or arm injury may be only part of the patient's need for skin coverage. The disadvantage of meshing is possibly a less cosmetically pleasing result, with the potential for this problem increasing with an increased size of the mesh. Usually a 1.5:1.0 ratio is used.

Graft edges are held against normal skin with absorbable or nonabsorbable sutures or staples. Immobilizing the graft itself on the vascular bed is best accomplished using tie-over dressings. Sometimes K-wires or splints are needed if the graft crosses a joint. I usually leave these dressings on for 4 to 5 days unless signs of infection (e.g., odor) develop and necessitate earlier removal. Others, however, recommend earlier dressing removal to allow evacuation by "rolling" of any subgraft collections of blood or serum. I have not found subgraft fluid collections to be a problem but have seen the delicate vascular and fibrous connections between the graft and bed disturbed by early uncovering. I therefore prefer to wait until inosculation is well established at the fourth or fifth day postoperatively before uncovering the graft.

To wait, however, means that a dressing that retains moisture for an extended period must be used: A mixture of one-third glycerine, one-third saline, and one-third Betadine applied in soaked cotton balls over Adaptic nonadherent gauze is satisfactory when incorporated into a tie-over dressing.

Postoperative care of the donor site for the STSG is best accomplished by coverage with Op-site or some other clear, plastic membrane, but Xeroform or scarlet red gauze and Duoderm have also been used successfully.

Extended splinting and massage of the graft is most often needed for the 3 to 6 months after the graft is applied to maintain suppleness and minimize contracture. The patient should also be warned about the discoloring effect of sun exposure to the healing graft for the 6 months immediately after application. This problem is best avoided by using a sunblock (more than No. 15 block) on a routine basis for this time period.

Full Thickness Skin Grafts
Full-thickness skin grafts include the entire dermal layer and therefore are less prone to contracture, provide more padding, and have the potential to regain more sensation at the recipient site, as it

includes more of the main nerve trunks of the skin than does split skin. Donor sites for FTSGs, however, are limited. Most commonly the hairless area of the groin is used, but other potential donor sites include the volar wrist crease, medial aspect of the antecubital fossa, and hypothenar area. In particular, one should again remember the significant color variation between palmar skin in black patients and the skin at these various donor sites, therefore using plantar instep skin for a better color match. Finally, do not forget the possibility of using skin from a nonsalvagable part for more severe injuries (this tissue can also serve as a split-thickness graft donor).

An FTSG is harvested with a scalpel, defatting the undersurface as much as possible using small, curved scissors before application to allow inosculation of vessels. The graft is held in position and immobilized as outlined above for the split-thickness skin grafts. The donor site is usually closed primarily but can be closed with an STSG if large areas of full-thickness skin are needed. Again, a massage and splinting regimen for 3 to 6 months may be necessary to obtain optimum results, and use of a sunblock is recommended.

Local Flaps

Situations not amenable to skin grafting are those where the underlying bed does not have the vascular supply to reperfuse the grafted tissue, or when the need for mobility in the reconstructed area (e.g., loss across a joint) dictates the use of a flap instead of a graft given the graft's variable but unavoidable shrinkage. Again, *tendon without paratenon and bone without periosteum cannot support skin grafts.*

When skin grafts are not appropriate one should next consider local flaps, which can be broadly classified as random or axial flaps. Random flaps depend on the subdermal plexus of blood vessels for perfusion and classically have been limited in size by the 1:1 width/length ratio. Axial pattern flaps are perfused by a longitudinally oriented vascular system that permits much longer length/width ratios (Fig. 11-4). The following sections discuss some of the more commonly used random and axial pattern flaps in the hand and arm.

Local Flaps in the Hand
Many hand flaps used today are random in nature. The following is a list and brief discussion of some of the possibilities.

1. *V-Y Volar (Atasoy) and lateral (Kleinert) flaps.*These advancement flaps for fingertip injuries are discussed elsewhere (see Chapter 5).
2. *Local Z-plasties.*These procedures are discussed in Chapter 1.
3. *Cross-finger flaps.* These flaps are sections of the dorsal skin usually situated over one phalanx (but extendable if needed) that are raised on a radially or ulnarly derived subdermal plexus and transposed to an adjacent finger (Fig. 11-5). The flap is raised at the level of the extensor mechanism, leaving the paratenon on the tendons to support a skin graft (usually a full-thickness graft). It can be used to resurface volar surface deficits by direct application or turned over like

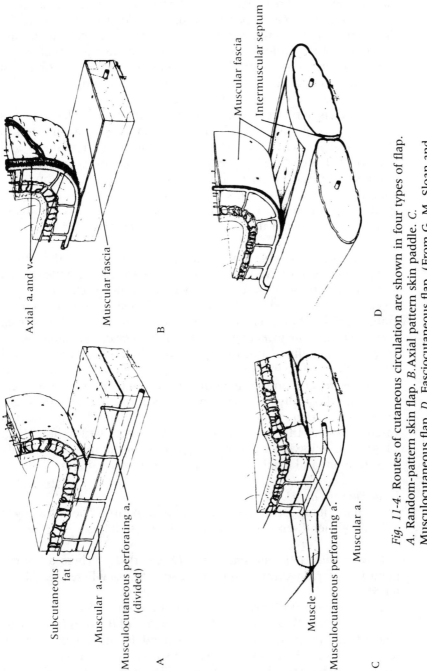

Fig. 11-4. Routes of cutaneous circulation are shown in four types of flap. *A.* Random-pattern skin flap. *B.* Axial pattern skin paddle. *C.* Musculocutaneous flap. *D.* Fasciocutaneous flap. (From G. M. Sloan and J. F. Reinisch. Flap physiology and the prediction of flap viability. *Hand Clinics.* Philadelphia: Saunders, 1985. With permission.)

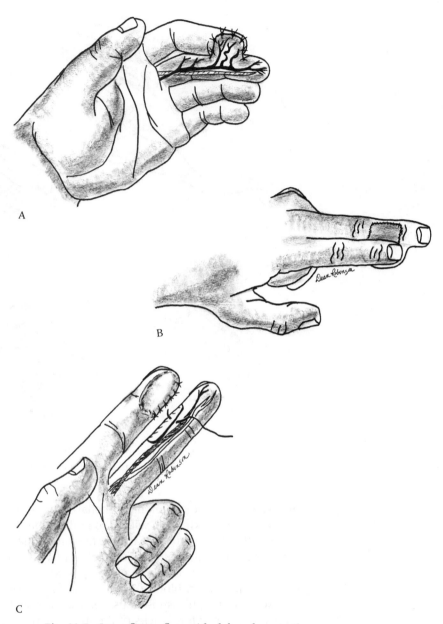

Fig. 11-5. Cross-finger flap with delayed separation.

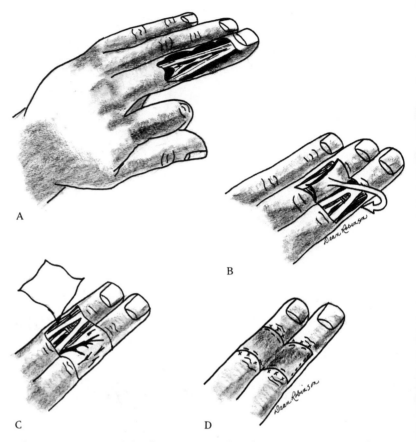

Fig. 11-6. Dorsum of the finger is treated with a "reversed" cross-finger flap. The donor defect and wound are covered with a skin graft.

the page of a book after deepithelializing the external surface to replace a dorsal skin loss, with skin grafts applied to both the donor site and the deep surface of the dermis on the flap (Fig. 11-6).

Using a cross-finger flap necessitates a two-stage procedure, with division of the pedicle taking place approximately 2 weeks after the initial raising when blood flow into the flap from the recipient site can support the transposed tissue. Classically, the middle finger serves as a donor for deficits of the index or ring finger and thumb, the ring finger for small finger losses, and the thumb for middle finger deficits; however, any digit adjacent to the injured one can serve as a donor.

Problems with this procedure include donor site visibility, the need for two operations, and the potential for joint stiffness with the two fingers joined together for 2 weeks in a position that allows joint capsule contraction (see section on splints, Chapter 19). One must especially consider this last problem when the patient is elderly and may have significant difficulty overcoming joint contractures.

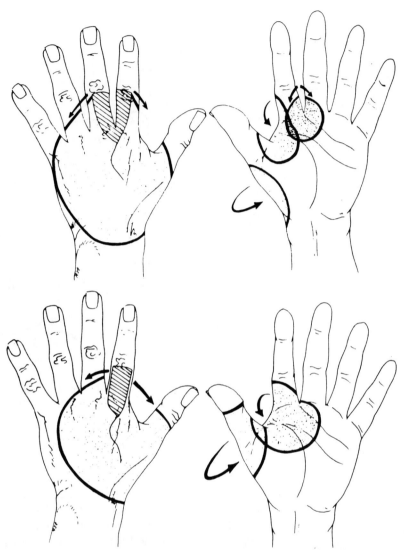

Fig. 11-7. Areas covered adequately by the first dorsal metacarpal artery flaps. (From Earley, M. I. and Milner, R. H., Dorsal metacarpal flaps. *Br. J. Plast. Surg.* 40:340, 1987. With permission.)

4. *Thenar Flaps.* These flaps are discussed in Chapter 5.

There are a few axial pattern local hand flaps, that is, flaps that have a longitudinally oriented vascular system that permits longer length/width ratios.

1. *First dorsal metacarpal artery neurovascular island flap.* This flap incorporates dorsal skin over the proximal phalanx of the index finger (Fig. 11-7). Its vascular supply is the first dorsal metacarpal artery (FDMA), which arises from the radial artery as it courses between the heads of the first dorsal interosseous muscle. Dissection

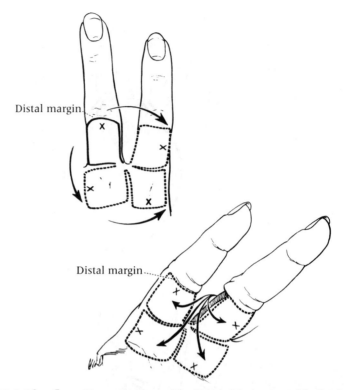

Distal margin

Distal margin

Fig. 11-8. Flag flap. (From G. Lister. *The Hand: Diagnosis and Indications,* 2nd ed. New York: Churchill Livingstone, 1984. With permission.)

is started dorsally over the first interosseous space and deepens along the radial side of the second metacarpal close to its periosteal surface to the level of the first dorsal interosseous muscle fascia on which the FDMA lies. The fascia is then incised, and the artery on a bed of fascia is elevated by dissecting in a plane between the fascia and the muscle. Finally, the skin unit over the proximal phalanx of the index finger is raised at the level of the extensor paratenon.

The FDMA can be followed proximally back as far as its origin from the radial artery depending on the rotational needs of the flap. The flap reaches as far as the metacarpophalangeal (MCP) joint of the small finger and covers defects over the wrist. It can also be used on the palmar surface and reaches almost all areas except the ulnar border of the hand. It covers the dorsum of the thumb and has the added advantage of containing a branch of the radial nerve and can therefore function as a neurosensory flap.

The donor site on the index finger is grafted with full-thickness skin. The visibility of this donor site is the main disadvantage of the flap.

2. *Flag flap variant of cross-finger flap.*This flap, originally described over the middle phalanx (Fig. 11-8), depends on a proximal extension of the flap of one-third of its width with its associated subdermal plexus. It can, however, be an axial flap when raised over

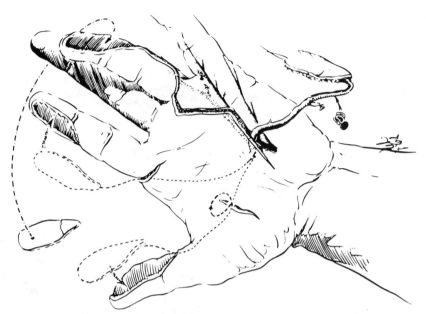

Fig. 11-9. Neurovascular island flap coverage. (From J. W. Littler. Principles of reconstructive surgery of the hand. In J. M. Converse, ed. *Reconstructive Plastic Surgery*, 2nd ed. Vol. 6. Philadelphia: Saunders, 1977. With permission.)

any of the proximal phalanxes of the fingers, when the proximal extension can include a branch of the common digital or dorsal metacarpal artery to that finger. The value of this flap is its greater mobility because of its narrow pedicle, which allows it to reach both the dorsal and the volar surfaces of adjacent fingers and even the volar surfaces of the same finger. It is raised like a standard cross-finger flap at the level of the extensor paratenon and is usually divided at 2 weeks. Full- or split-thickness skin grafts are used to resurface the donor site. Its drawbacks are the same as those discussed above.

3. *Neurosensory island flaps.* Occasionally a situation arises where the need for good sensation on a key functional area (e.g., radial side of the index finger) justifies sacrifice of a normally perfused and innervated finger surface (often the ulnar side of the ring finger). This area of skin is elevated with its neurovascular bundle and followed back to the superficial arch; then it is rotated and inset into the area needing sensation (Fig. 11-9). The obvious drawback of this procedure is the loss of sensation on the donating finger. Because a common digital artery serves as the pedicle for this flap one must be sure that the other digital artery on the donating finger *and the adjacent finger* is intact (e.g., the radial digital vessel of the ring finger and the ulnar digital vessel of the small finger when using the ulnar side of the ring finger as the flap.)

4. *Moberg flap (palmar advancement flap).* This flap utilizes the volar skin of a digit (usually the thumb) and advances it, including the

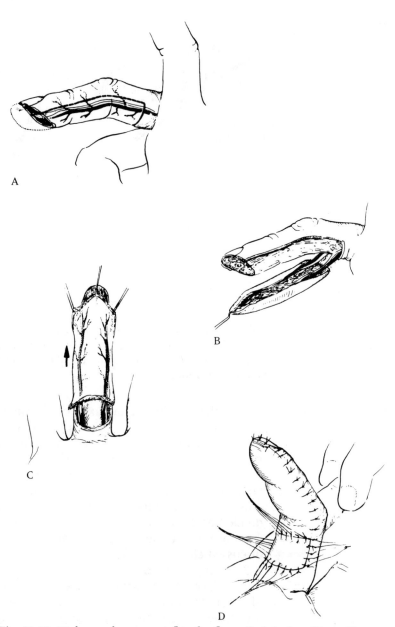

Fig. 11-10. Moberg advancment flap for fingertip injuries. (From R. Chase. *Atlas of Hand Surgery*. Philadelphia: Saunders, 1973. With permission.)

digital arteries and nerves, in the flap. The advancement is usually limited to 1.5 to 2.0 cm; and to obtain this amount of movement one may have to make the flap a true island and skin graft behind it (Fig. 11-10). It is most often used for tip defects of the thumb (see Chapter 5).

5. *Filet flap.* Sometimes a bony hand injury occurs that is not reconstructable, yet some of the soft-tissue envelope is viable. In this

situation one can use the skin as a donor for a full- or partial-thickness skin graft (see Skin Grafts, above) or as an axial pattern flap by removing the bone and leaving the skin covering with its digital artery and nerve (Fig. 11-11). This flap can then be used to resurface other injured areas. It epitomizes one of the dictums of reconstructive surgery, i.e., always think ahead and never waste any resource.

Local Flaps of the Arm

There are two basic flap designs one can employ using arm tissue: fascial (or fasciocutaneous) flaps and muscle (rarely musculocutaneous) flaps. These flap types are axial pattern flaps and are discussed separately below.

Fascial and Fasciocutaneous Flaps. There are two types of arm flap perfused via the fascial blood vessel architecture running in the deep fascia of the arm. The first depends on small, longitudinally oriented vessels that allow flaps with length/width ratios of up 3:1 to be successfully employed. These flaps can be raised on virtually any surface of the upper and lower arm but must include a broad fascial base to maintain perfusion and drainage via unnamed but dependable vessels. Usually the donor site must be skin-grafted (which may be a drawback cosmetically). The versatility of using this system is great, however, and fasciocutaneous units can be raised to cover virtually any defect in the upper forearm and elbow region (see Fig. 11-4).

The other type of fascial vascular pattern flap employs the same small, longitudinally oriented vessels as described above but also utilizes named, deeper situated vessels and fascial septal pathways to perfuse tissue. The well defined architecture of these systems allows more precise identification of pedicle structures, enables island flaps to be elevated, and thus improves the rotational abilities of the flap and its cosmetic inset. These flaps are discussed below.

RADIAL FOREARM FLAP. The radial forearm flap is one of the most versatile and frequently used flaps in arm and hand reconstruction (Fig. 11-12). It can be raised as a fasciocutaneous unit (most often) or as a fascial flap alone without skin. Its vascular pedicle is the radial artery, and it can be elevated with a proximal or distal base (the latter ability depending on the presence of a complete palmar arch as demonstrated by Allen's test) or as a free flap.

To elevate this flap one first outlines the needed tissue over the volar surface of the forearm either proximally (to rotate based on the radial artery at the wrist) or distally (to rotate on the proximal radial artery near its origin from the brachial artery). One first must confirm the patency of the ulnar circulation by performing Allen's test (i.e., sequentially opening and closing the fist compressing both radial and ulnar arteries at the wrist and releasing each artery in turn to check for contribution to the hand circulation). I do not routinely

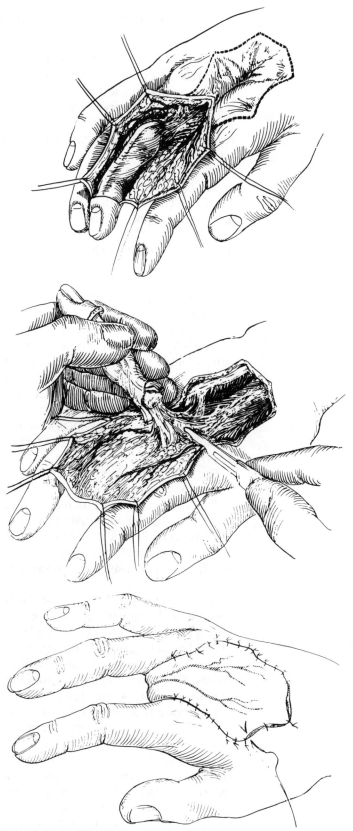

Fig. 11-11. Salvage fillet flap coverage of injured finger. (From R. Chase *Atlas of Hand Surgery*. Philadelphia: Saunders, 1973. With permission.)

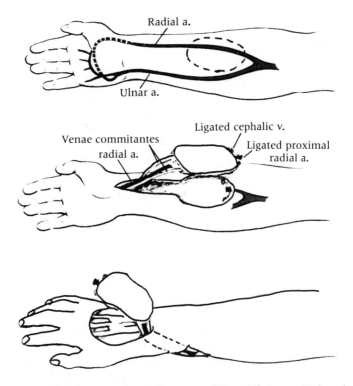

Fig. 11-12. Radial forearm flap. (Courtesy of Dr. Neil Jones, University of Pittsburgh.)

reconstruct the radial artery when there is good ulnar circulation; but if Allen's test suggested poor ulnar flow, a vein graft to reestablish vascular supply to the hand would have to be used. In addition, if the palmar arch is not complete, one cannot safely raise a distally based flap. *Note:* The perforators to the skin and fascia from the radial artery are significantly reduced in number in the proximal forearm compared to the distal forearm.

The flap itself is then incised down to and through the fascial layer, and the flap is then elevated leaving only the paratenon on the volar wrist tendons to support an STSG. I usually begin the elevation on the ulnar side of the arm, and one must be careful when dissecting the radial artery from under the ulnar edge of the brachioradialis muscle not to injure the delicate mesentery of vessels leading up from the artery to the overlying fascial and skin. As noted above, because the proximally situated flaps have fewer perforators present the dissection must be exceptionally delicate when raising a flap in this area. One should also protect any sensory branches of the radial or lateral antebrachial cutaneous nerve encountered (unless they are intentionally to be included in the flap to maintain sensation).

The donor site is then reconstructed by covering exposed tendons and median nerve with adjacent muscle and applying an STSG.

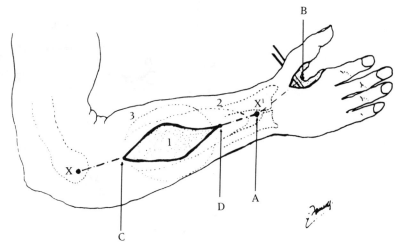

Fig. 11-13. Posterior interosseus flap. (From Zancolli, E. A., and Angrigiani, C. Posterior interossei island forearm flap. *J. Hand Surg.* 13(2):132 1988. With permission.)

Usually I splint the arm to avoid any shearing of the graft from its bed by unwanted hand and arm motion.

This flap is dependable, relatively simple to raise, and can include virtually the entire forearm skin and fascia (with proximal limits as noted above). It thereby provides a good amount of reconstructive tissue for upper arm losses, olecranon and antecubital fossa deficiencies, and forearm and hand reconstruction. Its main drawback is its donor site appearance and possible volar tendon loss if the skin graft does not take (usually because the paratenon was not left over the tendons at harvest).

POSTERIOR INTEROSSEOUS FLAP. The posterior interosseous artery lies in the intermuscular septum between the extensor carpi ulnaris and extensor digiti quinti. It supplies the overlying skin and fascia of the dorsal forearm after branching off the common interosseous artery in the proximal one-third of the forearm. This flap can be used for proximal or distal defects in a manner similar to the radial forearm flap.

To raise this flap one draws a line between the lateral epicondyle and the ulnar head with the forearm pronated (Fig. 11-13) using a point 9 cm distal to the lateral epicondyle as the center point for the flap. After incising the skin and fascia, dissection is carried down between the extensor carpi ulnaris and extensor digiti quinti, being careful to preserve the septum carrying the perforating vessels from the underlying posterior interosseous artery. The flap is raised from the transected end (either distal or proximal) to the pedicle end and can reach as far as the elbow or the level of the MCP joints and first web space. One advantage it has over the radial forearm flap is that this donor site usually can be closed directly, but the amount of transferable tissue is much smaller.

Table 11-2. Regional arterial supply

Artery	Muscle
Posterior humeral circumflex	Coracobrachialis
Profunda brachii	Triceps brachii
	Anconeus
Brachial	Biceps brachii
	Brachialis
Anterior interosseous	Flexor digitorum profundus
	Flexor pollicis longus
	Pronator quadratus
Posterior interosseous	Abductor pollicis longus
	Extensor pollicis brevis
	Extensor pollicis longus
	Extensor indicis proprius
	Extensor digitorum communis
	Extensor carpi ulnaris
Radial recurrent	Brachioradialis
	Extensor carpi radialis longus
	Extensor carpi radialis brevis
Posterior ulnar recurrent	Palmaris longus
	Flexor carpi ulnaris
	Supinator
Anterior ulnar recurrent	Pronator teres
Radial	Flexor carpi radialis
Ulnar	Flexor digitorum superficialis

Source: Parry, S. W. Ward, J. W. and Mathes, S. J. Vascular anatomy of the upper extremity. *Plast. Reconstruct. Surg.* 81:361, 1988. With permission.

RADIAL AND ULNAR RECURRENT FASCIOCUTANEOUS FLAPS. The anatomy of the radial and ulnar recurrent arteries has been delineated and employed to design medial and lateral fasciocutaneous flaps of the lower portion of the upper arm. These flaps are based around the elbow using the radial recurrent (lateral) or ulnar recurrent (medial) arteries as pedicles and can rotate anteriorly to cover the antecubital fossa or posteriorly to cover the olecranon. The donor site can be closed primarily. The method of harvest as described by Hayashi and Maruyama [2] should be reviewed.

REVERSE ULNAR ARTERY FOREARM FLAP. Like the radial forearm flap the skin and fascia of the volar forearm can be raised to a certain degree on the ulnar artery. Use of this flap often requires ulnar artery reconstruction using vein grafts, as it depends on the major artery supplying the hand. It should be used only as a last resort in select cases.

Muscle Flaps. There are many muscles in the arm available for covering arm defects if one considers only the vascular anatomy (Table 11-2). These possibilities are drastically reduced, however, when one recognizes that there is a functional price to pay when using each of these muscles. This price is often considered too high to allow the use of any but a few.

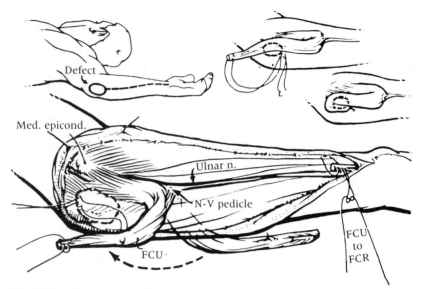

Fig. 11-14. Flexor carpi ulnaris flap. (From J.G. Kenney et al. The "fold back" flexor carpi ulnaris muscle flap for repair of soft tissue. *Contemp. Orthop.* 7:63, 1983. With permission.)

FLEXOR CARPI ULNARIS. The dominant proximal ulnar recurrent vessel blood supply to the flexor carpi ulnaris coupled with its location in the superficial group of volar arm muscles permits this muscle to be used to cover defects about the elbow, antecubital fossa, and upper forearm. It is often used to cover exposed vascular access structures in dialysis patients. It is usually taken without overlying skin and is grafted with an STSG.

It originates with two heads (between which runs the ulnar nerve): one from the common flexor origin of the superficial flexor muscles from the medial epicondyle of the humerus and one from the posterior border of the upper ulna. It inserts into the pisiform bone and surrounding ligaments and is one of the most powerful wrist flexors and adductors, with a work capacity of 2.0 Mkg. This loss must be considered when choosing to use this muscle for arm coverage.

Elevation of this flap (Fig. 11-14) is accomplished using a longitudinally oriented incision on the ulnar side of the volar forearm. The distal tendinous insertion of the muscle is identified and transected, being careful to first identify the underlying ulnar nerve and artery. With careful preservation of this important neurovascular bundle the flexor carpi ulnaris is then elevated from distal to proximal and rotated into the defect. The vascular pedicle consists of the ulnar recurrent vessels from the ulnar artery and enters the radial side of the muscle approximately 5 cm distal to the antecubital fossa, making it the point of rotation. Of note is the fact that this muscle in many patients becomes tendinous well up in the forearm, making the effective mass available for rotation small.

BRACHIORADIALIS. The brachioradialis is the most superficial muscle on the radial side of the forearm and has a dominant proximal pedicle from the radial recurrent vessels, which enter the muscle approximately 5 cm distal to the antecubital fossa. The muscle originates from the supracondylar area of the humerus and inserts into the lower end of the radius; it functions in flexing the arm and placing the arm in the mid-prone position. It has a work capacity of 1.9 Mkg. It is raised from distal to proximal, like the flexor carpi ulnaris flap, being careful to protect the underlying superficial branch of the radial nerve. It is best raised alone and skin-grafted, although there have been reports of using it as a musculocutaneous flap. It can cover defects about the elbow, antecubital fossa, and upper forearm.

ANCONEUS. The anconeus is a small muscle arising from the lateral epicondyle of the humerus and inserting onto the ulna. It has a vascular pedicle from the profunda brachii but is so small that it is useless except for the smallest of elbow defects (which are probably better handled with fasciocutaneous flaps).

Alternative Tissue Sources for Flaps

When tissue available in the upper extremity is not adequate in character or amount for reconstruction, one must resort to tissue expansion or employ distal tissue sources.

Tissue Expansion
As outlined by Van Beek and Adson [3], expansion of skin in the arm and hand has been used but infrequently. Compression of nerves and a significant number of complications, including deflation, expander exposure, and ischemic flaps, have tempered enthusiasm for this reconstructive modality. For selected patients, however, expansion can be a valuable adjunct.

One must avoid damage to major cutaneous nerves during expander placement and avoid positions over areas of potential nerve entrapment. The choice of expander shape, location, and mode of inflation does not differ markedly from expansion in other body areas.

Distal Tissue Sources
Skin grafting is obviously the most commonly used method of transferring tissue from other areas of the body to the upper extremity. Occasionally, however, the reconstructive need demands more than a simple graft, and one must employ distant flap sources, most often as a pedicled flap, which is attached at the first operation and subsequently divided and inset (e.g., groin flap) or as free tissue transfer employing microsurgical techniques.

Pedicled Flaps.

GROIN FLAP. The groin flap is an axial-patterned, fasciocutaneous flap based on the superficial circumflex iliac artery (SCIA), which arises

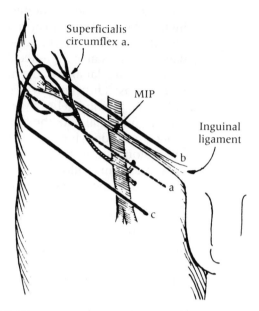

Fig. 11-15. Groin flap. (From P. J. Smith et al. The anatomic basis of the groin flap. *Plast. Reconstr. Surg. 49:41,* 1972. With permission.)

from the common femoral artery just below the inguinal ligament (Fig. 11-15). It then runs parallel to the inguinal ligament and approximately 2 cm below it as it travels to the area of the anterior superior iliac spine (ASIS). It starts out deep to the deep fascia of the thigh but then passes to a plane superficial to the fascia as it travels over the sartorius muscle. At the ASIS the artery arborizes; therefore skin raised beyond this point is considered random in nature.

Designing this flap begins by outlining the needed area of tissue centered around a line drawn 2 cm inferior and parallel to the inguinal ligament. The course of the artery can be checked with a Doppler examination. The flap can extend beyond the ASIS (i.e., into the random area) if the length of this extension is kept equal to the width of the base at the ASIS. The choice of which groin to use depends on the area of the hand to be reconstructed and which orientation allows maximum shoulder motion and pronation/ supination during the 3-week maturation period.

The flap can be raised from distal to proximal or proximal to distal. Raising it from distal to proximal is easier, but going from proximal to distal allows one to visualize the pedicle before incising the flap and thus allows more accurate flap design as there is some aberrency of this vascular system.

To go from distal to proximal, the dissection is started by incising the flap edges through skin, subcutaneous tissue, and superficial fascia. The flap is then elevated at this superficial fascial level heading toward the femoral artery until the lateral edge of the sartorius is reached. Here one must elevate the muscular fascia over the sartorius with the flap to ensure that the artery remains with the flap, as it is this area where the artery passes from below to above the deep fascia. Once the medial edge of the sartorius is reached, the vascular pedicle is usually visible and can be followed to its origin at the femoral vessels.

To raise this flap from proximal to distal, a transverse incision is made between the medial edge of the sartorius muscle and the femoral vessels. The superficial circumflex iliac artery and vein are identified before raising the fasciocutaneous portion of the flap. Usually the medial portion of the flap is then tubed and left in position for 2 weeks, at which time the SCIA is ligated, leaving the skin of the tube intact for another week before final inset and division.

Problems with this flap include the need for two procedures and stiffness that often results from having the patient's arm tethered to the groin for 3 weeks. Furthermore, there is donor site visibility and a general reluctance of most patients to be tethered to the groin for this period of time.

OTHER FLAPS. Other axial-pattern, fasciocutaneous flaps described to provide arm and hand coverage include the *hypogastric flap* based on the vessels, the *deltopectoral flap* based on perforators from the internal mammary artery, and the *Taylor flap* based on periumbilical perforators from the deep epigastric system. In addition, for upper arm problems the *latissimus dorsi* muscle or musculocutaneous flap based on the thoracodorsal artery and the *pectoralis major* muscle flap based on the thoracoacromial artery can provide coverage. Finally, in select circumstances a free vascularized flap of muscle, muscle and skin, or fascia and skin may be needed.

SUMMARY

Soft-tissue deficits of the upper extremity can appear, deceptively, to need only a simple solution. As during a good game of chess, however, the treating physician must be thinking three moves ahead to get the best result for the patient. This chapter has provided a brief outline and guide to choosing the best reconstructive option for many of these commonly treated situations.

REFERENCES

1. Rank, B. K., and Wakefield, A. R. *Surgery of Repair as Applied to Hand Injuries*, (2nd ed.). Edinburgh: Livingstone, 1970.
2. Hayashi, A., and Maruyama, Y. Anatomical study of the recurrent flaps of the upper arm. *Br. J. Plast. Surg.* 43(3):300, 1990.
3. Van Beek, A. L., and Adson, M. H. Tissue expansion in the upper extremity in tissue expansion. L. C. Argenta and E. D. Austad, (Eds.). *Clinics of Plastic Surgery* Philadelphia: Saunders, 1987.

Commentary on Chapter 11

Neil Ford Jones

Although open injuries of the hand are common, actual full-thickness loss of skin occurs much less frequently. However, because of the close proximity of the flexor and extensor tendons and the bones and joints underneath the overlying skin envelope, loss of skin invariably results in exposure of the flexor tendons within the digits, exposure of the extensor tendons over the dorsal aspect of the hand or the digits, and open MCP or interphalangeal joints. Many options are available to provide soft-tissue coverage of the hand, but logical selection depends on several factors, including: (1) the site of the defect; (2) the underlying tissues exposed; (3) the age of the patient; and (4) the necessity for providing sensate skin.

Because skin grafts do not "take" on bare tendon or bone, if the flexor or extensor tendons are exposed, if the metacarpals or phalanges are devoid of periosteum, or if there is an open joint, flap coverage is mandatory. If, however, these structures are not exposed, skin grafts are usually the best option. Generally, split-thickness skin grafts are used on the dorsum of the hand and full-thickness skin grafts over the volar aspect of the digits and the palmar aspect of the hand.

The site of skin loss may be simply classified as: (1) fingertip injuries (see Chapter 5); (2) palmar digital skin loss; (3) dorsal digital skin loss; (4) dorsal aspect of the hand; (5) palmar aspect of the hand; (6) the thumb.

1. *Skin loss over the palmar surface of the digits.* This situation usually leads to exposure of the flexor tendons or an open interphalangeal joint. For small defects at the base of the proximal phalanx, the "flag" flap, based on branches of the dorsal metacarpal arteries, can be transposed through the web space. Random lateral flaps provide coverage of small defects over the palmar aspect of the proximal interphalangeal (PIP) joint. However, the flap of choice for coverage of the flexor tendons or the volar aspect of the PIP joint is the cross-finger flap. Obviously it entails a two-stage procedure with the possible complication of a flexion contracture of the PIP joint of the donor finger and the conspicuous appearance of a skin graft on the donor finger, especially in a woman.

2. *Skin loss over the dorsal aspect of the digits.* These injuries usually result in an open PIP joint or are associated with injuries to the underlying extensor tendon system. Random lateral flaps can occasionally be used for coverage of the PIP joint, but the reversed deepithelialized variant of the cross-finger flap is reliable for dorsal coverage. The flap is deepithelialized and then covered with a split-thickness skin graft. "Flow-through" venous flaps may also be considered in this area. They are small flaps of forearm skin centered over a vein that can be revascularized by microsurgical anastomosis of the vein to a vein on the distal and proximal perimeters of the defect.

3. *Degloving injuries of the dorsal aspect of the hand.* Skin may be completely avulsed from the dorsum of the hand, exposing the underlying extensor tendons, or it may be incompletely detached, resulting in proximal- or distal-based flaps. The vascularity of distal-based flaps is more tenuous than proximal-based flaps; and should either flap be stretched back into its original position, it inevitably results in necrosis of a significant area of the flap. Intravenous fluorescein can sometimes be helpful for delineating the viable portion of these flaps. Alternatively, the flaps can be allowed to adopt their relaxed position so that no tension is placed on the skin edges. The remaining defect can then be skin-grafted.

For dorsal skin avulsions in which the extensor tendons are exposed or those that require secondary extensor tendon grafting, the pedicled groin flap based on the superficial circumflex iliac artery has been the preferred choice. The flap should be defatted primarily and a formal delayed procedure performed at 14 days by ligating the superficial circumflex iliac artery at the base of the pedicle. This maneuver allows the flap to be divided and inset completely at 3 weeks.

Two other excellent choices for coverage of dorsal hand defects are the reverse radial forearm flap and free skin or free fascial flaps. The reverse radial forearm flap supplied by retrograde flow through the radial artery obviously requires an intact palmar arch and is probably contraindicated if there has been concomitant injury to the palmar surface of the hand. The donor defect of the radial forearm flap has been criticized by some surgeons but may be minimized by using a thick sheet of nonmeshed split-thickness skin graft and by immobilizing the wrist and hand to ensure "take" of the graft over the flexor carpi radialis tendon.

The advent of the reverse radial forearm flap and free flaps has eliminated the need for immobilization of the hand in a groin flap for 3 weeks. The latter method is detrimental in elderly patients, as it results in stiffness of the shoulder. Single-stage coverage of dorsal defects of the hand using a free flap may therefore be advantageous in such patients but obviously requires microsurgical expertise.

If the skin over the lateral aspect of the upper arm is thin, the ipsilateral free lateral arm flap based on the posterior radial collateral artery is one of the two preferred donor flaps. The other alternative is the free temporoparietal fascial flap, which is a thin sheet of fascia underneath the scalp based on the superficial temporal artery, which then requires coverage with a thick split-thickness skin graft. The free temporoparietal fascial flap allows simultaneous extensor tendon grafting with reconstruction of the soft tissue defect.

4. *Degloving injuries of the palmar surface of the hand.* The skin of the palmar surface of the hand is much thicker than the dorsal aspect of the hand, and the flexor tendons are better protected by the palmar fascia and the bulk of the thenar and hypothenar muscles. For these two reasons, full-thickness skin defects of the palm may be amenable to coverage with a split-thickness or full-thickness graft. With exposure of the flexor tendons in the distal palm or at the level of the carpal tunnel, flap coverage becomes necessary, and the best options are similar to those discussed for dorsal hand defects, that is the groin flap, reverse radial forearm flap, free lateral arm flap, or free temporoparietal fascial flap.

5. *Soft-tissue coverage of the thumb.* With full-thickness loss of volar skin over the distal phalanx of the thumb, every effort should be made to replace it with sensate skin to preserve the critical function of the thumb in pulp pinch and key pinch. The Moberg advancement flap should be considered for tip amputations of the thumb, as advancement of sensate skin based on the two neurovascular bundles can be accomplished with slight flexion of the interphalangeal joint. With more extensive defects of the volar surface of the distal phalanx, sensate skin can be provided either by an innervated cross-finger flap from the index finger or by a neurovascular island pedicle flap from the dorsal aspect of the proximal phalanx of the index finger based on the first dorsal metacarpal artery. With the conventional cross-finger flap, sensation is provided by a branch of the superficial radial nerve. Occasionally, dual innervation can be provided by incorporating the dorsal branch of the radial digital nerve of the index finger. When the cross-finger flap is transposed, this dorsal branch of the radial digital nerve is sutured to the stump of the ulnar digital nerve of the thumb. The obvious disadvantage of the cross-finger flap is the necessity for a secondary division of the flap. Consequently, the advantage of the first dorsal metacarpal artery island flap is that it is a single-stage procedure.

For extensive degloving injuries of the thumb, the standard technique used to be a pedicled groin flap followed by a second stage neurovascular island flap from the ulnar aspect of the middle or ring fingers. It is now being superseded by two microvascular free flaps based on the big toe. The Morrison "wrap-around" flap may be used acutely or semiacutely for degloving injuries of the thumb in which the proximal and distal phalanges and the flexor and extensor tendons are preserved. A free first web space neurosensory flap incorporating skin from the lateral aspect of the big toe innervated by the lateral digital nerve can be considered for secondary reconstruction, especially for defects involving the important ulnar aspect of the thumb.

12 ACUTE INFECTIONS OF THE UPPER EXTREMITY

Richard J. Greco

Infections in the hand and upper extremity are common, and until the advent of antibiotics they were often devastating to limb function and were life-threatening. The first major textbook of hand surgery was written by Allen Kanavel of Chicago in 1912 and dealt exclusively with infections of the hand. The expectations in the treatment of severe hand infections have shifted from simple resolution of the infection to resolution of the infection with minimal residual functional deficit.

This chapter deals only with the more common acute infections of the hand. It stresses the diagnosis of these problems and the timing and need for operative intervention when appropriate, and it warns against sole reliance on antibiotics, which is often detrimental to the patient.

ANATOMY

The anatomic limits of the pulp are the distal interphalangeal (DIP) joint crease proximally, the edge of the nail distally, the junction of the volar and dorsal skin laterally, and the distal phalanx dorsally (Fig. 12-1). The pulp is rounded in all directions, and the overlying skin is supple but firmly attached to the distal phalanx by fibrous cones. The nail provides a solid support where the distal phalanx ends. True Cooper's ligaments, disposed radially, divide the fatty panniculus into compartments.

The dorsum of the fingertip is composed of the nail, nail bed, and perionychium (Fig,. 12-2). The proximal nail plate fits into a depression called the nail fold. This fold is separated into the dorsal roof and the ventral roof by the nail. All of the soft tissue underneath the nail that is responsible for nail generation and migration is called the nail matrix. The cuticle or eponychium is the thin membrane extending from the skin overlying the nail onto the dorsum of the nail. This area surrounds the lateral and proximal portions of the nail. The hyponychium is the thickened skin underneath the distal nail.

The tendon sheath is discussed in detail in Chapter 8. Lining the fibrosseous tunnel is a synovial sheath with a visceral and a parietal

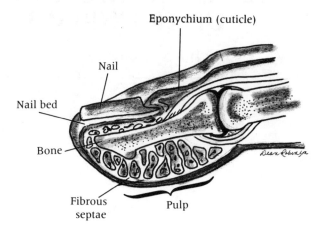

Fig. 12-1. Anatomy of distal fingertip. Note that the distal pulp is separated into compartments by the septal bands.

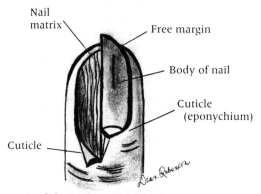

Fig. 12-2. Anatomy of the nail and nail bed.

layer. There is a space between these layers in which lubricating synovial fluid exists. The sheaths extend from the DIP joint to the metacarpolphalangeal (MCP) joint in the index, middle, and ring fingers. The thumb has a sheath from the interphalangeal joint through a radial bursa into the distal forearm surrounding the flexor pollicis longus. The little finger's synovial sheath extends from the distal phalangeal joint into a large ulnar bursa, which surrounds the superficial and profundus tendons of all four digits from the mid-palm proximally to the proximal margin of the pronator quadratus (Fig. 12-3). In nearly 85 percent of the patients there are interconnections between the radial and ulnar bursae in the palm.

Two important deep spaces of the palm may become infected. The thenar space is a potential space anterior to the adductor muscle and directly underneath the flexor tendon of the index finger. Its ulnar border is separated from the midpalm space by fascia arising from the metacarpal of the long finger and attaching to the palmar fascia called the mid-palmar ligament. The mid-palm space is the potential

Synovial Sheaths

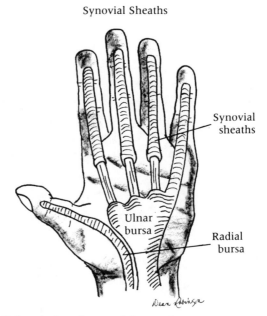

Fig. 12-3. Radial and ulnar bursa of the tendons.

space anterior to the fascia covering the third, fourth, and fifth metacarpals and their intervening interosseous muscles and deep to the flexor tendons of the long, ring, and little fingers (Fig. 12-4). Its medial border is the mid-palmer ligament attached to the metacarpal of the long finger.

EVALUATION

Patients with upper extremity infections may have a localized process or systemic manifestations. It is important to evaluate patients' overall health when evaluating them for treatment.

One should attempt to identify the probable source of contamination. A large number of varied organisms can cause infection of the hands and can penetrate the protective integument in a number of ways. Often a history of inadvertent skin puncture, animal or human bites, crush injury, prosthetic joint implants, systemic sepsis, needle injections, or traumatic lacerations can be obtained. The mode of inoculation is important in order to determine the most probable organism and the best empiric therapy.

After a thorough history of the mechanism of injury is obtained, the subsequent course of events should be detailed. How long ago did the injury occur? What types of treatment have been administered thus far? Does the patient have a fever, chills, or other systemic symptoms? Patients with a history of intravenous drug abuse should be questioned about their needle-sharing practices and history of hepatitis or AIDS. Chronic diseases such as diabetes, cancer, vascular disorders, and immunologic incompetence should be elicited.

Physical examination is performed, and often the classic signs of

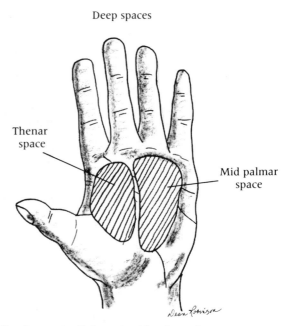

Deep spaces

Thenar
space

Mid palmar
space

Fig. 12-4. The thenar (radial) and mid-palm (ulnar) spaces often become infected.

infection — erythema, tenderness, swelling, and warmth — are present. Because of the relatively loose attachment of the dorsal skin and superficial fasica to the underlying structures and deep fascia, a potential space is present that can accumulate significant amounts of lymphedema. Therefore, despite the fact that the dorsum of the hand may not be involved in the infectious process, it is the location of the most prominent swelling.

Erythematous streaking up the arm, lymphangitis, is a significant sign of invasive infection, and palpation of the involved area may detect an area of fluctuance. Axillary lymph adenopathy is not uncommon with significant hand infections.

Most patients should have radiographic evaluation of the involved areas looking for foreign bodies or evidence of osteomyelitis in subacute wounds. This evaluation is not necessary in patients with acute paronychia.

It should be remembered that the flexion creases of the finger are almost directly contiguous with the tendon sheaths, and there is little subcutaneous tissue at these levels. Minor wounds in these areas have a significant potential for penetrating the tendon sheath and creating a purulent tenosynovitis.

The "cardinal signs" of acute suppurative tenosynovitis are the same as those described by Kanavel in 1912: flexed position of the finger, symmetric enlargement of the entire finger, excessive tenderness over and limited to the entire course of the flexor sheath of the involved digit, and severe pain created by passively extending the finger. The pain, most markedly felt in the proximal portion of the sheath, may be the earliest and most important sign of early purulent tenosynovitis.

The differential diagnosis of early tenosynovitis versus local cellulitis caused by an injury or animal bite is often difficult. Two helpful tips are useful here.

1. When a process involves the finger and it is swollen and painful, any motion including passive extension is painful. (1) The examiner's thumb nail is interlocked with the nail of the involved finger, after which the patient is asked to attempt to flex his or her finger against the resistance of the examiner's thumb nail. If the maneuver causes severe pain, the finger flexion test is positive. (2) The examiner can support the dorsal proximal phalanx from hyperextension with one hand while extending the involved finger with the interlocked nails. If this maneuver creates significant pain the passive extension test is positive.
2. If tenosynovitis is present, the entire flexor sheath should be infected and inflamed, pain should be elicited when pressing down on the A-1 pulley region (at the level of the MCP joint). If this area is not tender, the process is more likely to be a local process limited to the soft tissues of the finger.

ACUTE PRECAUTIONS

The medical personnel caring for patients with infections anywhere in the body should take special precautions when examining the patient, performing any procedures, and effecting dressing changes. Each patient should be treated with the same precautions. The risk of a concomitant disease, e.g., AIDS or hepatitis, is particularly a problem in intravenous drug abuse patients.

Tetanus prophylaxis should be verified, and it is important to obtain an accurate drug allergy history because of the likelihood of treating this patient with antibiotics. Any jewelry on the involved hand should be removed because of possible vascular compromise as the extremity becomes more edematous.

When operative procedures are necessary, they should be performed with adequate anesthesia and good facilities. Regional anesthesia can be used only in areas proximal to any area of infection. Axillary blocks should not be used in patients with lymphangitic spread up into the arm. Tourniquets can be used, but an Esmarch wrap should not. The tight wrapping increases the possibility of spreading infection proximally.

TREATMENT

The first therapeutic decisions confronting the physician are whether the patient requires hospitalization or outpatient therapy and if operative drainage is indicated at this time.

1. After appropriate cultures are obtained (if possible), empiric systemic antibiotics in appropriate dosage are administered. The

empiric therapy is based on the most likely organism. Actual tissue specimens from necrotic or nonvital tissues should be obtained, if possible, and sent to the laboratory for aerobic and anaerobic cultures. Results from specimens are more accurate than those from swabs and should be the basis for continued antibiotic therapy (see Empiric Therapy below).

2. Elevation of the affected part decreases the edema and helps to decrease the eventual stiffness of the part.

3. Immobilization in the position of safety is important during the acute phase (see Chapter 19). As the infection resolves, early mobilization is important to decrease the loss of hand function.

4. The use of water or saline soaks is controversial. Xenon flow studies performed by Gahhos and Aryiyan [1] showed a 50 percent decrease of blood flow to an infected hand after warm soaks. Others believe that in many patients warm soaks lead to complacency and needless delay in operative drainage. In my experience, the warm soaks are soothing to the patient and may indeed help the spontaneous drainage of paronychia. They are also useful for mobilizing the hand as the infection resolves.

EMPIRIC THERAPY Most infections of the upper extremity are caused by penetration of the skin. Virtually any organism can cause infection of the hand, but 65 percent are caused by *Staphylococcus aureus* and 15 percent by β-hemolytic streptococci. Empiric therapy therefore must be aimed at methacillin-resistant *S. aureus* and any other common potential organism based on the nature of the injury and the patient's general health (discussed below). Tetanus prophylaxis should be ensured for all injuries.

Hand injuries caused by a *human bite* may be caused by mixed organisms in up to 70 percent of the patients. *Staphylococcus, Streptococcus, Eikenella corrodens* (anaerobic gram-negative rod), and anaerobic bacteria are frequently found. *Eikenella* is sensitive to penicillin but not to synthetic penicillins or first generation cephalosporins. The use of a combination of penicillin and a synthetic penicillinase-resistant penicillin (i.e., dicloxacillin), penicillin plus a cephalosporin, or second or third generation cephalosporin with anaerobic coverage (i.e., cefoxitin or piperacillin) are recommended empiric therapy for human bites (Table 12-1).

Dog bites are covered adequately by dicloxacillin or cephalexin. Erythromycin is adequate if the patient is penicillin-allergic. *Pasteurella multocida* is found in up to 50 to 70 percent of the wounds caused by *cat bites* and is best covered with dicloxacillin. Dicloxacillin is preferred to cloxacillin and oxacillin because it produces higher serum levels and is the least expensive effective antibiotic. Oral second generation cephalosporins, cephalexin, or cefuroxime can also be used. If the patient has an allergy to penicillin, erythromycin can be given. If erythromycin is ineffective and the culture grows *Pasteurella,* tetracycline is a good alternative antibiotic.

Table 12-1. Empiric therapy

Mode of injury	Likely organism	Empiric antibiotics
Industrial accident	*Staphylococcus, Streptococcus*	Discloxacillin; Cipro or Keflex; erythromycin
Human bites	*Staphylococcus, Streptococcus, Eikenella*	Penicillin + dicloxacillin; penicillin + cephalosporin; 2nd or 3rd generation cephalosporin; penicillin (all) + tetracycline
Cat bites	*Pasteurella*	Penicillin or dicloxacillin; penicillin (all); erythromycin; if erythromycin fails, tetracycline
Dog bites	Mixed	Dicloxacillin; cephlexin; penicillin (all); erythromycin
Intravenous drug abuse Proximal to wrist	*Staphylococcus,* gram-neg. rods + *Pseudomonas*	Vancomycin/ aminoglycoside; 3rd generation cephalosporin
Distal to wrist	*Staphylococcus/ Streptococcus,* anaerobes	Vancomycin/ clindamycin; 3rd generation cephalosporin
Diabetes	Gram-neg. rods	Aminoglycoside; 3rd generation cephalosporin; Cipro

Diabetic patients frequently have gram-negative organisms as the infecting agent. They should be treated by a parenteral aminoglycoside, cefoxitin, or a third generation cephalosporin. Cipro, as an oral agent, is theoretically an excellent choice, but clinical studies are pending.

Farm injury wounds contain mixed gram-positive and gram-negative organisms in more than 80 percent of the cultures obtained. Appropriate wound débridement is the first line of therapy, and antibiotic prophylaxis is controversial. If prophylaxis is chosen, a new third generation cephalosporin and an aminoglycoside or the standard triple antibiotic regiment (ampicillin/clindamycin/aminoglycoside) are required.

Intravenous drug abusers have a high propensity for gram-negative and anaerobic organisms. Smith et al [2]. showed that anaerobes were more frequently found in the hand and enteric gram-negative bacilli and *Pseudomonas* in the upper extremity. Vancomycin and clindamycin or a third generation cephalosporin with adequate anaerobic coverage would be appropriate for distal infections; and vancomycin and an aminoglycoside or a third generation cephalosporin with adequate *Pseudomonas* coverage would be appropriate empiric therapy for proximal extremity infections in this group of patients.

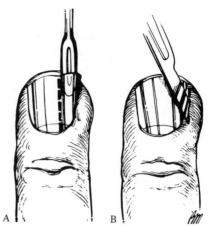

Fig. 12-5. A. Elevation and removal of one-fourth of the nail to decompress the perionychium. B. Incision of the perionychial fold with the blade directed away from the nail bed. (From R. J. Neviaser. Infections. In D. Green, ed., *Operative Hand Surgery,* 2nd ed. New York: Churchill Livingstone, 1988. With permission.)

SPECIFIC HAND INFECTIONS
Paronychia

A paronychia is an infection of the soft tissue around the fingernail that usually begins as a "hangnail." It spreads around the nail eponychium — thus the term "run around." It is red, swollen, and painful, with purulent drainage around the margin. The pain is usually described as throbbing and frequently prevents sleep. One must establish by palpation and physical examination if an abscess is located in the eponychial fold and if there is a subungual component of infection. The nail usually separates easily from the nail bed at the level of the hyponychium when a subungual abscess is present.

Paronychia make up approximately 30 percent of the infections seen in the upper extremity. The infection usually starts as cellulitis and progresses to a subcutaneous abscess if untreated. The offending organism is typically *Staphyloccocus aureus,* but there may be a mixed flora.

Treatment during the early stages consists in soaks in warm saline and pHisoDerm (30 minutes six times a day), oral antibiotics with *Staphylococcus* coverage, rest of the affected finger, and close supervision. Elevation of the eponychial fold may allow spontaneous drainage of superficial collections. Small, superficial abscesses can be drained without anesthesia: The thin layer of skin over the abscess is opened with a sharp blade or the sharp edge of an 18-gauge needle directed away from the nail bed and matrix.

Larger, more extensive lesions require digital block anesthesia with plain lidocaine at the metacarpal level. If the paronychial fold and the adjacent eponychium are involved, one-third of the nail is separated from the nail bed with a flat Freer elevator on the appropriate side. This portion of the nail is then excised with sharp-pointed scissors (Fig. 12-5). If this measure does not allow

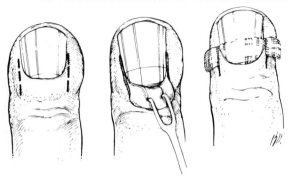

Fig. 12-6. Incisions and elevation of the entire eponychial fold with excision of the proximal one-third of the nail. Gauze helps prevent immature dihiscence of the repair. (From R. J. Neviaser. Infections. In D. Green, ed., *Operative Hand Surgery*, 2nd ed. New York: Churchill Livingstone, 1988. With permission.)

drainage of the collection, an incision is made in the eponychial fold with a No. 11 blade. Care is taken not to injure the nail matrix and bed. The area is irrigated, Xeroform gauze is placed to keep the nail bed covered and the skin edges open, and warm soaks are continued. Antibiotics are not necessary if significant cellulitis is not present.

If the entire eponychium and lateral fold are involved the lesion is called an *eponychia*. This problem is usually associated with a collection under the lunula. It is not necessary to remove the entire nail, and one can attempt to elevate the dorsal roof of the nail fold off the nail and excise the proximal one-third of the nail without a perionychial fold incision. If it is not possible, a single or double incision at the corners of the fold proximally can be made for better exposure of the proximal nail plate (Fig. 12-6). Xeroform gauze is placed under the fold, and soaks are begun. The gauze is removed at 48 hours.

Felon (Pulp Abscess)

A felon is a deep infection of the pulp space. It involves multiple compartments separated by fibrous septae. The anatomic limits of the pulp space are the DIP joint crease proximally, the edge of the nail distally, the junction of the volar and dorsal skin laterally, and the distal phalanx dorsally (Fig. 12-1).

The distal segment is red, swollen, and painful. The patient complains of severe throbbing pain, and the finger pad is tender. Frequently a history of a puncture injury to the finger pad can be elicited. Because of the unyielding character of the pulp space, venous congestion and subsequent vascular compromise can lead to necrosis of the pulp of the finger and even osteomyelitis. The center of the fat pad offers the least resistance to the infectious process. The infecting organism is usually a *Staphylococcus* and can involve the distal phalanx with osteomyelitis, septic arthritis, or tenosynovitis if there is no spontaneous or operative drainage.

If the lesion is found in the early stages consisting of cellulitis only, appropriate parenteral antibiotic coverage for *Staphylococcus* and

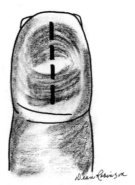

Fig. 12-7. Preferred incision for drainage of pulp space infection.

Streptococcus organisms, elevation, immobilization, and close observation every 4 to 6 hours may be adequate therapy. If there is any evidence of fluctuance, if the process has been present for 48 hours or longer, or if the patient has not responded to 24 hours of conservative therapy, a direct operative approach, as recommended by Bailey[3], is utilized for drainage.

The lesion should be drained in an adequately equipped operating room with anesthesia and a tourniquet. The incision is made in a vertical direction at the site of maximum tenderness (Fig. 12-7). This incision may vary from a central pulp to a mid-lateral incision depending on the site of maximum fluctuance. Contrary to previous teaching, these pulp drainage incisions are not usually painful. All fibrous septae must be divided to ensure adequate drainage. Skin hook retraction reveals the slough, which should be sharply débrided. A Xeroform gauze is placed in the wound as a wick catheter, and soaks are begun. Fishmouth and through-and-through mid-lateral incisions should be avoided because they often lead to skin slough, decreased finger pad sensation, unstable fat pad, unsightly scars, and long-term pulp pain.

The wound is allowed to heal by secondary intention, and the packing is slowly removed. Postoperative elevation and early motion during soaks are encouraged. Intravenous antibiotics are continued until the surrounding cellulitis resolves.

Aseptic Felon

Herpetic whitlow is a viral infection of the distal phalanx and is commonly found in medical and dental workers. The lesion is caused by the herpes simplex virus and has a self-limited course. The clinical symptoms are similar to those of a purulent felon, but the treatment is different. The clinical picture differs from a felon in the following ways.

1. The involved digit is painful and then becomes erythematous. Patients appear more comfortable with this lesion than one would anticipate by the serious appearance of the digit. This observation alone should make one suspicious of a viral etiology.

2. Tenderness is present but is markedly less than with a felon.
3. Multiple, small vesicles appear early and may coalesce to form bullae. The fluid in the bullae is clear, not purulent. These lesions become encrusted and desquamate.
4. The herpetic lesion is self-limited, and the treatment is therefore expectant. Complete resolution can be expected within 3 weeks. Inappropriate incision and drainage are not productive and may lead to secondary infection, osteomyelitis, or prolonged, disabling fingertip problems.

If the diagnosis is uncertain, one can remove the vesicles by sharp dissection. One should take care not to penetrate the subcutaneous tissues. If clear fluid is found, a viral infection may be assumed and a nonoperative course taken. If purulent fluid is found, the lesion is treated as a felon.

Purulent Tenosynovitis

Purulent infections of the tendon sheath have been, and still are, the most feared infection of the hand. The infectious process destroys the gliding mechanism, creates significant adhesions that limit motion, and may even lead to tendon necrosis. *Streptococcus* and *Staphylococcus* are the most common infecting organisms.

The "cardinal signs" of acute suppurative tenosynovitis are the same as those described by Kanavel in 1912.

1. Flexed position of the finger.
2. Symmetric enlargement of the entire finger.
3. Excessive tenderness over and limited to the entire course of the flexor sheath of the involved digit.
4. Severe pain created by passively extending the finger and felt most markedly in the proximal portion of the sheath. Such pain may be the earliest and most important sign on which to base the diagnosis of purulent tenosynovitis.

The clinical diagnosis is based on these factors and positive findings on the finger flexion test, passive extension test, or A-1 pulley tenderness as described in the Evaluation section, above. If the tendon sheath of the little finger or thumb is involved, the infection may spread into the wrist through the respective bursa. If the bursae communicate, the classic "horseshoe" infection may develop. Untreated purulent tenosynovitis spreads from the index finger into the thenar space, from the middle finger into either the thenar or mid-palmar space, and from the ring finger into the mid-palmar space.

If the process is seen within the first 24 to 48 hours or if a definitive diagnosis is not possible, conservative treatment is undertaken, with observation and evaluations at least twice a day, looking for either progression of the process or its resolution. It is possible to abort the infectious process by elevating the finger, immobilizing it in the

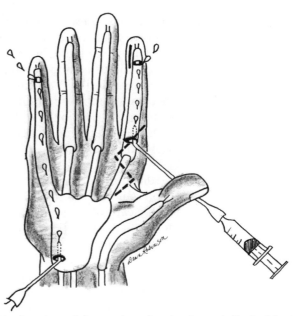

Fig. 12-8. Exploration of the tendon sheaths through limited incisions and copious irrigation.

position of safety, use of empiric parenteral antibiotics, and close observation. Any signs of progression should lead to operative drainage and irrigation.

Many combinations of incisions have been described for draining and irrigating the flexor sheath. An incision at the level of the distal palmar crease for access to the proximal end of the sheath plus a transverse incision at the DIP crease for access to the distal sheath have been the most beneficial for the index, middle, and long fingers (Fig. 12-8). Proximally, a soft rubber 16-gauge catheter is inserted into the flexor sheath and secured, with care taken not to injure the A-1 pulley. The tendon sheath is cultured and then irrigated copiously with saline until no more pus is encountered, after which antibiotic solution is instilled. Although it is unusual, the tendons may be necrotic and require débridement to resolve the infection.

Distally, a rubber drain is placed for efferent drainage and secured. The wounds can be loosely closed around the drain and catheter. Postoperatively, the sheath can be irrigated continuously (60 ml per hour) with antibiotic solution or saline or gently flushed with 50 ml every 2 hours for 24 to 48 hours.

When the signs of infection have resolved, the catheter and drain are removed and the patient is started on a range of motion program. With these limited incisions, compared to a completely open exposure technique, the long-term disability of healing by secondary intention is avoided and earlier rehabilitation efforts are possible.

In the thumb, the proximal exposure is created by an incision at the thenar crease. The distal 1 cm of the carpal ligament is incised to gain exposure to the flexor pollicis longus before entrance into the thenar eminence. The catheter is placed in this sheath.

The proximal portion of the radial and ulnar bursae need to be irrigated when the thumb or little fingers, respectively, are involved. If they are involved, an irrigation catheter can be left in through the palm exposure and directed toward drains in the proximal bursa. The ulnar bursa can be exposed through an incision in the volar forearm just radial to the flexor carpi ulnaris. The ulnar artery and nerve are retracted ulnarly and the flexor tendons radially to expose the ulnar bursa. The radial bursa is exposed just ulnar to the flexor carpi radialis tendon. After the bursa is irrigated thoroughly, a rubber drain is brought out through the bursa and secured. Postoperatively, the catheters are irrigated until the infection has resolved. They are subsequently removed, and range of motion exercises are begun.

It should be remembered that the flexion creases of the finger are almost directly contiguous with the tendon sheaths. There is little subcutaneous tissue at these levels, and any minor wound in these areas has a significant potential of penetrating the tendon sheath and creating a purulent tenosynovitis.

Palmar Space Infections

Mid-palm and thenar space infections are not common. When they do occur, the dorsum may be much more swollen than the palm of the hand. The usual findings of redness, tenderness, and fluctuance help define the abscess.

Mid-palm space infections present with throbbing pain in the palm, dorsal edema, swelling of the palm, and inability to use the middle, ring, little, and sometimes index fingers. Three areas may be involved: pretendinous space, ulnar bursa, and mid-palmar space. The approach to the central palm is through an incision parallel to the palmar crease. Care must be taken to avoid damage to the digital nerves and vessels (Fig. 12-9).

Thenar web space infections present as an inflammatory process in the web space of the thumb. The thumb is held in an adducted position, and the web space is swollen and tender. This compartment is best approached through a dorsal incision parallel to the anterior border of the second metacarpal (Fig. 12-10). The space is entered between the first dorsal interosseous and the adductor pollicis to drain the thenar space, thereby avoiding a possible sensitive palmar incision. Occasionally, a second volar incision is made parallel to the thenar crease when required to further drain the space.

Human Bite Infections

Human bites commonly occur over the dorsum of the MCP joints. They are typically the result of the "knuckle" area striking a tooth during a fight. The patient, because of ignorance or embarrassment, may consciously or unconsciously attempt to misinform the examiner as to the nature of the injury. The important point is that the wound may appear benign initially but is usually inoculated with a potent mixture of bacterial flora. Radiographic evaluation (antero-

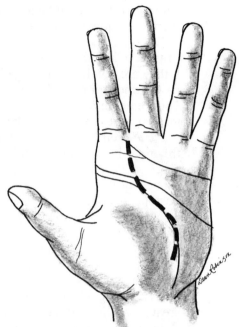

Fig. 12-9. Incision for drainage of a mid-palm collection.

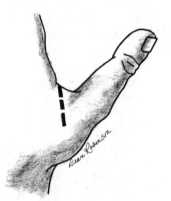

Fig. 12-10. Incision for drainage of a thenar space infection.

posterior, lateral, and steep oblique views) is valuable for signs of joint penetration, fractures, and foreign bodies.

If the wound is examined less than 24 hours after the injury and local exploration finds the extensor tendon intact, the wound is copiously irrigated, a culture obtained, and the wound left open. These patients may be treated as outpatients only if they are deemed totally reliable. The wound should be reexamined daily for 5 days. This injury is serious and may require extension of the laceration in order to evaluate the underlying extensor tendon and joint capsule.

When there is evidence of extensor tendon perforation without extensor lag or radiographic evidence of a fracture or foreign body, the patient is admitted to the hospital and started on empiric intravenous antibiotic therapy. The patient's wound is reevaluated every 6 to 8 hours. If local cellulitis persists, operative exploration is undertaken.

If the wound was initially untreated and subsequent purulent infection occurs, the patient should undergo immediate operative exploration, irrigation, and débridement. A soft drain should be left for 48 hours and the patient kept immobilized. Continuous irrigation of the wound can be utilized if a significant collection is drained.

Although it is not proved, Callaham [4] recommended that *bite wounds inflicted by human immunodeficiency (HIV)-positive assailants* be thoroughly irrigated with povidone-iodine because of its viricidal properties. Typically, there are antibodies to the virus in the HIV assailant's saliva, but the infectious nature is undocumented. A baseline and 6-month follow-up HIV titer should be ordered for medicolegal purposes.

REFERENCES

1. Gahhos, E. N., Cariles, V. J., Arygan, S., and Arons, M. S. Effects of local heat on blood flow in infected and normal hands. *Plast. Reconstr. Surg.*
2. Smith, D. J., Busuito, Mc. J., Velanovich, V., Spotts, J., Haggers, J. H., and Robson, M. Drug injection injuries of the upper extremity. *Ann. Plast. Surg.* 22:1, 1989.
3. Bailey, D. *The Infected Hand* London: Lewis, 1963.
4. Callaham, M. Controversies in antibiotic choices for bite wounds. *Ann. Emerg. Med.* 17:12, 1988.

Commentary on Chapter 12

Mary H. McGrath

A review of the incidence of acute hand infections highlights four infectious processes: Cellulitis, lymphangitis, nail fold infections (e.g., paronychia, eponychia), and subcutaneous infections (e.g., localized abscesses). These four account for more than 90 percent of all hand infections, comprise almost all infections treated on an outpatient basis, and make up over 50 percent of cases of hand infections requiring hospitalization for treatment [1]. Mainstays in the management of these infections are immobilization, elevation, antibiotics, and selective use of surgical drainage.

1. *Immobilization and elevation.* The purpose of immobilizing the infected hand is twofold: to prevent dissemination of infection by muscular action and to splint the hand in a moderate intrinsic-plus position to help prevent secondary joint contractures. A bulky or well padded dressing incorporating plaster should immobilize the hand in the position of "safety," which is 30 to 50 degrees of extension at the wrist joint, 50 to 90 degrees of flexion of the MCP joints, 0 to 10 degrees of flexion at the interphalangeal joints, and the thumb maximally abducted palmar to the line of the index metacarpal. A long arm cast may be needed to keep the arm at rest in children or uncooperative adults, but the dressing must be removable to inspect the hand at intervals, particularly to monitor swelling.

Elevation of the hand above heart level is critical for gaining control of the edema and swelling, which compromise venous return and contribute to early ischemia and late stiffness of the infected hand. In the hand, tissue reaction and swelling cause early venous and lymphatic congestion and local arterial insufficiency. Tissue tension quickly becomes crucial as tissue necrosis results from microvascular thrombosis. The newly devitalized tissue further promotes infection, whereas measures that improve circulation hasten resolution of the infection: hence the emphasis on elevating the infected extremity to improve venous return and the avoidance of constricting dressings.

Good drainage is obtained in the supine patient with the hand and forearm supported on pillows. Some manufacture a sling with stockinette, pins, and tape for suspending the arm from a bedside pole, but judgment is required here because some patients cannot maintain such a sling properly, and suspension with a potential noose that may become constricting is not advisable.

2. *Antibiotics.* Antimicrobial therapy is part of the treatment of established hand infections, and appropriate antibiotic selection must be based on the results of wound culture and sensitivity testing. Unfortunately, the treating surgeon may not yet have this bacteriologic data on hand at the time antibiotic treatment must be initiated. It is in this setting that information about the usual causative organisms is helpful for guiding antibiotic choice. Fortunately, it does not require as much information as it did several years ago, and antibiotic selection has actually become less complex.

Studies suggest that aerobic gram-positive, aerobic gram-negative, and anaerobic organisms in a mixed flora are cultured in a significant number of hand infections, particularly those caused by human and animal bites, and that a broad-spectrum second generation cephalosporin is a good choice for initial empiric therapy.

Prior to the availability of penicillin, the microorganism most feared in hand infections was the rapidly spreading β-hemolytic streptococcus. When it proved highly vulnerable to antibiotics, its preeminent place was taken by *Staphylococcus aureus,* the most common pathogen isolated in hand infections. By 1970 it was clear that much of the community-acquired *S. aureus* had become penicillin-resistant and from these findings came the recommendation for a penicillinase-resistant penicillin, such as nafcillin, for the treatment of hand infections. For some 10 years or more, a standard empiric antibiotic used while awaiting culture results was nafcillin or a first generation cephalosporin such as cephalothin or cefazolin.

With improved culture techniques and increased awareness of the pathogenicity of anerobic organisms, a clearer picture of the bacterial spectrum in hand infections began to emerge during the 1980s. Anaerobes had been cultured in as many as 60 percent of a small series of cases of clenched-fist injuries [2]. A subsequent prospective study of 200 established hand infections showed that 74 percent of the patients grew aerobes, most commonly *S. aureus* (35 percent) and *Streptococcus viridans* (29 percent), but that 26 percent of the patients grew anaerobes, most often *Bacteroides melaninogenicus* (10 percent) and *Peptostreptococcus anaerobius* (6 percent). There was a strong relation between human bite wounds and the presence of anaerobes. More than 60 percent of the patients grew multiple organisms, and 95 percent of the organisms were sensitive to cefamandole, a second generation broad-spectrum cephalosporin effective against both aerobes and anaerobes [1]. A second study appearing at the same time had an even larger proportion of infections due to anaerobes (42 percent), with 21 percent of the patients growing *P. anaerobius.* Among the 58 percent with aerobic infections, *S. aureus* (21 percent) and *Streptococcus viridans* (19 percent) remained the most common organisms. A mixed flora was cultured in 33 percent of the patients, and cefamandole was effica-cious in all but one case [3].

In wounds from animal sources, *Pasteurella multocida* is frequently encountered and has been the focus of attention particularly in cat bites. However, as with human bites, the incidence of anaerobes in animal bites is proving to be as high as 75 percent of cases and a broad-spectrum antibiotic such as cefamandole is recommended for initial empiric antibiotic therapy [3].

3. *Surgical management.* Surgery may be undertaken for several reasons: therapeutic evacuation of pus; therapeutic relief of tissue tension or decompression to abort a peripheral neuropathy; and diagnostic recovery of an organism. As a broad generalization, cellulitis and lymphangitis are treated nonsurgically with elevation, immobilization, and antibiotics, whereas almost all other acute infections in the hand require surgical treatment.

Severe hand infections remain relatively uncommon, but surpris-ingly the incidence has not changed dramatically since the 1940s. It is curious that the increasingly sophisticated culturing techniques and more recently available antibiotics have not had more impact on the overall incidence of serious hand infections. It has been suggested that an overreliance on antibiotics and the emergence of resistant organisms may be contributing factors to maintaining this stable population of patients. Perhaps the continuing growth in the pool of patients with diminished host resistance plays some role as well, as evidenced by the reports of uncommon bacterial and fungal infec-tions in diabetic and immunosuppressed patients.

REFERENCES

1. Stern, P. J., et al. Established hand infections: a controlled prospective study. *J. Hand Surg.* 8:553, 1983.
2. Goldstein, E. J. C., et al. Infections following clenched-fist injury: a new perspective. *J. Hand Surg.* 3:455, 1978.
3. Robson, M. C., Schmidt, D., and Heggers, J. P. Cefamandole therapy in hand infections. *J. Hand Surg.* 8:560, 1983.

III MAXILLOFACIAL TRAUMA

13 BASIC EVALUATION AND MANAGEMENT OF MAXILLOFACIAL TRAUMA

Timothy R. Jones

Maxillofacial injuries are the second most common type of injury seen in the emergency room, the first being hand injuries. Although these injuries are often striking, they are rarely life-threatening; and careful evaluation and appropriate treatment can minimize the final cosmetic and functional deficiencies.

ANATOMY
Scalp

The scalp and forehead are composed of five layers: skin, subcutaneous tissue, galea aponeurosis, loose connective tissue, and periosteum. The thick skin and subcutaneous layer contain the hair follicles and sebaceous glands. Within the subcutaneous layer are the arteries, veins, and lymphatics, which are divided into multiple lobules by interlacing fibrosepta. These septa limit the vessels from retracting after laceration. The galea serves as the origin of the frontalis muscle anteriorly and the occipitalis muscle posteriorly. The subgaleal layer, which contains the loose connective tissue, allows free movement of the scalp over the cranium. The periosteum of the skull is adherent to the skull and attaches to the sutures.

The scalp is richly supplied by multiple vessels that freely anastomose with each other (Fig. 13-1). The supratrochlear and supraorbital arteries, which represent branches of the internal carotid artery, exit the supraorbital area and travel superiorly to supply the forehead and vertex. The superficial temporal artery is a branch of the external carotid artery and supplies the frontoparietal portion of the scalp. The postauricular and occipital arteries also arise from the external carotid artery and supply the scalp in the area of their anatomic name. These vessels communicate freely with each other, cross the midline to communicate with contralateral vessels, and penetrate the calvaria to communicate with the intracranial cavity and supply the calvarium.

Sensation to the scalp is provided by nerves that travel with the arterial supply of the scalp (Figs. 13-2 and 13-3). The supratrochlear and supraorbital nerves are branches of the trigeminal nerve (V_1). The auriculotemporal nerve is a branch of the trigeminal nerve (V_3)

285

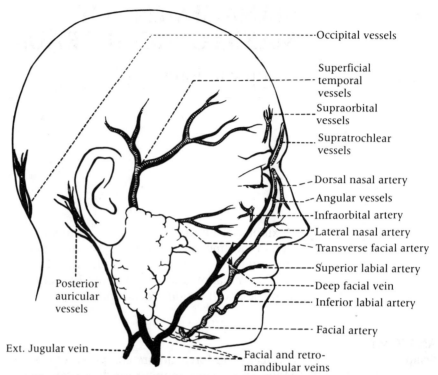

Occipital vessels

Superficial temporal vessels

Supraorbital vessels

Supratrochlear vessels

Dorsal nasal artery

Angular vessels

Infraorbital artery

Lateral nasal artery

Transverse facial artery

Superior labial artery

Deep facial vein

Inferior labial artery

Facial artery

Posterior auricular vessels

Ext. Jugular vein

Facial and retro-mandibular veins

Fig. 13-1. Vascular supply of the face and scalp. (From W. H. Hollinshead and C. Rosse. *Textbook of Anatomy,* 4th Ed. Philadelphia: Harper Medical 1985. With permission.)

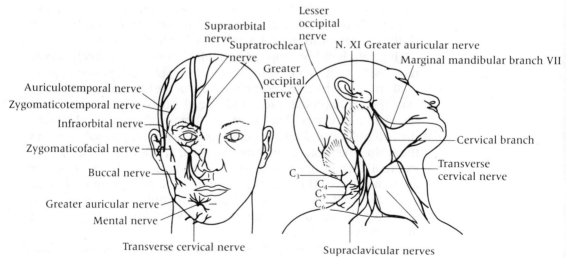

Supraorbital nerve

Supratrochlear nerve

Lesser occipital nerve

Greater occipital nerve

N. XI Greater auricular nerve

Marginal mandibular branch VII

Auriculotemporal nerve

Zygomaticotemporal nerve

Infraorbital nerve

Zygomaticofacial nerve

Buccal nerve

Greater auricular nerve

Mental nerve

Cervical branch

Transverse cervical nerve

C_3

C_4

C_5

C_6

Transverse cervical nerve

Supraclavicular nerves

Fig. 13-2. Sensory nerves of the head and neck region. (From J. Krmpotic-Nemanic, W. Draf, and J. Helms. *Surgical Anatomy of the Head and Neck.* Berlin: Springer-Verlag, 1988. With permission.)

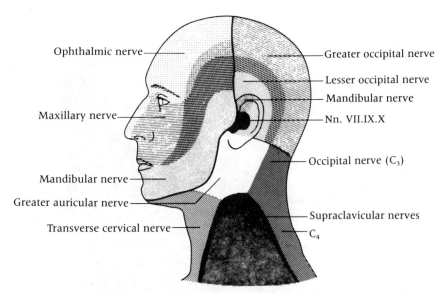

Fig. 13-3. Sensory dermatomes of the head and neck region. (From J. Krmpotic-Nemanic, W. Draf, and J. Helms. *Surgical Anatomy of the Head and Neck.* Berlin: Springer-Verlag, 1988. With permission.)

and runs with the superficial temporal vessels. The lesser occipital nerve (C_2, C_3) provides sensation to the postauricular area, and the greater occipital nerve and third occipital nerve (C_3, C_4) supply sensation to the occipital and nuchal areas of the scalp, respectively.

Skull

The calvarium is composed of four bone segments: Frontal, parietal, temporal, and occipital. The frontal, parietal, and occipital bones are membranous bone and have an inner and outer cortical table and a middle marrow space referred to as the diploë. The temporal bone is an endochondral bone and does not have an inner and outer table. (Figs. 13-4 and 13-5).

The base of the skull is formed by six bones that make up three cranial fossae: anterior, middle, and posterior. The anterior cranial fossa is formed by the frontal, ethmoid, and sphenoid bones. The middle cranial fossa is formed by the sphenoid and temporal bones. The posterior cranial fossa is formed by the temporal, parietal, and occipital bones.

Face

Eyelids
The upper and lower eyelids are similar anatomically and are divided into the anterior lamella, which is composed of skin and orbicularis muscle, and the posterior lamella, which is composed of the orbital septum, tarsus, and conjunctiva (see Fig. 17-2). A fine gray line along the free edge of the eyelid represents the junction between the anterior and posterior lamella. The lacrimal punctum of each eyelid is located at the medial aspect of the eyelid along the free edge.

Eyelid skin is thin and connected to the orbicularis oculi muscle by

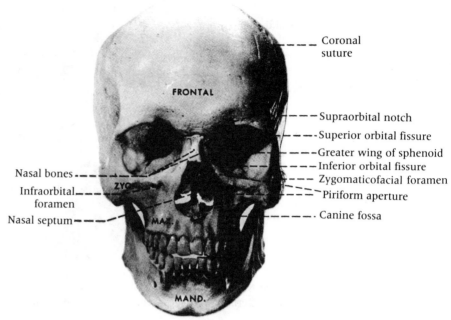

Fig. 13-4. Anterior view of skeletal anatomy. (From W. H. Hollinshead and C. Rosse. *Textbook of Anatomy,* 4th ed. Philadelphia: Harper Medical, 1985. With permission.)

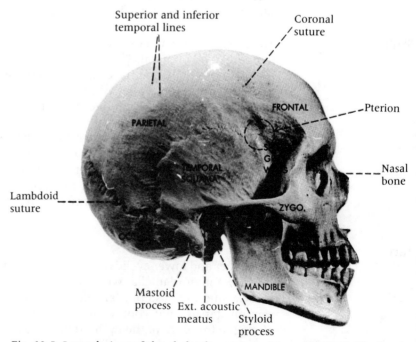

Fig. 13-5. Lateral view of the skeletal anatomy. (From W. H. Hollinshead and C. Rosse. *Textbook of Anatomy,* 4th ed. Philadelphia: Harper Medical, 1985. With permission.)

loose connective tissue. The orbicularis oculi muscle is a sphincteric muscle that serves to close the eye. Deep to the orbicularis oculi muscle is the orbital septum and tarsus (tarsal plate). The orbital septum is a continuation of the skull and face periosteum and extends from the inferior and superior margins of the bony orbit to the tarsal plate where it attaches. The tarsal plate forms the main structural support of the eyelid and is anchored to the bony orbit by the medial and lateral canthal tendons. The conjunctiva forms the posterior layer of the eyelid and is intimately attached to the posterior surface of the tarsus. It starts at the free margin of the eyelid and is reflected onto the eye, except over the cornea.

The upper eyelid has two muscles not present in the lower eyelid that serve to elevate the eyelid. The leavator palpebrae superior muscle attaches to the tarsal plate and acts as the primary elevator of the upper eyelid. Müller's muscle is a smaller, autonomically innervated muscle that also elevates the upper eyelid.

Lacrimal Apparatus

The lacrimal apparatus comprises a secretory and drainage system. The secretory apparatus consists of the lacrimal gland with its ducts. The drainage apparatus consists of the lacrimal canaliculi, lacrimal sac, and nasolacrimal duct. The upper and lower puncta of the lacrimal canaliculi open in the free margin of the eyelid just lateral to the medical canthal angle. They travel medially to drain into the lacrimal sac, which continues as the nasolacrimal duct to empty into the inferior meatus.

Bony Orbit

The eyes are encased in two pyramid-shaped bony cavities called the orbits (Fig. 13-6). The orbital walls are made up of seven bones: maxilla, zygoma, sphenoid (greater and lesser wings), palatine, ethmoid, lacrimal, and frontal bones.

The thin medial orbital wall separates the orbit from the ethmoid sinus. At the anterior aspect of the medial wall is the lacrimal fossa, which houses the lacrimal sac. The inferior orbital wall, formed primarily by the maxilla, separates the orbit from the maxillary sinus. Extending anteriorly from the mid-portion of the inferior orbital fissure is the infraorbital groove, which transmits the infraorbital nerve. The lateral orbital wall separates the orbit from the infratemporal fossa. It is formed primarily by the zygoma and the greater wing of the sphenoid. Along the lateral orbital rim is a bony projection, the orbital tubercle of Whitnall, where the lateral canthal ligament attaches. The superior orbital wall (roof), which separates the orbit from the brain, is composed primarily of the frontal bone. On the medial aspect of the roof is the trochlear fossa, which represents the attachment of the pulley for the superior oblique extraocular muscle.

At the apex of the orbit is the optic canal, through which the optic nerve and the opthalmic artery are transmitted. Just lateral to the

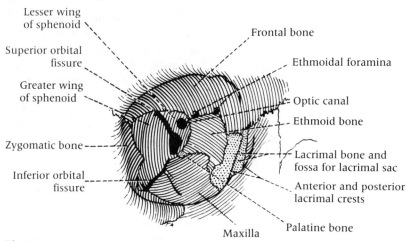

Lesser wing
of sphenoid

Superior orbital
fissure

Greater wing
of sphenoid

Zygomatic bone

Inferior orbital
fissure

Frontal bone

Ethmoidal foramina

Optic canal

Ethmoid bone

Lacrimal bone and
fossa for lacrimal sac

Anterior and posterior
lacrimal crests

Palatine bone

Maxilla

Fig. 13-6. Bony anatomy of the orbital apex. (From W. H. Hollinshead and C. Rosse. *Textbook of Anatomy,* 4th ed. Philadelphia: Harper Medical. 1985. With permission.)

optic canal is the superior orbital fissure, which transmits the oculomotor (III), trochlear (IV), and abducens (VI) cranial nerves; the lacrimal, frontal (V_1), and nasociliary branches of the ophthalmic nerve; the superior opthalmic vein; and small meningeal arteries (Fig. 13-6).

Extraocular Muscles
There are six extraocular muscles that coordinate eye movement (Table 13-1). All of the extraocular muscles insert on the globe and originate from the apex of the orbit except for the inferior oblique muscle, which originates from the anteromedial aspect of the orbital floor. The superior oblique tendon passes through the trochlea on the medial aspect of the orbital roof before taking an acute turn laterally to insert on the globe.

Ear
The framework of the auricle consists of a single elastic cartilage. It has little subcutaneous tissue, which allows the skin to be closely adherent to the underlying perichondrium. Blood supply to the auricle is abundant and is supplied by the superficial temporal and postauricular arteries (see Fig. 13-1). Cutaneous sensation to the auricle and external auditory canal is provided by the greater auricular nerve (C_2/C_3) and cranial nerves (CN) V (auriculotemporal nerve), VII, IX, and X (see Figs. 13-2 and 13-3).

Facial Skeleton and Muscles
The primary skeleton of the face is formed by the frontal, nasal, maxillary, zygomatic, palatine, and mandibular bones (see Fig.

Table 13-1. Extraocular muscles

Muscle	Cranial nerve	Gaze to test muscle
Superior rectus	III	Upward and outward
Inferior rectus	III	Downward and out-ward
Superior oblique	IV	Downward and inward
Inferior oblique	III	Upward and inward
Medial rectus	III	Inward
Lateral rectus	VI	Outward

13-5). The muscles of facial expression are superficial muscles located within the layers of subcutaneous fascia and act to move the mouth, nose, and eyes. They receive motor innervation from branches of the facial nerve (CN VII), which enters the muscles on their deep surfaces (Fig. 13-7).

Parotid Gland
The parotid gland is deep to the skin and the superficial fascia; and it spans vertically from the zygomatic arch to below the angle of the mandible, and horizontally from the mastoid to the masseter muscle (see Fig. 17-8). Saliva from the parotid gland is delivered to the oral cavity via the parotid duct. The parotid duct, also called Stensen's duct, exists from the anterior portion of the parotid gland and travels across the superficial surface of the masseter muscle to enter the oral cavity in the area of the second upper molar. At the anterior border of the masseter, where the duct enters the oral cavity, the buccal branch of the facial nerve is just superficial to the parotid duct.

The extratemporal portion of the facial nerve divides the parotid gland into superficial and deep lobes. The facial nerve exits the stylomastoid foramen and enters the parotid gland at its posterior edge. Within the gland the nerve divides into five branches: temporal, zygomatic, buccal, marginal mandibular, and cervical. As the branches of the facial nerve proceed distally, they arborize extensively. Consequently, lacerations of the facial nerve branches medial to the lateral canthus of the eye generally do not need primary repair to achieve good facial motion.

Located on the lateral side of the face are two muscles of mastication: temporalis and masseter. The masseter muscle is anterior and medial to the parotid gland. It originates from the zygoma and zygomatic bone and inserts onto the lateral surface of the mandible. The temporalis muscle arises from the temporal fossa and runs inferiorly, medial to the zygomatic arch, to insert on the coronoid process of the mandible. Both of these muscles receive their motor innervation from the mandibular division of the trigeminal nerve (CN V). Sensation to the face is through the maxillary and mandibular division of the trigeminal nerve (CN V).

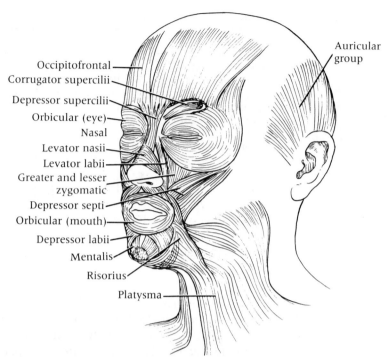

Occipitofrontal

Corrugator supercilii

Depressor supercilii

Orbicular (eye)

Nasal

Levator nasii

Levator labii

Greater and lesser
zygomatic

Depressor septi

Orbicular (mouth)

Depressor labii

Mentalis

Risorius

Platysma

Auricular
group

Fig. 13-7. Muscles of facial expression. (From C. W. Cummings. *Otolaryngology, Head and Neck Surgery.* St. Louis: Mosby, 1986. With permission.)

Oral Cavity

The boundaries of the oral cavity include the lips anteriorly, cheeks laterally, palate superiorly, anterior tonsillar pillars posteriorly, and the tongue and floor of the mouth inferiorly. Projecting from the roof and floor of the anterior part of the oral cavity are the alveolar ridges of the maxilla and mandible, respectively. The sulcus formed between the alveolar process and the lips is referred to as the gingivobuccal sulcus. Posterior and continuous with the oral cavity is the oropharynx. Inferior to the oropharynx are the hypopharynx and larynx. The anterior part of the hypopharynx opens into the larynx, and the posterior part of the hypopharynx opens into the esophagus. Directly posterior to the posterior pharyngeal wall is the cervical spine. The seven cervical vertebrae extend from the level of the soft palate to the level of the cricoid cartilage.

Neck

The neck is divided into various "triangles" by the sternocleidomastoid muscle and its prominent, midline framework: the hyoid bone, thyroid cartilage, and cricoid cartilage (Fig. 13-8). Situated directly behind the thyroid cartilage is the larynx. The carotid sheath is situated laterally, deep to the sternocleidomastoid muscle, and contains the carotid artery, internal jugular vein, and vagus nerve.

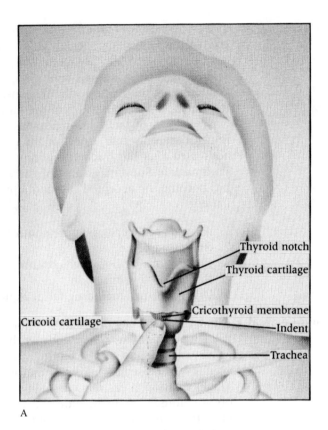

A

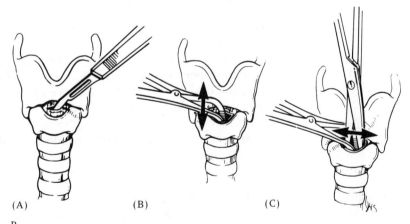

(A)   (B)   (C)

B

Fig. 13-8. A. Anatomy of the larynx and trachea. (From American
College of Surgeons. *Advanced Trauma Life Support Course for Physicians,*
1983. With permission.) *B.* Cricothyroidotomy. (A) Transverse puncture
of the membrane. (B) Vertical spread with hemostat. (From K. Mattox,
E. E. Moore, and D. V. Felaciano. *Trauma.* Norwalk, CT: Appleton &
Lange, 1988. With permission.) (C) Adequate transverse spread with
second instrument.

EVALUATION

The complexity of craniofacial injuries requires the cooperation and consultation of many specialists: general surgeons, neurosurgeons, ophthalmologists, otolaryngologists, oral surgeons, plastic surgeons, and dentists. In a trauma center the general surgeon serves as the "captain" of the team and is responsible for the initial evaluation, treatment, and stabilization of the patient.

Evaluation of facial injuries starts with the assumption that the injuries are only one aspect of the mutiply injured patient and are addressed after life-threatening injuries. The ABCs of the Advanced Trauma Life Support Course of the American College of Surgeons has become the accepted standard approach to the multiply injured patient.

1. Airways and cervical spine control
2. Breathing
3. Circulation: hemorrhage control
4. Neurologic examination
5. Other injuries, including facial injuries

Airway and Cervical Spine

Airway control has the highest priority in the initial assessment of the trauma patient, particularly with maxillofacial injuries. Upper airway obstruction can be produced by the tongue, blood, dentures, vomitus, collapsed mandible, hematoma, or laryngotracheal injuries. The evaluation is entirely clinical because of its urgency. Important observations to note include the position of the head and neck, anxiety, movement of air through the nose and mouth, stridor, ability to phonate, deviation of the larynx or trachea, presence of subcutaneous crepitus, motion of the chest, breath sounds, and the use of accessory respiratory muscles.

Hemorrhage

Hemorrhage from facial injuries can cause significant blood loss, but it rarely leads to shock. Shock in these patients is usually the result of associated injuries. However, hemorrhage from facial injuries can result in upper airway obstruction. Careful inspection of the face, scalp, and oral cavity may reveal active arterial bleeding that requires closer intervention. Brisk bleeding from the lateral pharyngeal wall or tonsillar area may indicate injury to the internal carotid artery. Arteriography is rarely used for evaluating craniofacial hemorrhage but is commonly used for evaluating neck trauma when there is concern about carotid artery injury.

Neurologic Examination

The face serves as a "shock absorber" for the cranium. As such, the more severe the facial injury, the greater is the likelihood of head injury. Thorough neurologic examination is of utmost importance.

The initial part of the neurologic examination begins with observation of the patient's level of consciousness and classification by the Glascow Coma Scale. If the patient is conscious, details about the events of the injury are obtained. If the patient is unconscious, details should be obtained from the witnesses, paramedics, or police. Information that helps direct the physical examination includes mechanism of injury, previous injuries, loss of consciousness, change in vision or hearing, areas of numbness or tenderness, and change in bite (occlusion).

Carotid pulses should be palpated and auscultated over the carotid bulb and the orbits. The size and reactivity of the pupils provide information about supratentorial compression, CN III function, and globe injury. Evaluation of spontaneous eye movements provides information about CN III, IV, and VI.

Special attention must be given to the cervical spine, as it is commonly injured in association with facial injuries. The neck is inspected for swelling or discoloration and palpated for alignment and tenderness. Radiographs of the entire cervical spine ($C1-C_7$) should be performed on unconscious patients, those with signs or symptoms of cervical spine injury, or those with severe facial trauma.

Craniofacial Examination

After stabilizing the more severe, life-threatening injuries, a secondary survey of the craniofacial area is performed. The area from the scalp to the clavicles is inspected, observing for asymmetry, local edema, discoloration, flattening, widening, or elongation of the face, lacerations, areas of tissue loss, exposed bones, and loss of function. If a penetrating injury is present, entrance and exit wounds are noted.

After the general inspection the craniofacial area is carefully palpated in a systematic fashion, comparing one side to the other. This examination can be organized into the following pattern: upper face, mid-face, lower face, and neck.

Upper Face

The cranium and forehead are examined for edema, ecchymosis, lacerations, and contour deformities. A depressed skull fracture may be concealed by overlying edema. Lacerations should be throughly palpated with a gloved finger to evaluate the underlying bone and search for foreign bodies.

The forehead area is evaluated for sensation and motion. The presence of crepitus in this area may indicate a frontal sinus fracture. The presence of clear fluid in the wound may represent a cerebrospinal fluid leak. A lateral skull radiograph is helpful for demonstrating both anterior and posterior tables of the frontal sinus and the frontal bone, but a computed tomography (CT) scan is more sensitive and is indicated to fully evaluate skull fractures, frontal sinus fractures, and intracerebral injuries.

Mid-face

Orbits. The presence of periorbital edema, ecchymosis, crepitus, and lacerations are noted. The height of the palpebral fissures and position of the medial and lateral canthi are compared to those on the opposite side. The orbital rims should be palpated for tenderness, depression, or angulation. The presence of subconjunctival hemorrhage, ocular proptosis, enophthalmos, or anesthesia of the cheek skin are observed. The eyes are examined for pupil size and reactivity to direct and indirect light stimulation. Visual acuity, visual fields, and eye movements are tested, and diplopia in certain directions of gaze is noted. The Waters view is the best single view for demonstrating fractures of the floor and inferior rim of the orbit. The Towne view can also be helpful for showing the orbital floor. A lateral view of the skull demonstrates the roof of the orbit. The CT scan is far superior to plain radiographs for evaluating the orbit and should be obtained when optimal imaging is necessary.

Zygoma and Zygomatic Arch. Injuries to the zygomatic complex often present with periorbital and orbital signs and symptoms. The eyelids should be examined for change in height, width, or inclination of the palpebral fissure. Flattening of the malar eminence may be difficult to perceive when looking directly at the patient, but examination from above, looking tangentially, may reveal a deformity. The orbital rim (especially inferiorly and laterally) and zygomatic arch should be thoroughly palpated. The integrity of the zygomatic arch can be further evaluated by having the patient open the mouth widely. Limitation or pain with opening the mouth (trismus) may indicate a zygomatic arch fracture. Numbness of the cheek and upper teeth on the affected side may indicate injury to the infraorbital nerve. The plain radiographs most helpful for assessing the zygomatic complex include Waters and submentovertex views. CT scans should be used for evaluating complex injuries.

Nasal bones. Injuries to the nasal bones, frontal processes of the maxilla, or nasal septum commonly result in periorbital edema and ecchymosis, especially in the intercanthal areas. The nasal pyramid should be carefully palpated for crepitus, tenderness, depression, angulation, or loss of support.

The nasal cavity should be inspected for sources of epistaxis, lacerations, septal deviation, septal hematoma, and the presence of clear or blood-tinged fluid (cerebrospinal fluid, CSF). With a simple nasal fracture, a clinical diagnosis is generally sufficient and radiographs are not necessarily indicated. Even though treatment of nasal fractures is based on the clinical examination, some authors recommend nasal radiographs (anteroposterior and lateral views) for medicolegal documentation. If a complex nasoethmoidal fracture is suspected, a CT scan should be obtained (see Chapter 16).

Maxilla. The middle part of the face is inspected for periorbital edema and ecchymosis as well as elongation, depression, or flattening of the facial profile. The oral cavity should be examined for change in occlusion, lacerations of the hard palate, and ecchymosis in the upper gingivobuccal sulcus. Palpation of the maxilla should be performed by grasping the maxilla with a gloved thumb and forefinger (Fig. 13-9). An attempt is made to move the maxilla while

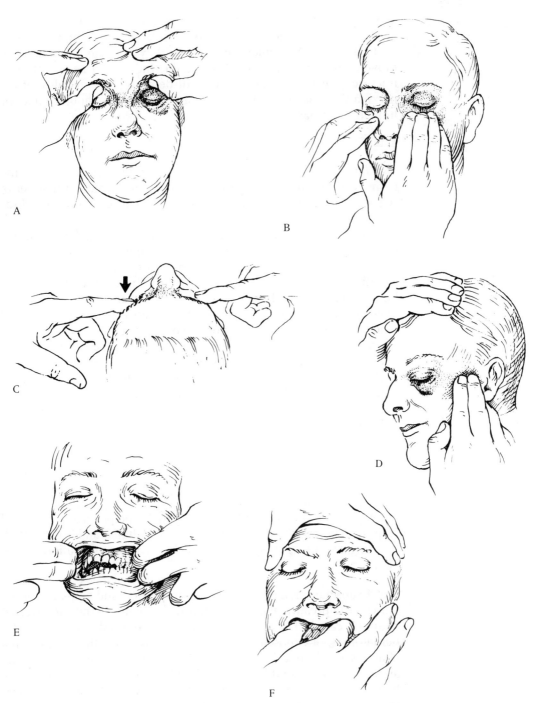

Fig. 13-9. A. Palpation for irregularities of supraorbital ridge. B. Palpation for irregularities of infraorbital ridge and zygoma. C. Comparing height of malar eminences. D. Palpation for depression of zygomtic arch. E. Visualization of gross dental occlusion. F. Maneuver to ascertain motion in maxilla. (From R. C. Schultz. Facial Injuries, 3rd ed. Chicago: Year Book, 1988. With permission.)

keeping the remainder of the face stable. Movement of the maxillary alveolus without movement at the nasofrontal area indicates a Le Fort I fracture. Movement at the maxillary alveolus in addition to movement at the nasofrontal suture line indicates a Le Fort II or III fracture (see Fig. 15-4). The lack of demonstrable mobility of the maxilla does not rule out a maxillary fracture, as mobility may be limited by impaction.

Lower Face

Mandible. Fractures of the mandible often produce malocclusion and trismus. Upper airway obstruction can be produced if the anterior segment of the mandible is free-floating and falls posterior to occlude the oropharynx.

Inspection and palpation of the mandible are initially performed externally. Gross deformities, skin lacerations, hematoma, edema, ecchymosis, and areas of local tenderness are noted. The mandible is examined intraorally for lacerations in the mucosa, ecchymosis, or hematoma in the floor of the mouth or gingivobuccal sulcus, deviation of the jaw, change in bite (occlusion), or areas of local tenderness. Injury to the inferior alveolar nerve can be evaluated by checking sensation to the lower lip. Plain radiographs are generally good for demonstrating the mandible, and a CT scan rarely adds useful clinical information. Panorex radiographs can provide a single view of the mandible and the supporting structures from one temporomandibular joint to the other. However, this film is often difficult to obtain in the multiply injured patient undergoing acute evaluation (see Chapter 14).

Neck. Examination of the neck starts with assessment of the airway. Stridor, hoarseness, or retractions may indicate a laryngotracheal injury. The midline prominences of the neck — hyoid bone, thyroid cartilage, and cricoid cartilage — should be palpated for pain and crepitus. The carotid arteries should be auscultated and bruits noted. If laryngeal injury is suspected, an ear/nose/throat evaluation should be done.

Ear. Examination of the ear includes inspection and palpation of the auricle, the preauricular and postauricular regions, and the external auditory canal. The auricle should be inspected for lacerations, hematomas, or exposed cartilage. Ecchymosis over the mastoid area (Battle's sign) may indicate a basilar skull fracture. The external auditory canal should be inspected with an otoscope for lacerations, hemotympanum, or CSF otorrhea. Hearing should be grossly tested by holding a wristwatch close to the affected ear to see if the patient hears the ticking sound.

Cheek. Wounds involving the lateral part of the face have the potential to injure the parotid gland, parotid duct, or facial nerve (see Chapter 17).

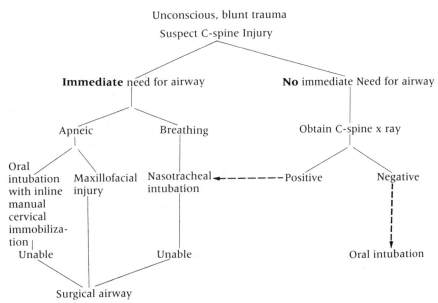

Fig. 13-10. Indications for intubation and surgical airways. (From American College of Surgeons. *Advanced Trauma Life Support Course for Physicians,* 1983. With permission.)

TREATMENT

In the unconscious patient, the most common cause of airway obstruction is the tongue. When the tongue is fully relaxed it falls against the posterior wall, occluding the upper airway. This situation can also occur with severe bilateral mandibular fracture, which creates a flail anterior mandibular segment. It can be treated by anterior traction on the tongue. In the unconscious patient with an intact mandible, a chin lift or jaw thrust maneuver is effective. If the obstruction is from a flail mandible, a towel clip or suture placed in the anterior part of the tongue can be used to pull the tongue anteriorly to relieve the obstruction.

Dentures, blood, gastric contents, or oral secretions can cause upper airway obstruction. These obstructions can usually be cleared quickly by sweeping with the index finger.

Oral and nasal airways are mechanical adjuncts to the above maneuvers. An oropharyngeal airway is not tolerated well in a conscious patient and can be used only with an unconscious patient. When the patient is conscious, a nasopharyngeal airway is more tolerable.

The disadvantages of the above airway adjuncts are that they do not isolate the trachea from the mouth and the patient can still aspirate. If the patient is conscious and can readily cough and clear secretions, all that may be needed is to provide the patient with a tonsil sucker. However, if the patient is unconscious, better control of the airway may be needed.

Endotracheal intubation by orotracheal intubation, nasotracheal intubation, or cricothyrotomy is necessary when control of the airway is mandatory (Fig. 13-10). Orotracheal intubation via direct laryngoscopy is the mainstay of airway management in nontrauma cardiopulmonary resuscitation. However, the possibility of a cervical spinal fracture in the trauma patient makes orotracheal intubation a higher risk. In the event that intubation is urgent and the cervical spine has not been "cleared," the physician must decide which poses the greatest risk: the obstructed airway or possible cervical spine fracture. Studies suggest that unconscious patients with an injury above the clavicles have a 20 percent incidence of fracture of the cervical spine. In this instance, the airway still has priority, as the possibility of a cervical cord injury is still relatively low [1]. In-line traction of the cervical spine is used during intubation.

Despite the concern about cervical spinal fractures, orotracheal intubation is advantageous because it can be performed under direct vision in both conscious (using local anesthesia) and unconscious patients. Moreover, it is safer with severe maxillofacial injuries, where a misdirected nasotracheal tube can be placed intracranially.

An alternative to orotracheal intubation is nasotracheal intubation. Advantages are that it is easier to perform in conscious patients, and it does not require hyperextension of the head or direct laryngoscopy. Nasotracheal intubation is limited by the fact that the patient must be breathing spontaneously so that breath sounds may be heard.

When access to the trachea cannot be gained by endotracheal intubation, cricothyrotomy is performed (Fig. 13-10). This procedure is most helpful in patients who have failed intubation attempts, or in those who have sustained destructive maxillofacial or cervical spinal injuries. McGill and Clinton [2] preferred cricothyrotomy over orotracheal intubation in patients who required airway control and for whom cervical spine radiographs were not available.

A useful technique for obtaining entrance into the airway in young children involves puncture of the cricothyroid membrane with a 14-gauge angiocatheter. Ventilation is then performed at 30 to 40 times per minute until a more secure airway is obtained.

Cricothyrotomy is preferable to tracheotomy in most emergency situations. The exception to this rule is when there is an acute laryngotracheal injury. In this instance there may be separation of the trachea from the larynx, and cricothyrotomy would not intubate the distally displaced trachea. Otherwise, tracheotomy should be performed "electively" after tracheal intubation has been established.

Hemorrhage

Hemorrhage from soft-tissue lacerations on the face or scalp can usually be controlled by direct pressure. Bleeding from scalp lacerations can be controlled by clamping or ligating the open vessel directly or by placing a suture through the skin, deep to the galea, and compressing the vessel. Bleeding vessels on the face should not be blindly clamped, as important nerves frequently accompany them. Rarely, extensive facial hemorrhage from gunshot wounds or uncontrolled epistaxis may require ligtion of the external carotid artery.

Intraoral bleeding from the floor of the mouth, tongue, or tonsil that does not stop spontaneously can be controlled by direct pressure using a folded gauze sponge on a Kelly forceps. If the site of the bleeding is thought to originate from the internal carotid artery (lateral pharyngeal wall/tonsillar area), arteriography, exploration, or both may be required.

Injuries to the mid-face often result in epistaxis. Epistaxis from a simple nasal fracture usually stops spontaneously or with pressure to the anterior septum, produced by pinching the alar rims against the septum. If this maneuver is unsuccessful in controlling the bleeding, an anterior nasal pack should be placed (see Chapter 16). More extensive mid-face injuries are often associated with bleeding from the posterior nasal cavity. Despite placement of an anterior nasal pack, bleeding continues posteriorly, and substantial quantities of blood can be swallowed. These injuries require anterior and posterior nasal packing. Conscious patients benefit from use of a tonsil sucker, but the unconscious patient may need to have the airway secured by endotracheal intubation or cricothyrotomy.

Scalp and Cranial Injuries

Scalp contusions, lacerations, and avulsions account for a high percentage of emergency room visits related to head trauma. Because of the scalp's rich blood supply, these injuries usually heal well, but they are also apt to bleed profusely.

Contusions of the scalp generally need no treatment. Hematomas resolve spontaneously and aspiration of a hematoma serves only to increase the chance of infection. The risk of necrosis of the scalp due to pressure is low because of the rich blood supply of the scalp, but an overly tight headwrap serves only to increase this risk. Particular attention should be paid to children with scalp hematomas that cross suture lines as they are often associated with an underlying skull fracture.

Simple scalp lacerations should be explored by palpation and skull radiography if there is a question of a skull fracture. Irrigation, débridement, and primary closure in layers can be done under local or regional anesthesia in the emergency room when the laceration is simple. Extensive or complex lacerations and lacerations associated with skull fractures may require closure in the operating room under general anesthesia.

Skull lacerations with significant tissue loss can be skin-grafted if the underlying periosteum is intact. If cortical bone is exposed, advancement, transposition, or rotational flaps can be used to close the wound.

Total scalp avulsions are rare. The point of dissection is usually between the galea and the periosteum. Replacement of the scalp as a free graft is not useful. If the periosteum is intact, a split-thickness skin graft can be used to cover the wound. If the periosteum is gone and the outer table exposed, the outer table can be removed down to the diploë, where a split-thickness skin graft can be accepted. Many times avulsed scalp can be replanted primarily with microvascular anastomosis. If the scalp is not available, other free tissue transfers (i.e., omentum, fasciocutaneous tissue, muscle) can be used to cover the skull.

Neurosurgical consultation should be obtained when there are signs or symptoms suggesting head injury. These include a history of lost consciousness, an abnormal neurological examination, the presence of a linear or basilar skull fracture, or evidence of a CSF leak.

Upper Face Lacerations and Fractures

Simple linear lacerations of the forehead can be irrigated, débrided, and closed primarily in layers. Whenever possible, forehead lacerations should be converted to horizontal lacerations by elliptical excision in the relaxed skin tension lines. Lacerations in the glabellar area should not be converted to horizontal lacerations because the relaxed skin tension lines are oriented vertically.

Stellate lesions on the forehead are often a result of a burst injury. These lacerations are more likely to become infected and to heal with uneven skin margins (trapdoor deformity). The likelihood of this posttraumatic deformity can be lessened by débriding the margins of the laceration so that the beveled edges are eliminated and the skin margins lie at right angles to each other.

Treatment of frontal sinus fractures depends on the extent of injury. Nondisplaced anterior wall fractures need no treatment. Displaced anterior wall fractures need to be explored and reduced to prevent a posttraumatic forehead deformity. Fractures involving the posterior wall of the frontal sinus usually require exploration. Exposure of the frontal sinus can be through the forehead laceration or via a number of incisions. A bicornal incision is preferred if there are complex facial fractures, the possibility of frontal craniotomy exists, or cranial bone grafts are needed. In a male patient with a receding hairline, a mid-forehead or brow incision may be preferred.

Fractures of the anterior wall of the frontal sinus pose only a cosmetic problem. Depressed fractures that are mildly comminuted can be stabilized with interosseous wire or plates. Occasionally, the anterior wall is too comminuted, and so cranial bone grafts are used to reconstruct the wall.

Fractures of the posterior wall of the frontal sinus are suggested by CSF rhinorrhea or pneumocephalus. These fractures often damage the nasofrontal ducts and cause impaired drainage of the sinus. If one nasofrontal duct is intact, the midline septum can be removed, allowing drainage of the affected side into the unaffected side. When both nasofrontal ducts are injured, the frontal sinus should be obliterated or cranialized. Neurosurgical consultation should be obtained when the posterior wall fracture is displaced or there is a CSF leak.

Infectious complications resulting from frontal sinus fractures can occur acutely or chronically. They include meningitis, sinusitis, or osteomyelitis. Mucoceles that result from inadequate sinus drainage may not become symptomatic for many years.

Mid-face Injuries

Orbit

Injuries to the globe and orbit are common with craniofacial trauma. Studies have shown that the incidence of eye injuries associated with blunt facial trauma is 30 to 60 percent [3–5]. Permanent eye impairment occurs in 10 percent of these patients, and blindness has been reported with 0.6 percent of mid-face fractures.

The urgency with which ophthalmologic consultation should be obtained depends on the severity of the injury. Problems for which immediate consultation is needed include blurred vision, blindness, scotoma, eye pain, afferent pupillary defect, hyphema, ruptured globe, and retrobulbar hematoma. Examination by an ophthalmologist with 24 hours is indicated for asymptomatic blunt trauma to the globe, Le Fort II and III fractures, orbital wall fractures, zygoma fractures, and corneal abrasion that is symptomatic after 24 hours. Patients with posttraumatic eyelid ptosis should be evaluated within 1 week of injury.

Eyebrows

The lacerated eyebrow should be carefully aligned and reapproximated in layers. The underlying muscle is reapproximated to prevent posttraumatic spreading and depression in the area. Skin edges that need sharp débridement should be done with oblique cuts in the angle of the hair follicles so as not to transect them.

Eyelid

Eyelid skin is relatively "forgiving," and lacerations in this area generally heal well. Simple eyelid lacerations, involving only the skin and underlying orbicularis oculi muscle, can be closed primarily with 6-0 sutures placed in the skin only. Lacerations with moderate amounts of skin loss can generally be closed primarily as well. Eyelid injuries that need further evaluation include lacerations with significant tissue loss or orbital fat protruding through the wound, or lacerations involving the free margin of the eyelid or lacrimal punta. (see Chapter 17).

Orbital Wall Fractures

Orbital wall fractures can be isolated or associated with fractures of the orbital rim, paranasal sinuses, or anterior cranial fossa. When the wall is displaced toward the globe, the fracture is referred to as a *blow-in fracture*. Blow-in fractures decrease the orbital volume and can produce exophthalmos or impingement on the extraocular muscles, especially the medial rectus. More commonly, when the orbital wall is displaced away from the globe, the fracture is referred to as a *blow-out fracture*. Blow-out fractures increase the orbital volume and can produce enophthalmos.

As might be expected, these patients commonly have periorbital edema, ecchymosis, and subcutaneous emphysema. The force transmitted to the globe can produce visual acuity and visual field disturbances, and all of these patients should be evaluated by an ophthalmologist.

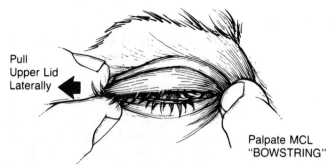

Fig. 13-11. "Bowstring test" for medical canthal ligament integrity. The test is performed by pulling the lateral lid laterally and palpating the integrity of the medial canthal ligament. (From C. A. Foster and J. E. Sherman. *Surgery of Facial Bones Fractures.* New York: Churchill Livingstone, 1987. With permission.)

Conventional radiographs do not demonstrate these fractures well and a CT scan should be obtained. CT scans image not only the bony orbit but also the optic nerve, extraocular muscles, and globe.

Treatment of orbital wall fractures depends on several factors: fracture location, associated facial or skull fractures, and visual symptoms. In general, open reduction/internal fixation is indicated for significantly displaced fractures that result in contour deformity of the orbit, entrapment of the ocular muscles, or injury to the suspensory structure of the globe.

Superior wall fractures are associated with fractures of the anterior cranial fossa, frontal sinus, and frontal bone. Fractures of the lateral orbital wall are rarely isolated but are associated with zygoma fractures. Medial wall fractures are common because the bone (the lamina papyracea) is thin. They can be treated conservatively when there is no significant orbital injury. Fractures associated with nasoethmoidal fractures should be treated by open reduction/internal fixation. Orbital floor fractures frequently injure the globe suspensory ligaments and inferior ocular muscles, producing diplopia. Conservative treatment is acceptable if there is no evidence of ocular muscle entrapment and the suspensory structure of the floor is intact. Entrapment of the inferior oblique rectus muscle or enophthalmos are indications for open reduction/internal fixation.

Nasoethmoidal Fractures
Comminuted fractures involving the medial orbital wall and nasal complex are referred to as nasoethmoidal fractures. These injuries produce marked periorbital edema and ecchymosis in the intercanthal area. Traumatic hypertelorism results from the medial canthal ligaments being laterally displaced. Integrity of the medial canthal ligaments can be evaluated by the lid traction test (Fig. 13-11).

As expected, nasoethmoidal fractures are frequently accompanied by severe head, orbital, and paranasal sinus injury. Consultation with a neurosurgeon and ophthalmologist should be obtained and the CT scan extended to include these areas.

Treatment goals for nasoethmoidal fractures are both functional and cosmetic. The frontal and ethmoid sinuses must be treated in such a way as to restore adequate drainage or be obliterated. The medial canthal ligaments must be repositioned medially to correct the pseudohypertelorism. The continuity of the lacrimal apparatus is restored and the bony integrity of the upper and mid-face reestablished.

Best results when treating nasoethmoidal fractures are obtained by open reduction/internal fixation. Comminuted or unstable fractures may need bone grafts at the time of immediate repair (see Chapter 15). Complications from nasoethmodial fractures include recurrent sinusitis, mucoceles, diplopia, enophthalmos, traumatic hypertelorism, epiphora, and change in facial profile.

Maxillary Fractures
High impact forces to the anterior face often result in fractures of the maxilla. Maxillary fractures are most easily understood by categorizing them according to the Le Fort classification (see Fig. 15-5). They all have fractures across the pterygoid plates — hence the potential for mobility of the maxillary alveolus, upper airway obstruction, epistaxis, malocclusion, and change in facial profile. Le Fort II and III fractures involve the orbital walls and produce periorbital edema and ecchymosis.

Maxillary fractures are reasonably demonstrated by plain radiographs. Waters view is the most helpful, but anteroposterior, lateral, and submentovertex views should also be obtained. Complex craniofacial fractures or mid-face fractures not satisfactorily demonstrated by conventional radiographs should be evaluated with a CT scan.

Treatment of maxillary fractures is aimed at restoring the original facial profile and dental occlusion. It is done by reestablishing the three structural pillars of the mid-face: the nasomaxillary buttress, the zygomatic buttress, and the pterygomaxillary buttress [6]. Fracture reduction and fixation depend on the severity of the fractures and the condition of the teeth. Available options range from closed reduction with mandibular-maxillary fixation to open reduction/internal fixation. Bone grafts are occasionally needed to reestablish the maxillary pillars (see Chapter 15).

Concomitant injuries to the cranial base or orbits are common and can produce CSF leak, enophthalmos, diplopia, and even blindness. Untreated maxillary fractures manifest as dental malocclusion and a facial profile that is shorter and wider than normal.

Mandibular Fractures
In comparison to other bones in the body, the mandible is unique in that it has the dual role of function and cosmesis. It plays a major functional role in eating, breathing, and talking, and it is a primary contributor to the facial profile. Its prominent position predisposes it to facial trauma. Studies report that the mandible is fractured in 50 to 67 percent of all facial fractures [7,8].

Mandibular fractures can be classified in several ways, but the most commonly used classification is based on location: alveolar, symphyseal, body, angle, ramus, coronoid, and condylar. Further classification of fractures include open versus closed, displaced versus nondisplaced, complete versus incomplete, and linear versus comminuted.

Treatment of mandibular fractures begins with evaluation of the upper airway. Obstruction of the upper airway can result from an unstable anterior mandible segment, bleeding, or fractured teeth. See Airway and Cervical Spine section, above, for airway management.

Most mandibular fractures are open to the oral cavity, and prophylactic antibiotics covering *Staphylococcus aureus* and anaerobes should be used. Definitive management depends on the condition of the teeth and the fracture location and severity. Although several methods are available for treating mandibular fractures, they are all based on the common premise of reestablishing the patient's original occlusion by immobilizing the fracture line by such methods as closed reduction, open reduction, mandibular-maxillary fixation, direct interosseous wiring, osteosynthesis with compression plates, intraoral splints including dentures, and external fixator devices. Suggested management of mandibular fractures is outlined in Table 13-2 [9]. Chapter 14 provides a more in-depth discussion of mandibular fractures.

Gunshot Wounds of the Mandible

Gunshot wounds involving the mandible produce a segmental mandibular defect. Initial treatment focuses on débridement of nonviable soft tissue and bone, intraoral closure, and maintenance of the mandibular arch. An external fixation device, such as the Morris-Biphasic Appliance, or a plate can be used to bridge the segmental loss until secondary reconstruction is performed.

Nonunion and malocclusion are the two most significant complications associated with treatment of mandibular fractures. Sound immobilization and proper alignment of the fractures minimize these problems. Dental problems arising from mandibular fractures may necessitate late endodontics or extraction of teeth.

Soft-Tissue Injuries

Parotid Duct

The parotid duct may be transected by lacerations that extend deep into the cheek. Injury to the buccal branch of the facial nerve should be suspected with a parotid duct laceration as it runs with the parotid duct toward the upper lip. Primary repair of the parotid duct should be performed (see Chapter 17).

Facial Nerve Lacerations

Lacerations across the cheek or temple can transect the facial nerve. Facial nerve branches transected lateral to the lateral canthus should be repaired by primary anastomosis or an interpositional nerve graft.

Table 13-2. Suggested management of mandibular fractures

Fracture and amount of displacement	Reduction/Fixation
Condyle	
Minimal	closed
Moderate	Closed
Severe	Open, preauricular or submandibular incision, plating or wiring
Ramus	
Minimal	Closed
Moderate	Closed
Severe	Open
Angle	
Minimal	Closed
Moderate	Open, intraoral incision, wiring or plating
Severe	Open, external incision, plating
Body	
Minimal	Closed
Moderate	Open, intraoral incision, plating
Severe	Open, external incision, plating
Symphysis	
Minimal	Closed
Moderate	Open, transoral incision, plating
Severe	Open, transoral incision, plating

Source: D. P. Sinn, R. A. Pollack, and R. J. Rohrich. Facial fractures. II. Mandibular, maxillary, and craniofacial (overview). *Selected Readings in Plastic Surgery* 5(26):6, 1989. With permission.

When the nerve is transected medial to the lateral canthus, primary repair is not necessary (see Chapter 17).

Nose
Lacerations on the nose should alert the physician to the possibility of an underlying nasal or septal fracture. The lacerations are repaired primarily in a layered closure with special attention to the alar rim alignment. The nasal or septal fracture can be treated immediately, or it can be postponed (see Chapter 16).

Ear
The excellent blood supply to the ear affords it "kind" healing. Extensive lacerations or avulsions, attached only by a small pedicle, commonly survive. Through-and-through lacerations should be closed in layers, preferably without cartilage sutures. Amputated ears can be treated in a number of ways, including microvascular reattachment, free grafting, and subcutaneous storage.

Hematomas may appear following blunt trauma to the ear. They can be treated by aspiration or incision and drainage. A pressure dressing is helpful in preventing recurrence, and prophylactic antibiotics are recommended (see Chapter 17).

Lips

Essential in the repair of lip lacerations is the accurate approximation of the vermilion–skin junction. Full-thickness lacerations of the lip should be closed in three layers: mucosa, muscle, and skin. Prophylactic antibiotic coverage against *Staphylococcus aureus* and anaerobes is indicated. Lip defects less than one-third of the lip length can be closed primarily.

Basilar Skull Fractures

Facial trauma significant enough to cause mid-facial or upper facial fractures are commonly associated with basilar skull fractures. These fractures occur most frequently along the floor of the anterior cranial fossa and the middle cranial fossa.

Fractures of the anterior cranial fossa classically present with CSF rhinorrhea. The fracture line can be at the cribriform plate, the fovea ethmoidalis, or the frontal sinus. Clinically, fractures of the anterior cranial fossa produce periorbital edema and ecchymosis, referred to as "raccoon eyes" or "panda bear eyes."

Fractures of the middle cranial fossa involve the temporal bone and may present with CSF rhinorrhea or otorrhea, hearing loss, vertigo, or facial nerve paralysis. Ecchymosis over the mastoid bone (Battle's sign) is the hallmark of a basilar skull fracture.

If facial nerve paralysis is immediate, surgical exploration and decompression of the nerve are indicated. Delayed facial nerve paralysis is initially managed with steroids. Neurosurgery and ear/nose/throat consultation should be obtained.

Most CSF leaks resulting from facial trauma stop within 1 to 2 weeks. Reduction of facial fractures may be all that is needed to stop a CSF leak. Use of prophylactic antibiotics is controversial, and packing the nose or ear canal is not indicated.

REFERENCES

1. Shaftan, G. W. The initial evaluation of the multiple trauma patient. *World J. Surg.* 7:19, 1983.
2. McGill, J, Clinton, J. E., and Ruize, E. Cricothyrotomy in the department. *Ann. Emerg. Med.* 11.17:361, 1982.
3. Holt, J. E., Holt, G. R., and Blodgett, J. M. Ocular injuries sustained during blunt facial trauma. Ophthalmology 90:14, 1983.
4. Javeley, M. E., Learman, M., and Sanders, H. J. Ocular injuries in orbital fractures — a review of 119 cases. *Plast. Reconstruct. Surg.* 56:410, 1975.
5. Smoot, C. E. When to call the ophthalmologist for facial trauma. *Resident Staff Physician* 34:89, 1988.
6. Manson, P. N., Hoopes, J. E., and Su, C. T. Structural pillars of the facial skeleton: an approach to the management of Le Fort fractures. *Plast. Reconstruct. Surg.* 66:54, 1980.
7. Ellis, E., Moosk, F., and El-Attar, A. Ten years of mandible fractures: analysis of 2,137 cases. *Oral Surg.* 59:129, 1985.
8. Natvig, T., and Dortzbach, R. K. Facial bone fractures. In W. C. Grabb and J. W. Smith, *Plastic Surgery*, (3rd Ed.) Boston: Little, Brown, p. 246, 1979.
9. Sinn, D. P., Pollock, R. A., and Rohrich, R. J. Facial fractures. II. Mandibular, maxillary, and craniofacial (overview). *Selected Readings in Plastic Surgery* 5(26):6, 1989.

Commentary on Chapter 13

Frederick R. Heckler

Basic evaluation and management of maxillofacial injuries are philosophically and technically similar to those for multisystem injuries in other anatomic areas. The facial area is, after all, a complex "multisystem" area with numerous composite tissue units having sophisticated and varying functions and interrelations. Packed into this relatively modestly sized arena are important musculoskeletal units, central and peripheral nervous system entities, critical sensory organs, and important segments of both the alimentary and respiratory tracts. It has always been our contention, therefore, that, like the trauma-trained general surgeon who oversees the global care of the trauma patient, the well trained plastic and reconstructive surgeon should function as the "general surgeon of the maxillofacial area." Involvement by representatives of many other specialties is clearly critical in the modern multidisciplinary approach to such patients, but the plastic surgeon, with his or her broadly based surgical background and training, seems uniquely qualified to best coordinate and steer the maxillofacial team toward the most positive outcome for the patient.

The care of patients with maxillofacial injuries has undergone significant evolution and change in recent years that has been concentrated in several areas: (1) timing of repair and, particularly, reconstruction; (2) strong tendencies toward single-stage primary or delayed primary repair/reconstruction; (3) greater appreciation of key functional bony architecture and its role in reconstruction; (4) major advances in diagnostic modalities centered around radiologic imaging; and (5) technologic advances in internal fixation modalities combined with emphasis on early rather than delayed bone grafting where indicated.

1. *Timing of repair.* Classically, repair of facial injuries played second fiddle in the multiple trauma situation to management of problems involving other organ systems with the obvious exception of life-threatening upper airway or central nervous system problems. These priorities are properly still observed, but modern life support systems and technical advances in monitoring have allowed a strong movement toward earlier definitive maxillofacial management. Our

current preference is to débride and close soft-tissue injuries, allow early systemic stabilization while diagnostic studies are completed, and proceed with definitive maxillofacial repair and reconstruction usually within 3 to 7 days. Our impression is that this approach has not increased complication rates and has shortened morbidity and hospitalization time while yielding improved overall functional and aesthetic results.

2. *Single-stage repair.* Most posttraumatic maxillofacial injuries are now managed with single-stage early definitive repairs, rather than delayed and multistaged approaches. This change is in part due to improvements in anesthesia and critical care units such that these already taxed patients can tolerate the additional stress of prolonged operative procedures. The other major factor leading to this emphasis on single-stage reconstruction is the modern ability to transfer large composite tissue masses, including bone, into areas with tissue deficits using regional axial, musculocutaneous, and fasciocutaneous flaps, as well as free microvascular flaps.

3. *Anatomic insights.* There has been stronger emphasis on appreciation of the major "bony pillars" of the face in terms of their roles in reestablishing and buttressing facial height and contour. With this emphasis have come the modern surgical incisions and approaches that allow full visualization of all skeletal injuries and complete anatomic restoration. This situation is in contrast to former techniques, which emphasized suspension of complex fractures to the cranium, and reliance on this nonspecific reduction combined with intermaxillary fixation to provide restoration of facial skeletal contour.

4. *Diagnostic techniques.* Modern CT and magnetic resonance imaging have revolutionized care of facial bony injuries. The surgeon is now able to completely visualize *all* injured areas, and therefore preoperative planning can be precise and thorough.

5. *Technologic advances in internal fixation.* The ability to proceed with early definitive intervention, aided and abetted by precise modern diagnostic imaging, would not be nearly as revolutionary if it had not been accompanied by the ready availability of plates and screws permitting rigid internal fixation. These "miniorthopedic" devices have permitted the reconstructive surgeon to accomplish the exact anatomic restorations desired while simultaneously permitting early mobilization of the temporomandibular joint, thereby curtailing morbidity. Incorporation of immediate bone grafting in areas of hopeless comminution or absence of bone has likewise been made far easier and more successful by these devices.

The modern approach to these potentially devastating injuries has therefore continued to evolve and advance. Our current "state of the art" makes management of facial injuries different in many aspects from that which was practiced a decade ago. Despite this fact, many of the classic rules and general approaches, as outlined in this chapter, remain valid and useful. Close attention to these concepts can maximize positive clinical outcomes.

14 MANDIBULAR FRACTURES

James M. Russavage

The mandible is a prominent and vulnerable bone. It forms the bony framework of the lower one-third of the face and plays an important role in the functions of eating, breathing, and speaking. Injuries to the mandible are best managed with careful attention to the restoration of form, function, and aesthetics.

Fractures of the mandible are common and second in frequency only to those of the nasal bones. The most common mechanism of injury in urban areas is aggravated assault, whereas motor vehicle accidents are the most frequent cause in rural areas. Gunshot wounds and sports injuries are also important, but less frequent, causes.

The mandible is a horseshoe-shaped bone with two vertical struts. The main anatomic divisions of the mandible are the body, angle, ramus, symphysis, and condylar and condyloid processes (Fig. 14-1). It has dense, stress-absorbing cortical bone at its inferior and posterior borders. The muscles of mastication attach to the mandible, as shown in Figure 14-2. Its blood supply comes primarily from the inferior alveolar artery (a branch of the internal maxillary artery), which enters the mandibular foramen, courses through the body of the mandible, and exits to the soft tissues of the face via the mental foramen. A second, smaller contribution comes from perforating periosteal blood vessels originating from the muscles of mastication.

Neural supply to the mandible comes from the sensory (mandibular) branch of the third division of the fifth cranial nerve (CN V), which provides sensation to the lips, teeth, and gums. Motor innervation to the muscles of mastication are provided by the motor branches of the third division of CN V.

EVALUATION

The clinical history of the injury provides important clues to establishing mandibular injury. Low velocity injuries usually have a fracture at the point of contact with little or no displacement and often a contrecoup, or contralateral, fracture. High velocity injuries usually have a displaced compound comminuted fracture at the point of impact with no contralateral fracture. Mandibular injuries

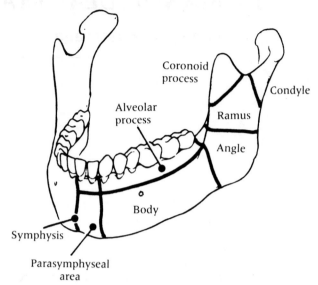

Fig. 14-1. Anatomy of the mandible. (From C. A. Foster and J. E. Sherman. *Surgery of Facial Bones Fractures.* New York: Churchill Livingstone, 1987. With permission.)

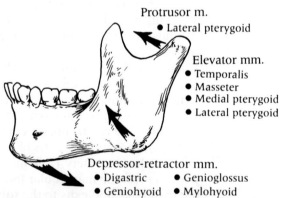

Fig. 14-2. Muscle groups that exert forces on the mandible to potentially distract fractures. (From R. H. Mathog. *Maxillofacial Trauma.* Baltimore: Williams & Wilkins, 1984. With permission.)

are commonly associated with other facial fractures and facial lacerations.

Symptoms expressed by a mandibular fracture are many. Pain may exist in the jaw due to nerve impingement from a bony segment, exposure of bone to air or oral secretions, or fracture movement. Malocclusion or alteration of bite is caused by movement of a tooth-bearing segment or bone by the force of injury or muscular contraction of unstable segments. A step-off, or vertical disparity, in the occlusal plane points to the site of the fracture. Most neurologically intact patients can determine an alteration in bite. Trismus, or inability to open the mouth due to muscular pain, is commonly exhibited with posterior mandibular fractures.

Edema and ecchymoses are commonly present over the site of the fracture. Hemorrhage may seep into tissue near the fracture site and migrate along facial planes. Direction of this movement is dictated by gravity and connective tissue anatomy.

An orderly systemic clinical examination is imperative. Surface injuries are assessed and may include contusions, lacerations, and excoriation. The patient is examined intraorally; and broken teeth, saliva, and blood are cleared from the oral cavity. An airway is guaranteed. An intraoral surface injury usually manifests mucosal disruption at the site of the fracture and hematoma in the floor of the mouth on the side of injury. Avulsed or loose teeth should be placed gently in their sockets. The level of occlusion should be assessed and recorded, and the type and degree of malocclusion noted. Bimanual mandibular palpation (with the thumb and forefinger of each hand) can reveal mobility, fracture edges, pain, incisal opening, and crepitation.

The temporomandibular joint (TMJ) in the preauricular area should be palpated with and without a digit in the external auditory canal. Pain suggests capsular damage, hemarthrosis, internal derangement, or condylar fracture. The mandible may deviate in right or left lateral excursions or protrude toward the side of the injury. One should accurately assess and document the function of the inferior alveolar, lingual, and mental nerves. Transection of the neurovascular bundle may exhibit paresthesia or anesthesia in the distribution of the inferior alveolar nerve, i.e., the lips, teeth, and gums.

RADIOLOGIC EXAMINATION

The mandibular plain film series — anteroposterior, right and left mandibular oblique, reverse Towne, and submental vertex (basal) views — is the preliminary examination of choice. The anteroposterior view visualizes the corpus, both alveolar arches, and lateral displacement of a posterior fracture. The right and left mandibular oblique views visualize the ascending ramus, coronoid process, and proximal corpus. The reverse Towne view visualizes the condylar neck and subcondylar areas; and the submental vertex view visualizes the corpus, ramus, and condyle.

The panorex radiograph is a tomogram of the mandible and provides the best overall view of the bone. It visualizes the bulk of the body and the condylar and subcondylar neck areas. It visualizes the maxillary and mandibular occlusal relation. However, the study lacks good definition of the anterior dentoalveolar segments because of cervical spine overlap. An occlusal radiograph is necessary to delineate the anterior dentoalveolar segments and symphysis areas.

Tomograms may be used to better visualize the degree of displacement of intracapsular and condylar neck fractures. Computed tomography (CT) scans are commonly used in the axial, coronal, and

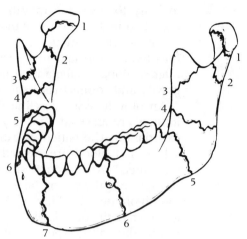

Fig. 14-3. Locations of mandibular fractures: (1) condylar, (2) subcondylar, (3) coronoid, (4) ramus, (5) angle, (6) body, (7) symphysis. (From C. A. Foster and J. E. Sherman. *Surgery of Facial Bones Fractures*. New York: Churchill Livingstone, 1987. With permission.)

three-dimensional formats for further evaluation of multiple and severely displaced injuries. Usually when a CT scan of the head is used to examine closed head injuries, lower axial cuts may be taken to assess the mandibular injury when clinical suspicion exists.

CLASSIFICATION

Mandibular fractures are classified by a number of criteria. The *location of the fracture* is the most common classification and includes the mandibular angles, mandibular symphysis, corpus, and subcondylar and condylar areas (Fig. 14-3). Open fractures are injuries in which bone is exposed to external elements through mucosa or skin. All fractures near the root of a tooth are considered open due to violation of the periodontal ligament. Segments may be displaced by the force of the injury or by muscular contraction. Unfavorable lines of fracture allow displacement of segments on muscular contraction of the muscles of mastication (Fig. 14-4).

Favorable lines of fracture allow segments to reduce with muscular contraction (Figs. 14-5–14-7):(1) horizontal favorable; (2) horizontal unfavorable; (3) vertical favorable; (4) vertical unfavorable. Fractures may also be classified by local characteristics. Simple fractures are those where the overlying skin and mucosa are intact. Compound fractures are exposed to the oral cavity or air via overlying mucosa or skin laceration. Linear fractures are single lines or straight fractures. Comminuted fractures have small curled segments with potentially compromised vascularity. Greenstick fractures are incomplete: One cortical plate is broken, and the other is bent. Complex fractures have fracture lines extending in multiple directions.

Further classification may be based on the *presence or absence of*

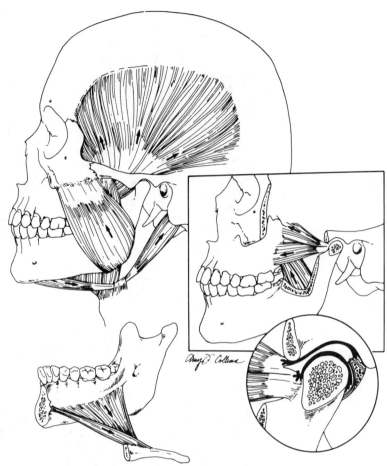

Fig. 14-4. Influence of muscles of mastication on fracture displacement. (From C. C. Alling and D. B. Osborn. *Maxillofacial Trauma.* Philadelphia: Lea & Febiger, 1988. With permission.)

teeth. Class III fractures are those with teeth in both sides of the fracture line. Class II fractures are those with teeth on one side of the fracture line. Class III fractures are those with no teeth on either side of the fracture line.

ACUTE CONSIDERATIONS

Patients with severe maxillofacial fractures often have many life-threatening injuries and are frequently unable to provide a history or to undergo a complete or cooperative examination. It is imperative that a physician trained in traumatology examines and manages the patient prior to considering management of the facial injuries.

Obtaining an adequate airway and beginning ventilation takes precedence during the initial management of patients with severe mandibular injuries, especially bilateral corpus or symphysis injuries. Prolapse or posterior positioning of the tongue may totally occlude the airway. Temporary management may include a towel clamp or

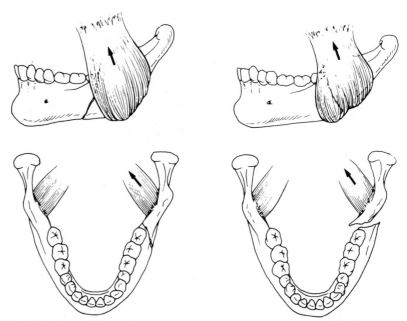

Fig. 14-5. Favorable and unfavorable fractures. (From C. C. Alling and D. B. Osborn. *Maxillofacial Trauma.* Philadelphia: Lea & Febiger, 1988. With permission.)

suture for anterior traction on the tongue prior to consideration for intubation. With concomitant severe soft-tissue injuries, hemorrhage, and multiple mid-facial fractures, tracheostomy should be considered. If respiratory embarrassment is acute, cricothyroidotomy should be done followed by a formal tracheostomy within 48 hours. In those patients with suspected cervical spine injuries and respiratory compromise, tracheostomy may be performed to prevent further neurologic sequelae by flexion or extension of the head during intubation.

Concomitant multisystemic injury is common and should be dealt with appropriately. Pneumothorax, hemothorax, and cardiac tamponade must be rapidly recognized and treated appropriately. Intravascular volume must be replaced. Visceral injuries, especially of the spleen, are not uncommon in multiply injured patients.

After appropriate stabilization of the patient, acute care of the mandibular injuries can be addressed. Oral debris, blood, and saliva should be suctioned and cleared in order that the injuries can be adequately assessed. Bleeding from fractures may be temporarily stopped by packing until further, permanent measures can be undertaken. Lacerations of the tongue and severance of the lingual artery are best treated with ligation and closure. Hemostasis should be obtained in a facility where appropriate lighting and equipment are available. Ligation of the internal maxillary, external carotid, or

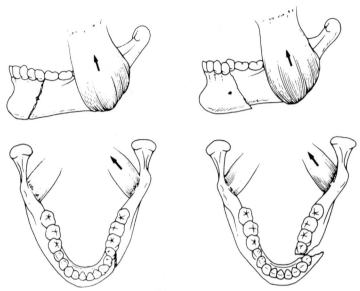

Fig. 14-6. Favorable and unfavorable fractures. (From C. C. Alling and D. B. Osborn. *Maxillofacial Trauma.* Philadelphia: Lea & Febiger, 1988. With permission.)

lingual artery in the neck is rarely required. Primary closure of wounds after proper irrigation and débridement is performed, and definitive fracture reduction is delayed.

THERAPY

Fractures with minimal displacement, greenstick fractures with an intact occlusion, or minimal trismus and discomfort may be treated with observation, soft diet, and close follow-up. Most mandibular fractures require some form of reduction and immobilization.

Closed reduction of mandibular fractures may be used as a form of definitive therapy, for temporary positioning intraoperatively, or as a postoperative adjunct. Maxillomandibular fixation is placement of the maxillary and mandibular teeth in correct relation and subsequent fixation with one of the many techniques available.

The *arch bar* is the workhorse of maxillomandibular fixation. These bars are bent around the buccal aspect of each tooth and do not extend past the last molar tooth. The bars are fixed to the segments with wires placed above and below the arch bar and passing around molar and premolar teeth below the height of the contour. Skeletal fixation of arch bars is recommended to prevent extrusion of teeth. It is accomplished by fixation to the upper and middle third of the bony skeleton via piriform aperture operative wires, circummalar wires, and circummandibular wires. Elastic bands are preferred to stainless steel wires for maxillomandibular fixation. Various interdental wire techniques can be used for max-

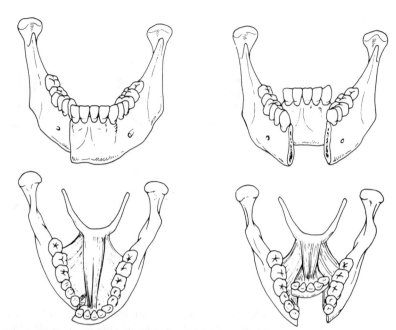

Fig. 14-7. Favorable and unfavorable fractures. (From C. C. Alling and D. B. Osborn. *Maxillofacial Trauma.* Philadelphia: Lea & Febiger, 1988. With permission.)

illomandibular fixation or to provide stability of dentoalveolar segments. Cap splinting, cast arch bars, lingual splints, and adaption prostheses are techniques that require a dental laboratory.

Treatment of mandibular fractures with maxillomandibular fixation forces the patient to maintain a liquid or blenderized diet. Weight loss is not uncommon, but with proper dieting, counseling, and compliance such loss can be minimized.

Permanent changes in tooth position, periodontium, short-term problems of poor hygiene and discomfort, and delayed return to work are potential complications of intermaxillary fixation being the sole therapy. Condylar changes may occur with prolonged maxillomandibular fixation. Open reduction and internal fixation of fractures with direct osseous wiring, plating, or lag screws with or without intermaxillary fixation is the most accurate method for reducing and immobilizing segments. Its advantages are that segments are directly visualized and rapidly returned to anatomic position; and the bony position is maintained with great security, so bone repair is hastened.

Virtually every fracture can be addressed by open means; however, there are certain fractures that definitely should be treated by open techniques. Fractures posterior to natural occlusion are better repaired with open reduction owing to the inability to control the position of the proximal segment with maxillomandibular fixation alone. Bilateral edentulous mandibular fractures are better repaired with open reduction and rigid fixation; they may require bone grafting.

Open reduction should be used when maxillomandibular fixation cannot be used successfully, as in severely uncooperative, mentally retarded, asthmatic, or myasthenia gravis patients. Open reduction is beneficial when therapy is delayed to better débride granulated tissue, approximate segments, and obtain more stable fixation. Open reduction of the mandible is used when the patient has suffered comminuted maxillary fractures, as it provides a stable base from which to build a normal occlusion.

CONSIDERATIONS BY A SPECIFIC LOCATION

Fractures in the condylar and subcondylar areas occur (1) high in the intracapsular area, (2) in the neck when the bone is thin and susceptible to fracture, and (3) in the subcondylar area from the sigmoid notch there to the posterior border of the ascending ramus (see Fig. 14-3). The lateral pterygoid pulls the proximal segment and may displace it anteriorly, medially, and inferiorly. The mandibular midline shifts toward the affected side upon opening. There may be an occlusion prematurely on the affected side, an open bite on the opposite side, or an anterior open bite with decreasing anterior facial height with bilateral fractures. Lacerations of the external auditory canal must be sought with these injuries.

They are further classified by the degree of displacement. *Minimal displacement* is when the condylar head is still present within the glenoid fossa. A *displaced fracture* is one that is out of the glenoid fossa but still within a range of normal movement. A *dislocated fracture* is one where the condyle is displaced out of the fossa and not in the range of normal movement (Table 14-1; Fig. 14-8).

Regarding therapy, the higher the fracture the more difficult is surgical and physiotherapeutic management. The lower the fracture,

Table 14-1. Temporomandibular joint fractures

Displacement	Head (intracapsular)	Neck (extracapsular)	Subcondylar (sigmoid notch)
Not displaced	Function movement[a]	Bony union (immobilization)	Bony union (immobilization)
Displaced	Function movement[a]	Bony union (manipulation, then immobilization) or Function movement[a]	Bony union (manipulation, then immobilization or open reduction)
Dislocated	Function movement[a] or excision	Function movement[a] or bony union (open reduction)	Bony union (open reduction)

[a] Initial immobilization to relieve pain.
Source: C. C. Alling and D. B. Osborn. *Maxillofacial Trauma*. Philadelphia: Lea & Febiger, 1989. With permission.

the greater is the need for open reduction. Adequate therapy includes closed reduction of minimally displaced and functional fractures with maxillary mandibular fixation for 8 to 14 days, followed by physiotherapy and oral opening exercises and elastics day and night for 4 weeks. Elastic rubber bands are then placed for a few months. Patients must be seen every 6 months for the first 4 years to monitor condylar position and resorption. If ankylosis, limitation of opening, or severe resorption with subsequent change and decreased facial height occurs, prosthetic reconstruction or costochondral grafting should be considered.

Open reduction may be accomplished by a Risdon (Fig. 14-9–14-11) incision with an extension in the low preauricular area for subcondylar fractures. The fracture may be rigidly fixed with compression miniplates accompanied by lag screws. Adoption plates are of inadequate strength for maintenance of position. Most fractures can be repaired by the modified Risdon approach. High condylar neck and intracapsular fractures may be addressed by a preauricular incision with or without a modified Risdon approach. This approach facilitates proper plate placement as well as direct repair of disc injury or displacement.

Neck fractures may be repaired with a single compression miniplate or a Kirschner wire placed as an intramedullary rod, from either above or below. Wire osteosynthesis to position the fragments prior to rigid fixation may facilitate fixation. It is important to attempt to maintain as much soft-tissue attachment to the proximal segment as possible to prevent aseptic necrosis of the condylar head. After rigid fixation, a blenderized diet should be maintained for 2 weeks followed by a soft mechanical diet for 4 weeks. Physiotherapy may be started after 2 weeks.

Mandibular angle fractures are best treated with open reduction through a Risdon incision followed by anatomic reduction after maxillomandibular fixation is accomplished. Rigid fixation with compression osteosynthesis at the inferior border and fixation with either a plate or wire in the tension band area is needed. Miniplates may be used only for those fractures with a favorable line and adequate bone edge adaptation. A mandibular compression plate should be placed at the inferior border; a four- to six-hole DCP or EDCP or a six-hole reconstruction plate followed by a 22- to 24-gauge wire, four-hole miniplate, or two- to four-hole DCP placed in the tension band area. When rigid fixation is obtained, the maxillomandibular fixation may be removed. Intraoral reduction and reduction with miniplates in the tension band area have been described and may be considered in selected cases. Proximal corpus and parasymphyseal fractures that are tiny and oblique may be approached by intraoral techniques, that is, an extended Risdon incision and rigid fixation, as described. In addition, long oblique fractures may be treated with multiple lag screws.

Parasymphyseal and symphyseal fractures may be treated via an

TMJ fractures

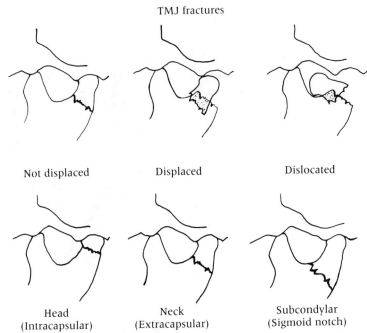

Not displaced   Displaced   Dislocated

Head   Neck   Subcondylar
(Intracapsular)   (Extracapsular)   (Sigmoid notch)

Fig. 14-8. TMJ fracture classification. (From C. C. Alling and D. B. Osborn. *Maxillofacial Trauma.* Philadelphia: Lea & Febiger, 1988. With permission.)

intraoral approach with fixation similar to that mentioned above.

Coronoid process fractures are unusual. They are not treated if little or no displacement is present. They are usually present in association with other mandibular fractures.

Multiple fractures of the mandible offer special consideration. Bilateral corpus fractures or corpus plus angle fractures have a tendency for the anterior segment to displace inferiorly and posteriorly with subsequent airway obstruction. Extraoral open reduction with rigid fixation is preferred. Body and condyle that may be displaced or dislocated is treated by rigid fixation and early mobilization. Comminuted fractures may be treated with a long stable fixation plate bridging the gap. Compression is *not* used in this area.

Extraoral skeletal fixation may not be used for injuries where there is a loss of bone stock or for comminuted fractures with multiple small fragments under unfavorable displacement forces. Grafting is necessary when it is difficult to attain internal fixation. Pins or screws are placed in bony fragments connected to bars connected by fixation clamps or set screws.

Fractures in children are treated as in adults with the following exceptions. Children's bones are more elastic and hence more resilient; greenstick fractures are thus more common. Intraosseous fixation has the increased risk of damaging developing tooth buds. Fixation is to be kept to a minimum. Condylar injuries with a

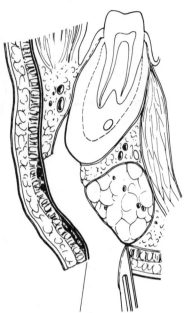

Superficial cervical fascia

Fig. 14-9. Risdon approach to the mandible. Dissection is carried through the skin, subcutaneous fascia, and platysma, preserving the marginal mandibular branch of the facial nerve, to the superficial layer of the deep cervical fascia. The dissection is carried superiorly along the fascia overlying the submandibular gland to the inferior border of the mandible. (From B. Spiessel. *Internal Fixation of the Mandible.* New York: Springer-Verlag, 1989. With permission.)

potential for altered growth and ankylosis are more likely to be treated with open operative surgery.

LAG SCREW PLACEMENT

The lag screw method is a compression technique that uses force generated by a screw perpendicular to the long arc of a fracture for stabilization. It uses the compressive force of the screw as well as the resistance to movement by the compressed segment. To use this technique, a hole is drilled in the outer cortex corresponding to the outer diameter of the screw. Using a paralleling device, a second hole is drilled into the inner cortex corresponding to the inner diameter of the screw and tapped with a tap of the same diameter as the hole in the outer cortex. This creates threads in the inner cortex only. A screw of the same diameter as the tap, and the hole in the outer cortex, is then placed.

For example, to place a 2.7 mm screw using lag technique, a 2.7 mm hole is drilled into the outer cortex, a 2.0 mm hole is then drilled into the inner cortex (corresponding to the 2.0 mm inner diameter of this screw) and the inner cortex is finally tapped with a 2.7 mm tap.

When using a 2.0 mm screw, the inner cortex is drilled with a

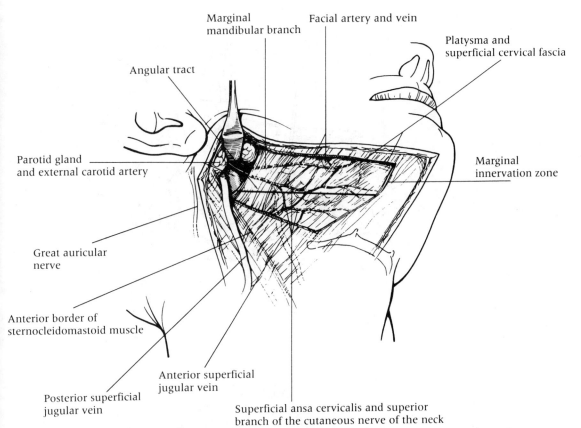

Marginal
mandibular branch

Facial artery and vein

Platysma and
superficial cervical fascia

Angular tract

Parotid gland
and external carotid artery

Marginal
innervation zone

Great auricular
nerve

Anterior border of
sternocleidomastoid muscle

Anterior superficial
jugular vein

Posterior superficial
jugular vein

Superficial ansa cervicalis and superior
branch of the cutaneous nerve of the neck

Fig. 14-10. Anatomy of the submandibular area. (From B. Spiessel.
Fixation of the Mandible. New York: Springer-Verlag, 1989. With
permission.)

1.5 mm drill and the outer cortex width a 2.0 mm drill, and the 2.0
mm tap is used.

COMPLICATIONS   Infection may be manifested by fever, purulent drainage, or an oral
cutaneous fistula. Adequate débridement, meticulous attention to
closure of wounds, and adequate stabilization of segments minimize
the risk. Any screw or fixation device that is loose creates an
increased risk of infection and should be removed. Preoperative and
interoperative antibiotics may be used in high risk cases. Penicillin is
the antibiotic of choice.

Malocclusion is not uncommon. Placing the patient in accurate
and rigid maxillomandibular fixation prior to rigid fixation of
osseous segments is imperative. Strict attention to detail during
plate-bending and screw placement prevents distortion of bone
segments and subsequent malocclusion. Rigidly fixed occlusal discrepancies are permanent unless the fixation is removed or the
occulsion is adjusted by movement of the teeth or sequential occlusal
adjustment.

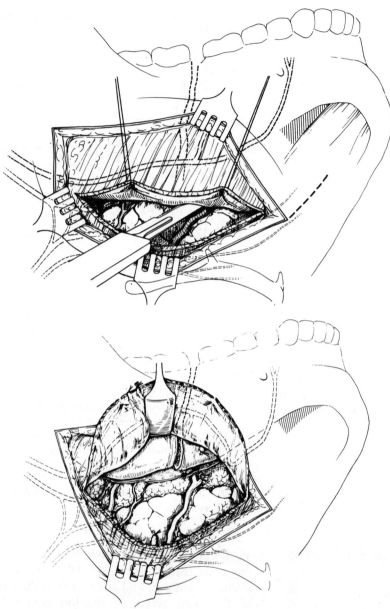

Fig. 14-11. Risdon approach to the mandible. (From B. Spiessel. *Internal Fixation of the Mandible.* Springer-Verlag, 1989. With permission.)

SUGGESTED READING

Alling, C. C., III, and Osborn, D. B. *Maxillofacial Trauma*. Philadelphia: Lea & Febiger, 1988. P. 259.

Bailey, B. J., and Halt, G. *Surgery of the Mandible*. New York: Thieme, 1987.

Converse, J. M., and Kazanjian, V. H. *Surgical Treatment of Facial Injuries*, Vols. 1 and 2. Baltimore: Williams & Wilkins, 1974.

Dingman, R. O., and Natvig, P. *Surgery of Facial Fractures*. Philadelphia: Saunders, 1964.

Foster, C. A., and Sherman, J. E. *Surgery of Facial Bone Fractures*. New York: Churchill Livingstone. 1987. P. 117.

Manson, P. N. (ed.), *Clinics in Plastic Surgery*, Vol. 16. Philadelphia: Saunders, 1989.

Rowe, N. L., and Williams, J. L. *Maxillofacial Injuries*, Vols. 1 and 2. New York: Churchill Livingstone, 1985.

Spiessel, B. *Rigid Fixation of the Mandible*. New York: Springer-Verlag, 1989.

Commentary on Chapter 14

Gary Patterson

The mandible, as we know, plays an important role in the vital oral functions of speech, mastication, and swallowing. During repair of mandibular injuries, let us not forget the simpler and adequately acceptable methods of fracture reduction and stabilization. Although not as popular as before, closed reduction techniques with the proper placement of arch bars or loop appliances continue to have a place in mandibular fracture repair. The use of interosseous wires, bone plates and screws, and crib trays are still widely used for open reduction techniques.

The advent of plate and screw fixation techniques is well covered in the literature, and Dr. Russavage covers the basic concepts regarding rigid osteosynthesis techniques. Although well behind the orthopedic surgical basic science and clinical aspects of rigid system design and use, the use of rigid techniques for facial trauma and maxillofacial reconstruction procedures has been running in "the fast lane." This concept of treatment has allowed the facial surgeon to more aggressively tailor the required treatment to the individual patient (adult and pediatric) during the initial repair and secondary revisions. The use of these systems enhances the patient's healing time and provides comfort during convalescence regarding the ability to communicate, masticate, and maintain oral hygiene. It appears that new instrumentation and methods of treatment are addressed daily. We must not be fooled that these methods are a panacea but must incorporate the ideas into our general knowledge store, thereby building on our *basic* foundation of delivering proper care and treatment.

The appearance of one's face is an important individual identity tag in our society, and the loss of facial form and function becomes a significant detriment. The goals of facial fracture (mandible) repair should include forming a proper diagnosis and establishing a workable treatment plan, achieving anatomic reductions, and establishing pretraumatic occlusion and facial form. Regardless of the technique and instrumentation used, the patient's well-being can be served if these rules are followed.

15 MAXILLA, ZYGOMA, AND ORBIT

James M. Russavage

People are identified by their own characteristic facial features. Society has unwritten standards of the features that are considered normal and those that are not. Successful communication with others from the basic act of speaking to the subtlest emotional expression depends largely on normal facial structure and function. The face is totally exposed, and any significant deformity is immediately noticeable. Therefore the preservation or restoration of normal facial structure and function is important.

MAXILLARY FRACTURES
Anatomy

The maxilla and associated facial bones are collectively the *mid-face*, or middle one-third of the facial skeleton. This complex area is bounded above by a line passing through the zygomaticofrontal, frontomaxillary, and frontonasal junctions, bound below by the occlusal table, and bound posteriorly by the sphenoethmoid junction superiorly and the pterygoid processes inferiorly. The facial skeleton in this region is composed of the paired nasal, lacrimal, zygomatic, inferior nasal conchae, palatine, and maxillary bones, as well as the unpaired vomer, ethmoid, and sphenoid bones (Fig. 15-1).

The *maxilla* is the principal bone of the mid-face and contributes to the structure of the orbit, nasal cavity, paranasal sinuses, and hard palate. It consists of a body and four processes. The body is hollowed by the pyramid-shaped maxillary sinus, with its base formed by the lateral nasal wall and its apex extending into the body of the zygoma. At birth the maxillary sinus is small, enlarging to its adult size at about 15 years of age. The growth of the sinus allows the maxilla to increase in size without a proportional increase in mass. The anterior wall becomes thin and is more easily fractured as it matures. The maxilla has four processes: alveolar, frontal, zygomatic, and palatine. The *alveolar process* contains the teeth, and with the loss of these teeth there is gradual resorption of this process. In the edentulous patient, resorption may be complete up to the nasal spine, leaving little bone between the sinus and the oral cavity. The

327

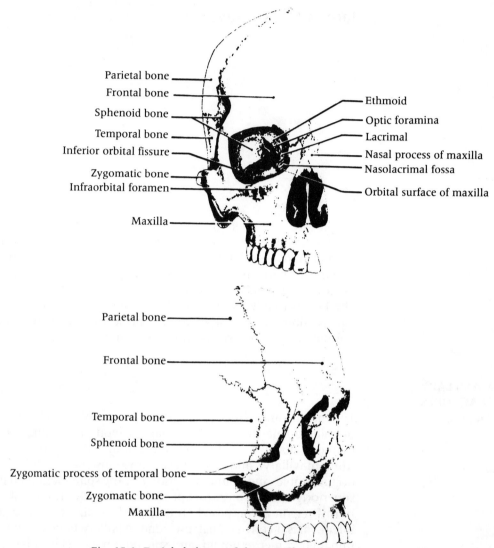

Fig. 15-1. Facial skeleton of the maxilla, orbit, and zygoma. (From C. C. Alling and D. B. Osborn. *Maxillofacial Trauma.* Philadelphia: Lea & Febiger, 1988. With permission.)

frontal process supports the nasal bones and articulates superiorly with the frontal bone at the frontomaxillary suture. The *zygomatic process* articulates laterally with the zygoma, and the *palatine process* articulates posteriorly with the vertical and horizontal plates of the palatine bone. The maxilla joins the vertical plate of the palatine bone to complete the pterygopalatine canal and with the horizontal plate of the palatine bone to form the posterior part of the hard palate.

The maxilla's anterior wall is thinned in the area of the canine fossa and thickened laterally at its junction with the zygoma. The posterior wall, formed by the maxillary tuberosity, faces the infratemporal space and forms the anterior boundary of the pterygopalatine fossa. The superior wall forms the greater portion of the anterior floor of the orbit and is traversed by the infraorbital groove containing the infraorbital nerve and vessels. The inferior wall of the maxilla is formed by the alveolar process containing the maxillary teeth.

The maxilla relates functionally and structurally to the mandible and cranium. Contact with the mandible occurs at the occlusal surface of the teeth. Although a normal class I occlusion is usually present, the incidence of class II and class III malocclusions is such that either may be the patient's pretraumatic occlusion. Loss of the maxillary teeth secondary to trauma or due to age may allow overrotation of the mandible, resulting in a pseudoprognathic appearance.

The *maxillary nerve*, the second branch of the fifth cranial nerve (CN V), exits through the foramen rotundum into the pterygopalatine fossa. It passes through the inferior orbital fissure to become the *infraorbital nerve*. Traversing the infraorbital canal and exiting through the infraorbital foramen, it supplies sensation to the upper lip and lateral aspect of the nose. Among its branches are the *anterosuperior alveolar nerve*, which arises from the infraorbital nerve and traverses the roof of the maxillary sinus to the anterior wall where it gives off branches to the incisor, canine, premolar, and first molar teeth; the adjacent gingiva; the maxillary sinus; and the floor, lateral wall, and septum of the nasal cavity anteriorly. The *posterior alveolar nerve* arises from the maxillary nerve in the pterygomaxillary fissure, where it lies along the posterior maxilla and then enters the bone to supply the molar teeth and join the anterior superior alveolar nerve in the plexus. The blood supply to the maxilla is rich and derives from the internal maxillary artery; its terminal branches are the greater palatine, infraorbital, and incisal arteries.

The middle facial skeleton is designed to resist the vertical forces of mastication and is reinforced by six vertical pillars, three on each side. These pillars — canine, zygomatic, and pterygoid — transmit the vertical forces generated by the teeth and distribute those forces over the cranial base.

Traumatic forces applied to the maxilla are distributed to the base of the skull through these pillars; and although they are effective in resisting forces exerted in a vertical direction, shear forces directed perpendicularly to the vertical pillars produce transverse oriented fractures of the maxilla (Fig. 15-2).

The zygomatic buttress begins in the alveolar bone of the anterior molar teeth and extends to the zygomatic process of the frontal bone. The zygomatic arch extends temporally to the cranial base. The pterygomaxillary buttress has two components. The pterygoid component extends from the posterior maxillary alveolus to the cranial base through the pyramidal process of the palatine bone, and the maxillary component relates the maxilla to the cranial base via the

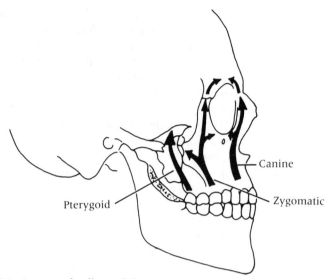

Fig. 15-2. Structural pillars of the mid-face protect the maxilla from vertical forces. (From C. C. Alling and D. B. Osborn. *Maxillofacial Trauma.* Philadelphia: Lea & Febiger, 1988. With permission.)

sphenoid. The structural pillars encircle the maxillary sinus, orbit, nasal cavity, and dental arch.

The zygoma articulates with four bones: maxilla, sphenoid, frontal, and temporal bones. This relation has often been confused by the misnomer "tripod" fractures, which is commonly applied to these injuries. There are three buttresses that resist significant displacement of the zygoma. The zygomatic process of the temporal bone buttresses the zygoma against forces that would displace it backward underneath the cranium. The greater wing of the sphenoid and the zygomatic process of the frontal bone provide resistance to vertical displacement. The usual pattern of zygomatic displacements bear out the infrequency with which fractures violate these buttresses (Fig. 15-3).

Knowing the zygoma's relation to the skull and familiarity with its surface anatomy allows one to appreciate and evaluate the extent of its injury more easily. There are three surfaces that comprise the zygoma: malar, orbital, and temporal surfaces. The malar surface forms the prominence of the cheek. The zygomaticofacial and zygomaticotemporal nerves exit through foramens on this surface to supply the sensation to the cheek and anterior temporal area, respectively. The orbital surface of the zygoma forms part of the floor and lateral wall of the orbit.

Teeth are largely formed from dentine, which is modified bone. However, the crown, which is normally the exposed part of the tooth, is covered by much harder enamel. At the neck (collum) of a tooth, the gingiva is attached, the enamel ceases, and the roots of the teeth extend into the alveolar process. When dentine is exposed through resorption of periodontal tissue, the entire exposed part of

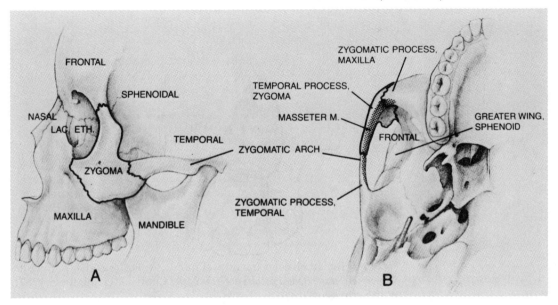

Fig. 15-3. A. Relation of the zygoma to the facial skeleton. *B.* Basal view. (From C. A. Foster and J. E. Sherman. *Surgery of Facial Bone Fractures.* New York: Churchill Livingstone, 1987. With permission.)

the tooth, regardless of whether it is covered by enamel, is known as the *clinical crown,* whereas the part deep to the gingival attachment is the *clinical root.* The incisors and canines have a single root each, the premolars have a single or double root or a single root with a bifid apex, and the molars have three roots. Each root is united by cementum to a periodontal ligament or membrane called *periodontium,* which represents the periosteal lining of the alveolus. The apex of each root presents a foramen that leads through a root canal.

The crown of each tooth has an occlusal (masticatory) surface, a vestibular or facial (outer) surface, a lingual (inner) surface, and, except for the third molar, two surfaces of contact — mesial (medial or anterior) and distal (lateral or posterior) — with other teeth. The occlusal "surfaces" of the incisors are more or less sharp incisal edges, and the canines end in blunted points. The upper canines or incisors sometimes show a marked thickening, the cingulum, on the lingual surfaces close to the gingiva. The occlusal surfaces of the premolars and molars are broad and have cusps (tubercles) that add to their grinding power but sometimes interfere with good occlusion between upper and lower teeth and may have to be reduced in height. The premolars have two cusps (hence "bicuspids"), the upper molars three or four, and the lower molars four or five.

The alveolar arch of the maxilla is typically somewhat larger than that of the mandible, and the premolars and molars of the upper jaw typically slant slightly outward toward their occlusal surfaces. The external walls of the alveoli, especially of the more anterior ones, are thin, but the medial walls are strengthened by the attachment of the palatine process. The third molar lacks this medial strengthen-

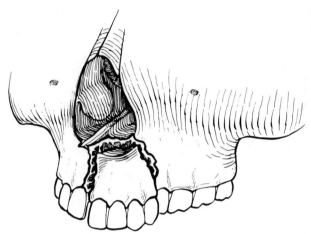

Fig. 15-4. Dental alveolar fracture. (From C. A. Foster and J. E. Sherman. *Surgery of Facial Bone Fractures.* New York: Churchill Livingstone, 1987. With permission.)

ing and is also close to the infratemporal (posterior) surface of the maxilla.

Etiology

Interpersonal violence accounts for most mandibular, zygomatico-maxillary complex, and nasal fractures. However, maxillary fractures occur more frequently in the young, mobile segment of the population in motor vehicle accidents, with men being affected three times more frequently than women.

Maxillary fractures in children less than 12 years old are uncommon because the maxilla is more elastic, more pneumatized, and more protected by the mandible and frontal bone in this group. Also, the child's lighter weight produces less inertial force when the head hits an object. The most common causes of maxillary fractures in the child are motor vehicle accidents, falls, and physical abuse.

Classification

An accurate clinical and radiographic appraisal of all the involved bones in mid-facial fractures is often difficult. One method of classifying fractures of the mid-face defines areas of the facial skeleton as *stable* and *not stable*. This designation is, however, descriptively inadequate; and in the clinical situation comminution and combinations of the various maxillary fracture types are the rule. Associated nasal, orbital, zygomatic, and nasoethmoid fractures are common, and a classification scheme allows a more systematic approach to these complex fractures.

Alveolar Fractures

The dentoalveolar process may be fractured alone or in combination with other maxillary fractures (Fig. 15-4). The mechanism is typically one of direct force applied anteriorly or laterally. The mandible may serve as an intermediary that directs the force of the blow upward and outward against the teeth of the maxilla. The fractured segment generally contains several teeth. The blood supply is usually secure and is based on the soft tissue of the labial-buccal sulcus or the palatal mucosa.

Sagittal Fractures

The sagittal fracture runs in a sagittal plane through the maxilla. The fracture may follow the transverse course of a Le Fort I type or cross the infraorbital rim into the orbit and down through the zygomaticomaxillary suture area. Many variations are possible. The fractures are caused by a force directed from the side; they are less common than the Le Fort fractures and are uncommon in pure form.

Le Fort Fractures

Rene Le Fort of Paris reported in 1901 his classic study of maxillary fractures in cadavers. By varying the degree and direction of blows to the maxilla, Le Fort found that fractures could generally be classified according to the highest level of fracture. Even today this monumental work forms the basis for the classification of fractures of the maxilla.

Le Fort I: Horizontal Fracture. The Le Fort I fracture (Fig. 15-5) begins at the lateral piriform rim, runs horizontally above the apices of the teeth, passes below the zygomaticomaxillary junction, through the pterygomaxillary junction, and passes through both pterygoid plates, usually at or below the pterygomaxillary fissure. The cartilaginous nasal septum is separated from the nasal spine and anterior palate, and a fracture extends through the base of the vomer.

Le Fort II: Pyramidal Fracture. The pattern formed by the lines of the Le Fort II fracture (see Fig. 15-5) resembles a pyramid. The fracture begins at a weak portion of the nasal bridge just below or at the frontonasal sutures and passes bilaterally through the frontal process of the maxillae and across the lacrimal bones to the anterior crest of the nasolacrimal canal. The fracture line then passes downward, laterally, and anteriorly across the most anterior aspect of the orbital floor and across the inferior orbital rim through or near the infraorbital foramen, then inferiorly along the anterior wall of the antrum. From here it runs under the zygoma (as does the Le Fort I fracture) and then extends along the tuberosity across the pterygomaxillary fissure and through the pterygoid plates at a higher level than does the Le Fort I fracture. Intranasally, the fracture runs through the upper one-third of the nasal septum, passing through the perpendicular plate of the ethmoid and across the middle of the vomer.

LeFort III: Transverse Fracture. A craniofacial disjunction is produced by the Le Fort III fracture (see Fig. 15-5). The fracture line is at the frontonasal and frontomaxillary junctions, passes bilaterally through the uppermost aspect of the nasolacrimal groove, and extends pos-

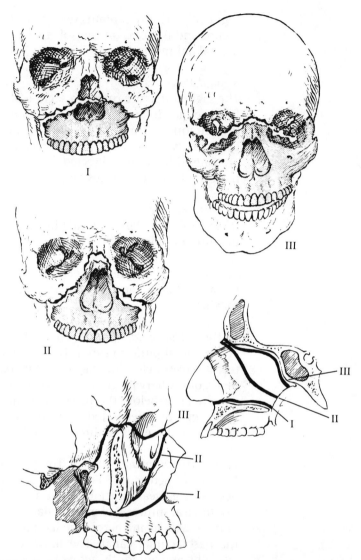

Fig. 15-5. Le Fort classification of maxillary fractures. (I) Transverse fracture of the maxilla. (II) Pyramidal fracture of the maxilla. (III) Craniofacial disjunction. (From R. B. Stark. *Plastic Surgery of the Head and Neck.* New York: Churchill, Livingstone, 1987. With permission.)

teriorly along the ethmoid to a point just anterior to the optic foramen. The thickness of the sphenoid bone surrounding the optic foramen is greater. Hence the incidence of fracture into the optic canal is reduced. The fracture then descends to the most posterior extent of the infraorbital canal and from there extends to the sphenopalatine fossa and then high across the pterygoid plates.

From within the orbit, a second fracture line passes anteriorly along the inferior orbital fissure and then extends superiorly along the lateral orbital wall at the junction of the zygoma and the greater wing of the sphenoid bone. It then passes through the zygomaticofrontal suture. A fracture through the zygomatic arches completes the extranasal course of the Le Fort III fracture.

Within the nose, the fracture line passes through the base of the perpendicular plate of the ethmoid, usually causing disruption and comminution of the cribriform plate. The fracture line finally passes through the connection of the vomer with the sphenoid bone, thus completing the disjunction of the mid-face from its cranial connection.

Comment. The Le Fort description provides a basis with which to identify and classify maxillary fractures. Though the fractures frequently occur as recognizable entities, combinations are also produced, and all three types of maxillary fracture can be present in the same patient bilaterally or unilaterally. The adjacent facial bones are commonly involved in maxillary fractures.

ZYGOMATIC FRACTURES

Because zygomatic fractures may be complex, classification systems have been proposed to aid in understanding the problem and facilitating treatment. A better understanding of specific fractures may be obtained by systematically grouping them into categories based on anatomic displacement. These groupings can then serve as a guide to management, leading to better and more predictable results.

The most widely accepted classification of zygomatic fractures was proposed by Knight and North in 1962 [1]. Modifications by Yanagisawa [2] have been added to include rotation around a longitudinal (anteroposterior) as well as vetical axis. Fracture *type I* represents nondisplaced fractures of the zygoma, and *type II* represents all fractures of the zygomatic arch. *Type III* fractures describe rotation around a vertical axis that is medial, lateral, or both. *Type IV* includes fractures around the longitudinal axis, again either medial or lateral. *Type V* fractures have displacement but no rotation; it may be either medial or lateral displacement. *Type VI* is the rim fracture, and *type VII* includes all complex fractures. Because the zygoma can rotate around a vertical or longitudinal axis, a complete classification should include this observation. In the modified Rowe and Killey classification [3], posterior displacement was added to type V because of its uniqueness and apparent frequency (12 percent of zygomatic fractures) (Fig. 15-6).

Initial Evaluation

Although facial injuries are often the most obvious, the patient must be evaluated and treated first for less obvious and more life-threatening injuries. The basic principles of trauma care must not be forgotten, and priority must be given to securing a clear airway, supporting respiration, and ensuring an adequate circulation. Only after the patient has been adequately evaluated and stabilized should the evaluation and treatment of the facial injuries begin. Many times

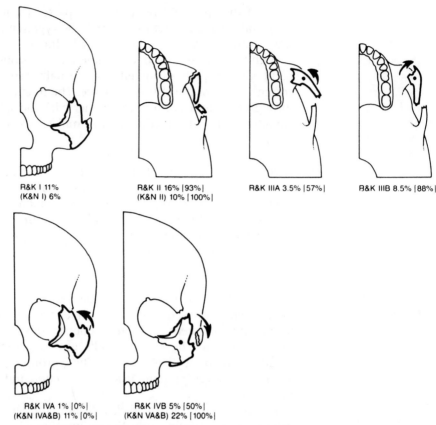

R&K I 11%
(K&N I) 6%

R&K II 16% |93%|
(K&N II) 10% |100%|

R&K IIIA 3.5% |57%|

R&K IIIB 8.5% |88%|

R&K IVA 1% |0%|
(K&N IVA&B) 11% |0%|

R&K IVB 5% |50%|
(K&N VA&B) 22% |100%|

Fig. 15-6. Classification of zygomatic fractures. (From C. C. Alling and D. B. Osborn. *Maxillofacial Trauma.* Philadelphia: Lea & Febiger, 1987. With permission.)

the definitive treatment of facial fractures can be postponed until the edema has subsided, although thorough early evaluation must not be neglected.

Evaluation should begin with a good history. Often it must be obtained from a family member or friend because the patient is unable to respond. Important facts include the cause of the injury (indicating type, amount, and direction of forces), the time of injury, and any previous facial injuries or preexisting abnormalities (e.g., malocclusion, blindness, deafness, facial asymmetry, or facial palsies).

Clinical Examination
The facial features of the patient who has sustained mid-facial trauma are often obscured by edema, ecchymosis, and hematoma. Soft-tissue edema forms rapidly, and areas of ecchymosis strongly suggest an underlying fracture.

The clinical examination should be detailed and systematic so that no areas are overlooked. The necessary instruments include a good light (preferably a headlamp), suction, dental and laryngeal mirrors,

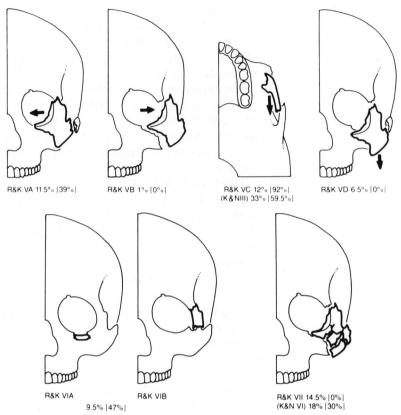

R&K VA 11.5% |39%| R&K VB 1% |0%| R&K VC 12% |92%| (K&NIII) 33% |59.5%| R&K VD 6.5% |0%|

R&K VIA   R&K VIB   R&K VII 14.5% |0%| (K&N VI) 18% |30%|
9.5% |47%|

Fig. 15-6. (continued)

tongue blade, small or medium nasal speculum, otoscope, and an ophthalmoscope. The examiner should closely observe the face, looking for asymmetry from the frontal and lateral views, as well as from the coronal view (looking over the face from above). Although swelling may obscure the underlying discrepancies, the observer can still note depressed fractures of the maxilla, zygoma, and zygomatic arch, as well as orbital rim and nasal fractures.

The entire head and neck is examined as described in Chapter 13. A thorough ophthalmologic examination is performed to rule out any injury to the eye prior to manipulation or treatment. The minimal eye examination includes carefully retracting the lids to examine for conjunctival or scleral lacerations, foreign bodies, corneal abrasions, and penetrating injuries of the globe; testing ocular movements and pupillary response; examining for enophthalmos, proptosis, and diplopia; and evaluating gross visual acuity. If edema and dried blood hamper the eye examination, gently retracting the lids with a lid retractor or moist cotton applicator sticks and washing the eye with sterile water can clear the field for a more unobstructed examination. If injuries to the globe, orbit, or periorbita are detected, an immediate ophthalmologic consultation should be requested.

The orbital rims are palpated. The examination begins in the medial canthal regions and progresses over the inferior, lateral, and superior borders of the rim. Lack of orbital integrity and displacement can be readily detected even when not apparent on radiographs.

The *medial canthal regions* should be palpated for crepitus and movement. The intercanthal distance should be measured (normal 33–35 mm); an increased distance may be the result of a displaced fracture of the frontomaxillary and lacrimal bones or of a tearing loose of the medial canthal ligament from the anterior and posterior lacrimal crests.

The *lateral canthal ligament* is attached to the frontal process of the zygoma. Inferior and medial displacement of the zygoma causes narrowing and inferior displacement of the lateral palpebral fissure. When there is a "step-off" of the inferior orbital rim, the integrity of the orbital floor must be tested. When the floor of the orbit is disrupted (blow-out fracture), orbital fat may herniate into the antrum, carrying with it the inferior rectus muscle. The patient is carefully tested for diplopia, enophthalmos, inferior rectus dysfunction, and infraorbital nerve hypoesthesia or anesthesia.

The zygomas are examined visually and tactilely for asymmetry. A depressed zygoma can be readily appreciated by viewing the face from a coronal position. The surgeon can better appreciate an asymmetry by displacing the edematous tissues over the zygoma. Another method to detect zygoma displacement is to place a tongue blade so that it contacts the bridge of the nose and the most prominent point on the zygoma and then compare the angle it forms with the frontal plane of the face with the opposite side. Palpation of the zygomaticoalveolar junction discloses the lack of continuity associated with the displaced zygoma. Displaced zygoma fractures can produce hypoesthesia or anesthesia over the infraorbital nerve and zygomaticofrontal and zygomaticotemporal nerve distributions.

A detailed examination of the maxilla begins with the dentition. Each tooth should be examined individually for fracture and mobility. A vertical alveolar or palatal fracture can be detected by manipulating the teeth. A tear in the palatal mucosa, a step deformity, or palatal ecchymosis may disclose a sagittal palatal fracture. Displaced or impacted maxillary fractures usually produce a malocclusion. To detect maxillary tipping, the lips are retracted and the teeth brought into contact so that the occlusion can be examined from a frontal view. Most horizontal maxillary fractures result in an anterior open bite.

The examining finger is next moved along the anterior and lateral sinus walls to detect a step or discontinuity in the bone. Attention should be directed to the junction of the zygoma and alveolar process, where a step or separation in the bone may be felt.

The presence of vestibular ecchymosis suggests an underlying fracture. Next, bimanual palpation of the facial skeleton is carried out to detect the type and extent of the maxillary fracture(s). The head is stabilized with one hand while the other hand attempts to move the maxilla. With Le Fort I fractures, the alveolar process of the maxilla and palate moves. With a sagittal fracture of the palate and alveolus, the two sides of the maxilla may move independently of one another. A finger placed in the vestibule while the maxilla is being manipulated can detect the fracture lines. If movement is noted at the frontonasal junction as well as at the inferior orbital rims, a Le Fort II fracture is present. With a Le Fort III fracture, the entire mid-face is movable, and palpation reveals separation and movement at the frontonasal and frontozygomatic junctions as well as movement over the zygomatic arches. These fractures are best detected with a second examiner stablizing the head while the primary examiner manipulates the maxilla and simultaneously palpates the bony junctions. If a Le Fort III fracture is identified, further manipulation of the maxilla should be avoided until radiographs have ruled out a fracture into the orbital apex.

The patient is also examined for cerebrospinal fluid (CSF) rhinorrhea. This problem may be obscured by nasal bleeding or because the CSF is escaping into the nasopharynx when the patient is observed in the supine position.

Trismus can occur if there has been impingement of the zygoma or the zygomatic arch on the coronoid process of the mandible. When fractures of the zygomatic arch are present, a noticeable depression in that area may be seen and confirmed by palpation. Fractures of the orbital process of the zygoma can result in disruption of the orbital floor and the suspensory ligament of Lockwood, and signs of entrapment may be noted. Examination of extraocular motion may demonstrate incomplete upward, lateral, or medial movement accompanied by diplopia. Confirmatory evidence of entrapment, especially of the inferior rectus muscle, can be obtained by a *forced duction test*. This test is performed by topically anesthetizing the area and putting forceps traction on the muscle.

An antimongoloid slant to the palpebral fissure can be caused by inferior displacement of the lateral canthus. The infraorbital nerve may be affected, and numbness or paresthesias in the distribution of this nerve may be present. Retraction of the lower eyelid may also result from downward displacement of the zygoma because of attachments of the orbital septum to the orbital rim.

To complete the mid-facial examination, the nose is examined externally and internally for nasal bone displacement, crepitation, obstruction, submucosal hematoma, septal displacement, and CSF rhinorrhea. With maxillary fractures or isolated nasal fractures, the septum is frequently displaced from the midline. The escape of CSF through the nose might indicate the presence of a pyramidal or transverse facial fracture in addition to a fracture of the cribriform plate. Nasal discharge can be identified as mucus rather than CSF if it starches a cloth when drying or by medical laboratory evaluation.

RADIOGRAPHIC EXAMINATION

Radiographs, computed tomography (CT) studies, or both are obtained for all patients with suspected or known facial injuries. In general, routine paranasal sinus (Waters) and lateral skull views are taken first, along with a lateral cervical spine film. If the neurologic and general status of the patient permit, special views of the skull, face, and mandible are obtained. The *Waters view* is the most informative film for maxillary fractures. The nasal septum, lateral nasal walls, lateral sinus walls, orbital rims, nasal bones, and frontozygomatic, frontomaxillary, and frontonasal junctions can be readily assessed from this view. The oblique view of the upper facial bones allows a relatively unobstructed view of the orbital rims, zygoma, and maxillary sinus. Occlusal views, although not generally part of the facial series, are useful for sagittal and alveolar fractures. The *panorex film* is useful not only for the mandible but for the lower maxilla as well. The use of tomograms, though occasionally helpful, has given way to the use of computed tomography, which more clearly shows the extent of the fractures, including intracranial and posterior orbital extensions. *Note:* A CT scan of the facial bones can be performed emergently at the same time intracranial injuries are investigated. The CT scan clearly displays and differentiates hard and soft tissues and shows distortion and displacement of bone, cartilage, and muscle.

The *axial view* is standard, but the coronal view may be helpful, particularly for looking at the orbital floor. The coronal cuts, however, require extension of the neck and are contraindicated in the presence of a suspected neck injury. Sagittal cuts can be reconstituted from axial views, and CT scans should be utilized in all patients with severe maxillary fractures, prior to exploration, in preference to any other radiographic technique.

In the patient with altered vision, a *CT scan* may be helpful for determining the need for optic nerve decompression. Soft tissues around the orbit can be displayed in detail as finely as bone structures, and a significant amount of information regarding the orbital contents and the optic nerve can be obtained. By altering the density and thickness of CT cuts, small bone fragments can be seen that are often missed by routine radiographs. Fractures associated with hemorrhage into the ethmoid and sphenoid sinuses could suffer optic nerve injury during reduction of the fractures.

Magnetic resonance imaging (MRI) is the latest advance in diagnostic cross-sectional depiction of the internal structures of the human body. Radiowaves, rather than ionizing radiation, are used to penetrate the tissues. MRI is sensitive to soft-tissue changes and shows good detail of fat and muscle planes. Excellent images of the orbits, paranasal sinuses, and cranial cavity are obtained from both sagittal and frontal planes. Currently the major drawbacks of using MRI in the traumatized patient are the length of time needed for the study and the absolute need for lack of motion during the imaging procedure.

The patient should never be sent to the radiography department of the hospital without a well trained attendant — one who is capable of monitoring the patient's level of consciousness, vital signs, and airway patency.

ORBITAL AND OCULAR INJURIES

Orbital and ocular injuries are produced by trauma directly to the orbit or indirectly from maxillary and zygomatic fractures. Although they do not occur frequently, when they are unrecognized or not managed appropriately the results can be disastrous for the patient. The signs and symptoms of fractures of the orbit include periorbital edema, ecchymosis, subconjunctival hemorrhage, ptosis of the lids, enophthalmos, exophthalmos, chemosis, and restriction of ocular motility. Ocular complications involving the globe include rupture of the globe, vitreous and anterior chamber hemorrhage, dislocated lens, choroid rupture, and late complications such as glaucoma and cataract formation. Any injury that involves the globe demands a pretreatment ophthalmologic consultation.

Le Fort III and nasoethmoid fractures involve the orbit and are associated with the highest incidence of orbital and ocular injuries. Le Fort III fractures disrupt the medial, lateral, and inferior orbital walls and may reach the orbital apex, producing several recognized syndromes.

Superior Orbital Fissure Syndrome

The superior orbital fissure syndrome is caused by pressure or disruption of the contents of the superior orbital fissure, that is, the oculomotor, trochlear, and abducent nerves, the three branches of the ophthalmic division of the trigeminal nerve, and sympathetic nerves from the cavernous plexus. The most common cause for this syndrome is pressure at the apex within the muscular cone formed by the common tendinous ring, the pressure being the result of edema or hemorrhage. Less commonly the fissure itself is disrupted, and fragments of bone impinge on the contents of the fissure. The results of this injury include varying degrees of exophthalmos, ophthalmoplegia, retroorbital pain, a fixed-dilated pupil, ptosis, and anesthesia over the distribution of the ophthalmic division of CN V, including loss of the corneal reflex (Table 15-1).

Orbital Apex Syndrome

Fracture through the optic foramen plus optic nerve injury are termed the orbital apex syndrome. Although the optic nerve is well protected by the body of the sphenoid bone, a fracture may nevertheless penetrate the foramen. Pressure from edema and hemorrhage may cause optic nerve damage without fracture. The results of optic nerve injury are neuritis, papilledema, or blindness.

Unilateral or bilateral loss of vision may accompany fractures of the frontonasal complex. On the rare occasion that unilateral vision loss occurs and fracture of the orbital apex on the opposite side is suspected, manipulation of the fractures should be delayed until fracture of the optic foramen is ruled out. Should there be loss of vision in one eye and fracture of the optic foramen in the other, the

Table 15-1. Manifestations of the superior orbital fissure syndrome

Signs and symptoms	Etiology
Gross and persistent edema of the periorbital tissues	Obstruction to venous and lymphatic drainage through the ophthalmic veins
Proptosis and subconjunctival ecchymosis	Intraconal and extraconal hemorrhage; loss of tone of extraocular muscles
Ptosis and ophthalmoplegia	Involvement of cranial nerves (CN) III, IV, VI
Dilation of the pupil	Involvement of parasympathetic supply carried in oculomotor nerve allowing unopposed sympathetic activity
Direct light reflex absent	Ipsilateral *efferent* arc blocked by lesion of CN III
Indirect (consensual) reflex present	Ipsilateral *afferent* arc intact; contralateral efferent arc also unaffected
Loss of accommodation reflex	Involvement of the motor (parasympathetic) root of the ciliary ganglion derived from the branch of the oculomotor nerve to the inferior oblique
Loss of corneal reflex	Anesthesia due to involvement of the nasociliary branch of the ophthalmic division of CN V
Loss of sensation over forehead extending to vertex	Involvement of frontal branch of ophthalmic division of CN V, mainly affecting supratrochlear and supraorbital nerves
Radiologic evidence of reduction in the dimensions of the superior orbital fissure	Medial displacement of greater wing of the sphenoid bone

Source: N. L. Rowe and J. L. Williams. *Maxillofacial Injuries.* Edinburgh: Churchill Livingstone, 1985. With permission.

fractures of the mid-face should be stabilized, but not reduced, in order to prevent possible bilateral loss of vision.

Diplopia

Diplopia, monocular or binocular, is a common sign of an orbital fracture. Monocular diplopia is caused by direct injury to the globe, such as hemorrhage into the anterior chamber or a detached lens. Binocular diplopia is usually caused by restriction of extraocular muscles, as is seen with orbital floor fractures, medial wall fractures, and blow-out fractures. Hemorrhage and edema causing increased intraorbital pressure can cause a transient diplopia, whereas a decrease in volume of the orbital contents (as seen with herniation of fat and muscle into the maxillary sinus) can result in permanent diplopia unless treated.

Blindness is usually a complication of the initial injury. The mechanism is thought to be an optic nerve laceration caused by displaced bone fragments.

ACUTE CONSIDERATIONS

Mid-facial fractures in themselves are seldom life-threatening unless they cause acute airway obstruction or significant hemorrhage. Life-threatening injuries are frequently associated with mid-facial fractures. Hence the management priority should be to rule out potentially lethal or permanently disfiguring injuries, and definitive management of the fractures can be delayed until the patient's overall condition is stabilized. Because of the frequency of associated injuries, the patient with facial trauma should primarily be under the care of a trauma team capable of the diagnosis and emergency management of these associated injuries. The principal aspects of acute management of the facial trauma patient are discussed in Chapter 13.

TREATMENT

The objectives in the treatment of mid-facial injuries are reestablishment of the functions of the oral cavity with the teeth in normal occlusion and correction of any facial deformity. Returning the teeth to their preinjury occlusion is the key for reducing maxillary fractures; on the basis of this reduction, other mid-facial fractures are reduced. The mandible is the structural pillar of the lower mid-face; it relates the mid-face to the cranium through the temporomandibular articulation. Bringing the maxillary teeth into occlusion with the intact mandible accurately establishes the maxillary position. If the mandible also is fractured, it must first be reduced and stabilized before treatment of maxillary and associated mid-facial fractures can proceed. It cannot be overemphasized that the *key to establishing the position of the mid-face is articulation of the teeth.* When the patient's natural teeth are missing, dentures or surgical splints can act as the key to reduction and provide sufficient stabilization.

Because mid-facial injuries produce a wide array of fracture patterns, no single treatment pattern or method can be applied to all patients. The principles of fracture treatment, however, are adequate reduction of the fragments, adequate immobilization of the fragments, and maintenance of the fragments in the immobilized position for sufficient time to allow the fracture to heal. The preferred method of treatment is the simplest one that satisfies the principles of fracture reduction and produces the best results.

An acceptable sequence of treatment is as follows.

1. Cleansing and débriding the oral cavity and face
2. Making dental impressions and pouring stone casts (optional)
3. Removing fractured, nonrestorable teeth and temporarily protecting injured, restorable teeth
4. Closing all oral and oropharyngeal lacerations, including lacerated major salivary gland ducts
5. Applying interdental wire ligature or arch bars
6. Reducing dental arch fractures
7. Reducing maxillary fractures and applying intermaxillary fixation

8. Performing transoral open reductions and fixation with miniplates or intraosseous wiring, when indicated

9. Reducing and fixating zygomatic, nasoethmoidal, orbital, and nasal fractures

10. Placing zygomatic, cranial, and extracranial suspension, if needed

11. Closing all facial incisions and lacerations

Initial Wound Care and Débridement

The oral cavity is cleansed by irrigation with copious amounts of sterile saline or an antiseptic solution using a 30- to 50-ml plastic syringe and a blunted 18-gauge irrigating needle. Use of solutions containing hydrogen peroxide should be discouraged. A toothbrush can be used to clean dried blood clots from the teeth, gingiva, tongue, and hard palate. If loose bone fragments are encountered, only those fragments that become dislodged with irrigation should be removed. All other bone fragments, no matter how minimally attached to soft tissue, must be retained. Likewise, all tissues must be retained unless they are obviously nonvital. The repair potential of the oral soft tissues is excellent; only crushed tissue or tissues without blood supply should be excised.

Injured and Fractured Teeth

Only teeth that are fractured beyond repair or impacted teeth that are displaced in a fracture line should be removed. Sound, fully erupted, functional teeth left in the line of fracture have not been shown to increase the incidence of infection or nonunion. Exposed dentin should be protected with intermediate restorative materials, and exposed pulps should be partially or totally extirpated and the pulp chamber sealed. Teeth with nonrestorable caries that will not aid in intermaxillary fixation are best removed at this time. Dental or oral surgical consultations are valuable here.

Closure of Oral Lacerations

A watertight seal of the oral mucosa is necessary to prevent continued contamination of underlying fractures. If a laceration can be used to gain access for an intraoral open reduction, its closure can be delayed until after fracture reduction and application of intermaxillary fixation. Gingival and mucosal lacerations are best closed with interrupted absorbable sutures such as 4-0 or 5-0 chromic gut. Lacerations of the tongue are closed before intermaxillary fixation is applied; all muscle layers of the tongue are closed with deep, widely placed absorbable sutures. If a laceration has passed through the areas of the parotid and submandibular ducts, the ducts should be probed; if they are found to be severed, their ends should be identified and closed with 5-0 or 6-0 nylon over a polyethylene tube with an inside diameter of at least 0.034 inch. The polyethylene tube is left in place for 2 weeks (see Chapter 17).

Alveolar Fractures

When there is an intact maxilla on either side, the displaced dentoalveolar segment is reduced and ligated to the adjacent teeth. This repair may be accomplished by utilizing an arch bar to fix the segment relative to the intact maxilla or intraosseous fixation with wire or miniplate. Associated soft-tissue injury is repaired. When there are other fractures of the maxilla that make secure immobilization of the segment impossible, temporary intermaxillary fixation should be performed. When the alveolar segment is large, added stability may be gained by fabrication of an acrylic splint. An alternative approach obviating the need for an open reduction is the use of rubber band intermaxillary fixation. The mandible gradually forces the segment into place over a period of hours. *Failure to achieve reduction by this technique requires open reduction.* Treatment of a fracture of the dentoalveolar segment requires immobilization for 3 to 4 weeks unless rigidly fixed.

Reduction of Maxillary Fractures and Intermaxillary Fixation

When the maxillary arch and dentition have been stabilized, the maxilla is then reduced. Le Fort I fractures that are nondisplaced need only to be placed in maxillomandibular fixation using 28-gauge stainless steel wires ligated to the previously placed maxillary and mandibular arch bars or interdental loops. The displaced maxilla is then brought into its proper position by manual manipulation. Adequate mobilization of the maxilla is essential prior to fixation. A wire placed around the arch bar near the midline can be used to pull the impacted maxilla forward and into occlusion. If the maxilla is so impacted or displaced that it cannot be reduced by the previous methods, disimpaction forceps should be used to reduce the maxilla with the patient under general anesthesia. The Rowe disimpaction forceps engages the palate bilaterally from the nasal and oral side and provides excellent leverage and control. The Tessier disimpaction forceps engages the tuberosity just below the fracture line and disimpacts the maxilla by rocking it slowly. At this point intermaxillary wires are applied, and the anterior and lateral maxillary walls are palpated to confirm anatomic reduction. Sudden bleeding from the descending palatine or transeptal arteries may occur during this maneuver.

Le Fort II fractures are managed in a similar manner. The surgeon should manually reduce Le Fort II fractures with great care, remembering that the medial orbital wall and anterior orbital floor are fractures and that excessive manipulation could damage the nasolacrimal duct and inferior orbital nerve. After intermaxillary fixation is applied, the frontonasal junction and inferior orbital rims are palpated to confirm fracture reduction. Ocular motility must be checked at this time to ensure that the inferior rectus has not been entrapped during the reduction procedure.

As with the Le Fort I and II fractures of the maxilla, the Le Fort III fracture is reduced by first placing the maxillary and mandibular teeth into occlusion and applying intermaxillary fixation. Disimpaction forceps may be needed to bring the fractured buttresses into anatomic position. As mentioned earlier in this chapter, the possibility of fracture into the optic foraminae should be ruled out before manipulating the mid-face. If there is any doubt about injury to the optic nerves, fracture reduction should be delayed. During manipulation of the mid-face the frontonasal and zygomaticofrontal junction should be palpated to confirm adequate mobilization and reduction. Nasal bleeding, if encountered, usually stops once the mid-face is fully reduced and stabilized to the mandible.

Skeletal Fixation and Open Reduction

Skeletal fixation of maxillary fractures can be achieved through the use of suspension wires, direct intraosseous wires, miniplates, or external cranial suspension devices. The sites commonly used for placement of suspension wires, compression plates and miniplates, or intraosseous wires are the anterior nasal spine, lateral piriform rim, inferior orbital rim, zygomatic buttress, zygomatic arch, and frontomaxillary junction. Suspension wires serve to prevent distraction of the maxilla in an inferior direction when the teeth are in occlusion. The surgeon must bear in mind, however, that suspension wires from the zygomatic arch and from the frontozygomatic junction when tightened are angled 30 to 45 degrees from the vertical and exert a backward and upward pull on the maxilla, which tends to displace the maxilla superiorly and posteriorly. Great care must be exercised not to tighten the wires such that the mid-face is shortened; also, the wires must be placed with equal tension on both sides so as not to cant the maxilla.

The use of suspension wires is contraindicated in cases in which intermaxillary fixation cannot be applied, for example in edentulous patients when splints or dentures are not available. In these cases, transosseous wires or bone plates are used. A headframe for external craniofacial support should be considered for (1) mid-facial fractures that require significant anterior traction for reduction and fixation, (2) mid-facial fractures with concomitant bilateral, dislocated condylar process fractures that are not amenable to open reduction, and (3) severely comminuted mid-facial fractures that do not provide the stable bone contacts at the fractured areas. The first intact bone above the fracture site ordinarily serves for wire suspension, although wires may be suspended from higher sites. If suspension wires are necessary for the treatment of a horizontal maxillary fracture (Le Fort I), the level of the fracture influences the site used for suspension. The anterior nasal spine can be used only if the fracture is below this point. The lateral piriform rim and zygomatic arch can be used as points of suspension for high or low horizontal fractures (Fig. 15-7A, B). Circumzygomatic wiring can also be used for the suspension of a pyramidal (Le Fort II) fracture (Fig. 15-7C). Other sites of suspension that can be used for the Le Fort II fracture are the lateral infraorbital rims and the zygomatic processes of the frontal bone. Intraosseous wire fixation in the infraorbital area can be accomplished concurrently, although it is needed infrequently because reestablishment of the occlusion and wire suspension when indicated usually restores the orbital rim contour. Suspension of the

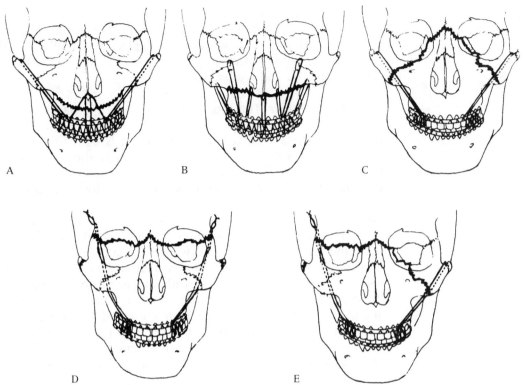

Fig. 15-7. Suspension wires. Midfacial skeletal fractures are usually comminuted, with unstable associated sections of bone. Suspending wires circumvent the fragmented fracture lines and preserve the nonyielding sling on the periosteal sheath and the periosteum attachments to bony fragments. A. Le Fort I, zygomatic arch suspension. B. Le Fort I, infraorbital suspension. C. Le Fort II, zygomatic arch suspension. D. Le Fort III, frontal bone suspension. E. Mixed fracture, mixed suspension. (From C. A. Foster and J. E. Sherman. *Surgery of Facial Bone Fractures.* New York: Churchill Livingstone, 1987. With permission.)

transverse facial (Le Fort III) fracture is accomplished by means of direct intraosseous wiring of the zygomaticofrontal separation and concurrent placement of suspension wires from the zygomatic processes of the frontal bones; the suspension wires are introduced into the oral cavity with a zygomatic passing awl (Fig. 15-7D). Combinations of fractures, such as a Le Fort I on one side and a Le Fort II on the other, may also require suspension. If so, the same suspension point should be used for both sides to avoid any difference in angulation or tension on the suspension wire (Fig. 15-7E). Mid-facial skeletal fractures are usually comminuted, with unstable associated sections of bone. Suspending wires circumvent the fragmented fracture lines and preserve the nonyielding sling of the periosteal sheath and the periosteal attachments to bony fragments.

Techniques for Placement of Suspension and Intraosseous Wires
Because all suspension wires communicate with the oral cavity, one might expect infection to be a complicting factor. Actually, infection occurs rarely, although prophylactic antibiotics are used when the wires are placed and removed.

Anterior Nasal Spine. The anterior nasal spine is approached through a 1.5-cm vertical mucoperiosteal incision directly over it. A sharp periosteum elevator or a large dental curet is used to expose the spine, after which a hole is drilled through the spine with a wire-passing bur. A length of 26-gauge stainless steel wire is threaded through the hole, and the incision is closed around it.

Lateral Piriform Rim. The lateral piriform rim is palpated, and a vertical mucoperiosteal incision is made just lateral to it so as not to enter the nose. The periosteum is elevated laterally, and the nasal mucosa is carefully elevated medially to allow insertion of a submucous elevator or a periosteal elevator under the nasal mucosa for protection from the bur. A bur hole is made from a lateral direction and placed at least 5 mm above the fracture and 5 mm lateral to the rim. A wire is then threaded through the hole and extended through the incision. The mucosa is closed around the wire. This wire provides strong, direct support to the anterior maxilla.

Infraorbital Rim. The infraorbital rim is approached through a 2 cm long horizontal incision made in the mucobuccal fold at the canine fossa. While a finger palpates the infraorbital rim externally, the mucoperiosteum is elevated lateral to the infraorbital foramen until the rim is reached. The periosteal reflection is then carried to the orbital side of the rim. An instrument protects the globe while a bur hole is started 3 to 5 mm below the rim, slanted superiorly, and carried until the bur perforates the anterior orbital floor and hits the protecting instrument.

With the protecting instrument still in place, a length of wire is placed through the hole, grasped, and brought through the incision. The incision is closed around the wire. The infraorbital wire provides direct support to the entire maxilla and avoids the posterior angulation seen with circumzygomatic wires. It can also be used for the pyramidal fracture, provided the zygoma is intact and the wire is placed lateral to the infraorbital fracture.

Zygomatic Buttress. The zygomatic buttress is approached through a horizontal mucoperiosteal incision placed in the buccal sulcus directly over the buttress. The buttress is exposed on its anterior and posterior surfaces. A bur hole is made through the buttress, passing from anterior to posterior, and is placed at least 5mm above the fracture line. A wire is then passed through both bur holes and brought through the incision. The mucosa is closed around the wire.

The zygomatic buttress wire provides strong, direct suspension for the Le Fort I fracture when the zygoma is intact. In the edentulous patient it also provides a direct method of securing the denture or splint to the maxilla.

A second method of passing the suspension wire involves use of a No. 18 spinal needle that has been slightly curved. The needle is passed medially to the zygomatic arch from the same point on the skin from which the awl is passed. After the spinal needle enters the oral cavity, a strand of wire is passed through the lumen of the needle into the mouth. The intraoral end of the wire is grasped with a hemostat, and the needle is then withdrawn superiorly and passed laterally to the arch, directing the wire ahead of the needle. The wire is carried over the arch and into the mouth. The end of the wire in the needle is pulled out of the needle, and the needle is removed inferiorly. Both ends of the suspension wire are grasped, and a sawing motion is used to ensure that the wire is securely placed over the arch.

The many variations for passing circumzygomatic arch wires and other circumferential wires include the use of autopsy needles, 18-gauge spinal needles, and intracatheter plastic cannulas. They may be introduced from a sterile cutaneous area into the oral cavity carrying the wire medially to the zygomatic arch, for example. The carrying instrument is discarded; and a second, sterile carrying instrument is introduced into the same cutaneous puncture site that carries the other end of the wire into the oral cavity.

Zygomatic Process of the Frontal Bone. The zygomaticofrontal suture is the landmark used to place a suspension wire from the frontal bone. The suture is not palpable unless it is separated. The suture is found directly under the lateral one-third of the eyebrow. The eyebrows are not shaved. A skin incision 1.5 cm long is made through the lateral one-third of the eyebrow. The incision should not extend to the outer canthus. The incision may be carried directly to bone. The periosteum is elevated to expose the zygomaticofrontal suture. A finger is placed along the orbital surface of the suture to protect the globe. The temporal fascia is incised, and the temporal muscle must be elevated slightly and protected from the bur. A bur hole is made through the zygomatic process of the frontal bone obliquely from the orbital to the temporal surface. The hole is placed 5 mm superiorly to the suture line. If the suture is separated, a second hole is placed inferiorly to the separation through the frontal process of the zygoma. A second wire, usually 26 gauge, is passed through both holes, tightened to reduce the separation, and twisted on the temporal surface of the frontal process of the zygoma. The suspension wire is then passed through the superior bone hole; and with a passing awl or other instrument, both ends of the wires are carried medially to the zygomatic arch and under the zygoma into the oral cavity in the region of the first molar. Before the craniofacial suspension wire is tightened it is inspected to make certain it is not under the transosseous wire, a condition that makes its removal difficult. The incision is left open until the contralateral wiring has been completed.

Extraoral Approach to the Inferior Orbital Rim. An extraoral approach to the inferior orbital rim is necessary when there is a displaced fracture through the inferior orbital rim that is unstable or not reducible by closed methods of treatment or when there is a fracture with disruption of the orbital floor.

A 5-0 nylon tarsorraphy suture is placed. The rim is palpated, and an incision is planned to center over the fracture. A subciliary or transconjunctival incision is made. The periosteum is then sharply incised over the rim and gently elevated anteriorly to expose the fracture and identify the infraorbital foramen and nerve. Small fragments of bone that are encountered should not be freed from their periosteal attachment but, rather, preserved and minimally repositioned. The periosteum is also carefully elevated from the anterior orbital floor. Great care must be taken not to perforate the periosteum or orbital septum, as perforation would result in the extravasation of orbital fat. The infraorbital fracture is reduced, and mini- or microplate or 28-gauge wire fixation is applied. The globe must be protected with an instrument during the drilling. If possible, the twisted end of the wire is placed into one of the holes so that it does not interfere with the orbicularis oculi function. The periosteum and muscle layers are closed separately, and a subcutaneous running suture of 6-0 nylon is used for skin closure.

As transosseous wires between fragments of mid-facial skeletal fractures are tightened, the wires may pull through or displace small, thin fragments. Miniplates or microplates are simpler to place than transosseous wires, but their use is limited to fragments sufficiently thick to hold the screws and large enough to maintain periosteal attachments.

External Cranial Suspension

The use of halo-type and box-type head frames has been well documented. They provide a stable base well above the fractures of the mid-face and allow anterior traction of the maxilla and mandible, which internal wire suspension cannot provide. They may be used for (1) severely comminuted mid-facial fractures that lack a solid bone base from which to suspend the maxilla or to wire or plate directly; (2) displaced mid-facial fractures associated with bilaterally displaced or dislocated mandibular condylar fractures; (3) patients whose associated injuries do not permit lengthy fracture reduction and fixation procedures; and (4) delayed treatment of impacted maxillary fractures that require continuous anterior traction for reduction. Because the need for a head-frame may arise suddenly, the surgeon responsible for treating maxillofacial fractures should have a head-frame set ready to use.

Le Fort Fractures

The Le Fort classification is used when planning surgical treatment, but variations of maxillary fractures are so common that treatment needs to be individualized more for those fractures than for any other facial fracture. Nevertheless, in the interest of simplicity, treatment is best discussed by considering each of the three classes of maxillary fractures separately.

Because of the need for access to both mid-face and teeth, particularly when intermaxillary fixation is indicated, nasotracheal intubation is necessary. Tracheostomy is helpful to the craniofacial surgeon if both mandible and maxilla are injured or if other injuries require it.

The concept of treatment of Le Fort fractures is evolving from one based on reduction, intermaxillary fixation, and craniomaxillary suspension to one based on open reduction, intermaxillary fixation, rigid fixation, and less use of craniomaxillary suspension wires. Mid-facial fractures are commonly comminuted. The impaction associated with suspension wires may lead to excessive shortening of the maxilla and premature contact of the molar teeth, which leads to an anterior open bite. Shortening of the maxilla (loss of vertical height), a difficult condition to correct later, is more common than lengthening of the mid-face following treatment. Recently, interest has been generated in the use of miniplate plus microplate fixation to eliminate the necessity of prolonged intermaxillary fixation. Reestablishment of the patient's pretraumatic occlusion and intermaxillary fixation remain, however, the foundation of Le Fort fracture treatment.

Le Fort I: Transverse Maxillary Fractures. The mandible is the key to reduction of the maxilla. All mandibular fractures are reduced and fixed relative to the cranial base. The maxilla is then reduced and placed in proper occlusion with the mandible. The incidence of pretraumatic malocclusion is significant and should be considered if any difficulty is encountered when placing the maxilla in class I occlusion. The *wear pattern* of the teeth can be a reliable guide to proper occlusion.

When vertical displacement is minimal, simple intermaxillary elastic fixation is sufficient to achieve the best possible dental occlusion. If there is segmental maxillary fracture, interdental fixation with a supporting metal arch bar usually suffices.

Although it is reported that the maxillary fracture heals without malunion or facial elongation with intermaxillary fixation alone, some additional means of stabilization is commonly added. A suspension wire may be passed percutaneously around the zygomatic arch and attached to the upper or lower arch bar. This route offers the *disadvantages of a posteriorly directed force* that may tend to retrude the maxilla. Alternatively, a hole may be drilled through the inferior orbital rim and used to anchor the suspension wires. Obviously, this procedure requires an open approach. Another approach is to explore the fracture through the labial-buccal sulcus with direct fragment wiring in the region of the zygomatic buttress and the piriform aperture. Additionally, from the same holes, suspension wire can be passed from the strong triangle of bone where the piriform aperture meets the maxillary sinus. This approach, however, may still lead to excessive shortening of the maxilla in cases of severe comminution. If this problem occurs, simple internal fixation is appropriate. Regardless of the method used for suspension, it is suggested that this loop be twisted closed just inside the labiobuccal sulcus with an auxiliary loop dropped from here to the upper or lower arch bar. Tightening of the stretched wire may be necessary for several weeks postoperatively. As this wire may break, it is easily replaced without jeopardizing the suspension wire. This suspension loop, visible in the upper sulcus, is easily removed after the period of intermaxillary fixation is over. Union is usually uneventful and nonunion rare. Intermaxillary fixation is maintained for 4 to 6 weeks.

Maxillary suspension is indicated when there is significant downward or lateral displacement of fracture fragments. It is accomplished as above. Le Fort I fractures in edentulous patients often require no therapy. On occasion, reduction and fixation of these fractures are necessary to reestablish and maintain normal maxillomandibular relations. The patient's dentures are ideal for use in this reduction. If dentures are unavailable, Gunning's splints may be constructed to maintain fixation.

When patients have concomitant mandibular fractures, the management becomes more complex. Establishing normal occlusion becomes a prime goal when planning treatment: The maxilla must be suspended and rigidly immobilized at just described. After interosseous fixation of the mandibular fracture, arch bars are ligated to the mandibular dental arch, after which the jaws are immobilized in occlusion, preferably with intermaxillary elastics. The suspension wires are well tolerated if the mouth is kept clean. The suspension is maintained for about 6 weeks until fibrous union of the fracture has taken place. The suspension wires can then be removed by cutting them within the mouth and pulling on one end. If difficulty is encountered, a small incision can be made under local anesthesia at the lateral orbital rim and the wire loop removed directly.

Le Fort II: Pyramidal Fractures. Pyramidal fractures and fractures of the zygoma have in common involvement of the maxillary antrum, the inferior orbital rim at the infraorbital foramen, and the orbital floor. With maxillary fractures, however, the central segment is displaced posteriorly with upward angulation so the patient has an anterior open bite. The apex of this fracture segment involves the nasal bones and often the bones making up the medial aspect of the orbit as well.

The surgical approach is similar to that for open reduction of zygoma fractures, with incisions in the lower eyelids and internal wire fixation of the reduced fracture fragments at the inferior orbital rims. Open or closed reduction of the nasal fracture is necessary to align the apex of this pyramidal segment.

The maxilla is usually retruded, and reduction is frequently facilitated with the use of Rowe or Hayton-Williams disimpaction forceps. Pretraumatic occlusion is reestablished, and the maxilla is placed in intermaxillary fixation. Commonly, craniomaxillary suspension wires are then dropped from the zygomatic arch or inferior orbital rim to complete treatment. However, open reduction of the upper maxilla is preferred to simple suspension wires for reasons already mentioned. Internal fixation is done at the nasofrontal suture, infraorbital rim, and zygomatic buttress. Superiorly, exposure is gained through any existing laceration, a local incision, or preferably through a bicoronal approach. The bicoronal exposure also allows for adequate visualization for the treatment of any nasoorbital fracture and traumatic telecanthus.

As with transverse maxillary fractures, when significant displacement or mobility of fracture fragments is present, the maxilla must be suspended from intact temporal bone. In cases of marked comminution and fragment instability, segments of split rib or cranial bone can be wired across the fracture sites to achieve rigidity. Occasionally this maneuver may even eliminate the need for maxillary suspension. As stated previously miniplates and microplates may be used in place of transosseous wires.

Le Fort III: Craniofacial Disjunction. Craniofacial disjunction is the most complex of all facial fractures. As the name describes, it constitutes separation of the mid-face from the cranium. With this injury the entire middle third of the face is fractured, with not only the maxilla but also one or both zygomas and the nose involved.

Patients with this injury have a bloated, edematous mid-face that in itself is rather typical. A "free-floating" maxilla is usually found. Malocclusion due to tilting upward and backward of the detached maxilla usually occurs and presents as an anterior open bite.

Numerous special instruments have been developed to treat these fractures, and special metal or plastic head caps have been devised for external support. Despite mechanical refinements, these skull-supported traction devices usually fail to fulfill completely their intended function. They are difficult to apply, uncomfortable for the patient to wear, and require constant adjustment. They do not usually remain in place for the length of time required.

Reduction and immobilization is approached as for the Le Fort II fracture. The maxilla is reduced and placed into intermaxillary fixation. Craniomaxillary suspension wires can be dropped from the superior lateral orbital rim after reduction and interosseous wire fixation of the frontozygomatic suture region of the fracture. However, direct wiring or open reduction/internal fixation of the major fracture is preferred. A bicoronal flap is raised. The nasofrontal region is wired. The lateral orbital rim is easily exposed and wired or plated through the bicoronal incision. In addition, this incision affords a direct approach to the zygomatic arch, which is difficult to achieve through local incisions because of the danger of injury to the temporal branch of the facial nerve. A lower eyelid incision allows inspection and treatment of orbital floor fractures. With extensive orbital floor fracture or nasoethmoid fracture, primary bone grafting may be indicated. The outer table of skull is preferred and is easily accessible through the bicoronal incision. The utility of bone grafts in the pterygomaxillary area is unproved. Intermaxillary fixation is continued for approximately 6 weeks. Rigid fixation with plates from the unfractured superiormost bone to the mobile segments may obviate the need for maxillomandibular fixation.

Sagittal Fractures

Simply placing the maxilla into intermaxillary fixation allows palatal rotation of the lateral maxillary segments toward the midline. To prevent this problem, a palatal splint is fabricated to hold the lateral segments in proper occlusion. In addition, it is suggested that an interosseous wire is necessary at the piriform aperture. Fractures that also extend laterally in the manner of a Le Fort I fracture are additionally wired in the zygomatic buttress area. Occasionally, posterior displacement of the palate is treated by raising a muco-periosteal flap and directly wiring the posterior palate with an interosseous wire. Intermaxillary fixation is maintained for 6 to 8 weeks if rigid fixation is not used.

TREATMENT OF ZYGOMA FRACTURES

Depressed fractures of the zygoma usually require open reduction/internal fixation. To do less invites a late depression deformity of the zygoma and enophthalmos with or without diplopia because of associated depressed orbital floor fractures that have been overlooked and untreated. There are numerous surgical techniques for open and "semiopen" reduction of these fractures.

Nonoperative Therapy

Nondisplaced malar fractures without signs of orbital floor disruption require no surgical treatment. However, these patients should be reevaluated once a week for 2 weeks and again at 4 to 6 weeks to check for any signs of fracture displacement. If at any time during the observation period changes in the status of the fracture are noted, appropriate therapy should be instituted. In patients with minimally displaced fractures of the zygoma and no functional problems, the presence of a slight contour deformity becomes the only complaint. Some of these patients may wish to forego corrective surgery, but this therapeutic compromise must be a mutual agreement between patient and surgeon. It is appropriate in all cases — but in this instance critical — that careful photographic documentation of the injury and deformity be obtained and kept in the record. Displaced zygomatic arch fractures not impinging on the coronoid process may be managed in a similar fashion. Nondisplaced zygomatic arch fractures require no therapy.

Operative Treatment

Zygomatic fractures exhibiting contour deformities or signs of displacement of the globe, with or without signs of nerve and muscle entrapment, should be treated. Treatment may proceed in an orderly fashion: Fractures should be operated on within 7 to 10 days after injury, as surrounding fibrous fixation may make later reduction difficult. This point is particularly true for children, in whom reduction within a week should be the goal. Many authors believe immediate reduction is the simplest and ideal approach.

When selecting the best approach for reducing a zygomatic fracture, the type of fixation required to maintain the bone in a stable position is the determining factor. Knight and North [1] as well as Larsen and Thomsen [4] have pointed out that 60 to 64 percent of zygomatic fractures are stable after reduction without fixation. Dingman and Natvig [5], however, observed that adequate reduction and continued stability usually require direct visualization and wiring because palpation alone is not always sufficient for determining adequacy of reduction, and initially stable fractures may become displaced later owing to masseter muscle pull or other factors. The latter observation implies that all displaced fractures requiring surgery should have some form of fixation. We suggest that once the decision for reduction has been made, adequate fixation is indicated, which lowers the incidence of late displacement and contour loss.

Antrum Approach

The antrum approach is made through an incision in the mucous membrane of the upper buccal sulcus. The maxillary antrum is entered above the first premolar tooth, and blood is aspirated from the antrum. To accomplish reduction of the zygoma through this approach, curved Mayo scissors are passed into the antrum to elevate the zygoma from below. Iodoform gauze, 1 inch wide, is used to pack the antrum and maintain the zygoma in reduction. As the pack is inserted, the surgeon palpates the inferior orbital rim with his or her free hand, thereby controlling the fracture fragments and preventing depression of the malar eminence. The latter is most commonly seen with untreated or inadequately reduced zygoma fractures. A depressed appearance can also occur months after reduction when marked comminution at the site results in late bony resorption.

Sometimes restoration of the malar prominence can be accomplished by late refracturing and reduction of the fractures using the open reduction technique described above. Internal wire fixation along the lateral and inferior orbital rim is essential to maintain this late reduction. When such a reduction is not attempted, some augmentation procedure is indicated. Adequate restoration of form seldom succeeds with soft-tissue alteration alone. Bony defects should be reconstructed with solid material such as autogenous bone grafts or alloplastic implants.

Direct Approach for Reduction and Fixation

With orbital floor involvement or comminution, indirect reduction with or without fixation does not suffice. If pin fixation is established and instability persists, a more direct means of stabilization is required. Local anesthesia with epinephrine for hemostasis is used in combination with general anesthesia. Dissection is performed to expose the fracture site while a malleable retractor holds orbital contents medially. An incision is then made through the lower eyelid skin 3 mm below the gray line. The skin is undermined a few millimeters, and the orbicularis muscle fibers are split horizontally, thereby avoiding scar inversion that may occur when muscle and skin incisions are placed at the same level. Access may also be accomplished through a subciliary or transconjunctival incision. It has been pointed out that the subciliary incision requires dissection over the pretarsal fibers and may result in vertical shortening of the lid. The transconjunctival approach is performed by making an incision through the conjunctiva and periosteum, exposing the orbital rim (Fig. 15-8). This technique is rapid, affords ready access to small blow-out fractures of the orbit, and has the advantage of a hidden scar. If more exposure is needed, a lateral canthotomy extension is required, thereby eliminating the advantage of a hidden scar. Once the orbital rim is exposed, the periosteum is incised and elevated to expose the orbital floor for inspection. After the fracture site has been identified, the superior orbital incision is retracted laterally. A sturdy elevator is placed behind and under the zygoma, and the bone is reduced under direct observation of the fracture site. The fracture lines are inspected directly, and an anatomic reduction is accomplished. Care is required, however, because although the fracture line may look reduced it is possible for the malar prominence to have been depressed when the bone was rotated.

In some cases, direct intraoral inspection of the maxillary buttress, for obtaining three-point alignment, is necessary for accurate reduction prior to fixation. Once normal anatomic position has been obtained, drill holes are placed on either side of the fracture lines and secured with 26- or 28-gauge wires. Miniplates or microplates work well here. If the fracture still feels unstable, a third point fixation can be established intraorally at the maxillary buttress or by passing a 2.0- to 2.5-mm Kirschner wire (K-wire) percutaneously. These additional procedures should alleviate most delayed loss of malar prominence after two-point fixation. If the orbital floor needs reconstruction, anterior maxillary sinus wall or conchal cartilage grafts may be used for defects up to 5 cm^2. With larger defects iliac bone grafts or preferably calvarial bone grafts can be used effectively. Our preference for calvarial bone grafts relates to the ease of harvesting this bone as well as to the reduced

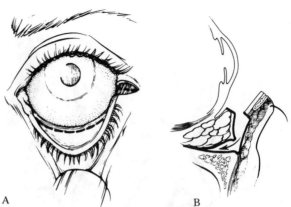

Fig. 15-8. A. Lateral canthotomy, lateral cantholysis, and subtarsal transconjunctival incisions. *B.* Cross-sectional view demonstrating the anterior septal approach to the inferior orbital rim. (From C. A. Foster and J. E. Sherman. *Surgery of Facial Bone Fractures.* New York: Churchill Livingstone, 1987. With permission.)

postoperative morbidity compared to the iliac bone graft site. Prosthetic materials such as thin Silastic sheets are effective, but foreign body implants with their associated problems are best avoided whenever possible.

Zygomatic arch fractures can also be reduced through the orbital rim or temporal approaches and rarely require fixation. If some form of stabilization is necessary, packing the temporal fossa with a Penrose drain or an inflated Foley catheter is effective. It can be removed within 7 to 10 days, once organization and early fibrosis around the fracture site has occurred. External support techniques have also been utilized by either K-wire fixation or transcutaneous suspension with a halo or biphase appliance.

To reduce zygomatic arch fractures, the arch is restored by a force opposite in direction to the fracturing force. It is mostly simply accomplished by a "semiopen" method known as the *Gillies technique* (Fig. 15-9). The scalp is shaved just anterior and superior to the superior margin of the ear, and an incision is made in a vertical direction through the scalp and temporalis fascia, care being taken not to injure the superficial temporal vessels. The Kilner elevator, a sturdy, blunt instrument with a "lifting handle," can then be passed through this incision, deep to the zygomatic arch, following the course of the temporalis muscle. With a lifting force, the bone fragments are reduced, restoring the arch. A "snapping" sensation is often felt by the surgeon as the arch is restored. The inherent stability of the arch form obviates the need for support from below or internal fixation. The small opening in the temporalis fascia need not be sutured, but the scalp incision is closed in a single layer with 3-0 or 4-0 nonabsorbable sutures. Pressure dressings are contraindicated.

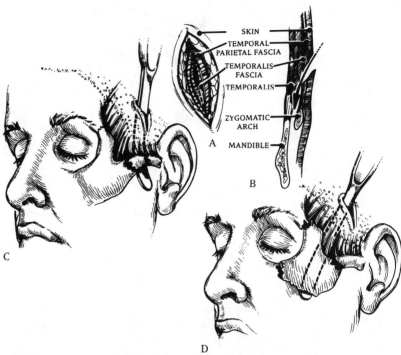

Fig. 15-9. Temporal (Gilles) approach for reduction of fractures of the zygoma and the zygomatic arch, as described by Killey. *A.* A small area posterior to the hairline and overlying the temporalis muscle is shaved and infiltrated with local anesthetic plus epinephrine. The vertical incision is carried down through both the temporoparietal and temporalis fascia. *B.* The elevator (arrow) is inserted behind the zygoma or the zygomatic arch. *C.* The elevator is shown in position for elevation of the arch. *D,* The elevator is shown in position for reduction of the zygomatic fracture. (From C. A. Foster and J. E. Sherman. *Surgery of Facial Bone Fractures.* New York: Churchill Livingstone, 1987. With permission.)

These fractures are best reduced immediately or as soon as the periorbital swelling subsides, as comminuted fracture fragments are more easily reduced before fibrous union takes place. The operative technique is as described above for treating the orbital floor portion of zygoma fractures by the open reduction method. Occasionally, when marked depression has taken place, it is difficult to elevate the fragments from above. In such a case, the orbital floor fracture can be reduced through the maxillary antrum. The bone fragments are positioned anatomically under direct vision and supported from below by an antral pack. Some type of subperiosteal support, as described above, is still advisable.

There is a growing tendency among some ophthalmologists to treat many "blow-out" fractures conservatively. The risks involved in exploration of the orbital floor are minimal, and the delayed reconstruction of traumatic enophthalmos is difficult. Direct observation is still the only certain means of determining the extent of the orbital floor injury.

OPEN FRACTURES

Open fractures of the zygomaticomaxillary complex are the result of severe trauma, such as that experienced in an automobile accident. Because of the possibility of foreign bodies in the open wound, thorough irrigation under pressure and débridement of devitalized tissue must be accomplished. Once the wound has been cleansed and the bony fragments located, direct reduction and fixation of the fracture can be undertaken, often through the wound. Access may be facilitated by extending the laceration with conservative incisions along expression lines. Packing the maxillary antrum for support of the orbital floor has been discouraged by some during elective procedures where "blind" packing through a Caldwell-Luc approach has been used. It may, however, be of particular benefit for open fractures. If an open fracture of the zygomaticomaxillary complex affords ready access to the maxillary antrum and there is comminution and disruption of the orbital floor, the sinus can be packed under direct vision with Vaseline- or antibacterial-impregnated gauze brought through a Penrose drain. The Penrose drain is then brought through a nasal antrostomy underneath the inferior turbinate and out the nares.

Packing brought out through the wound or through a Caldwell-Luc incision increases the risk of infection and fistulization. The Caldwell-Luc approach facilitates reduction of the orbital floor and is relatively safe when performed under direct vision. The volume of the maxillary antrum in an adult is about 17 ml. Overpacking or overinflation of a Foley balloon used to support the orbital floor should be avoided.

Once reduction and fixation have been established and wound margins conservatively débrided, the wounds can be closed in layers. If packing was placed in the maxillary antrum, it should be removed in stages 7 to 10 days postoperatively, when sufficient organization and early fibrosis around the fractures afford adequate stability. For open fractures involving the maxillary sinus and fractures into the oral cavity, prophylactic antibiotics are recommended. They should be given at the time of injury, prescribed specifically for oral organisms most likely to cause infection, and discontinued at 24 to 36 hours after injury. When antibiotics are used in this way, the incidence of infection can be reduced, and the emergence of resistant organisms is less likely to occur.

COMMINUTED FRACTURES

In cases where severe comminution and multiple fractures affect the zygomaticomaxillary complex and periorbital area, a bicoronal approach may afford the best access for anatomic reduction and fixation. After adequate exposure has been obtained, direct plating or wiring techniques are performed, beginning at the most stable point and reassembling bone fragments into monobloc fixation. If bony destruction or loss is substantial, direct fixation alone may be inadequate to establish skeletal integrity. Primary bone grafting may be required to achieve stability and restore bony contour.

COMPLICATIONS OF MAXILLARY AND ZYGOMA FRACTURES

Complications occur seldom if mid-facial fractures receive early and adequate treatment. Complications are usually the result of the injury itself but can also be secondary to delayed or improper treatment. One must be constantly alert for delayed manifestations of cerebral injury. CSF rhinorrhea is not uncommon with Le Fort II and III fractures and usually resolves spontaneously after fracture reduction. Persistent rhinorrhea has been reported to last as long as 105 days, and in such cases craniotomy and dural repair are necessary. Cranial nerve injuries are common. The most common nerve injury is to the infraorbital nerve in Le Fort II and zygoma fractures. With proper fracture reduction, nerve dysfunction usually resolves within months.

Occlusal and maxillofacial deformities after trauma include dental malocclusion, facial asymmetry, and limited jaw opening. They are almost exclusively the result of failure to restore proper dental occlusion at the time of initial fracture treatment and failure to adequately reduce associated facial bone fractures. If the dental occlusion is not restored to its preinjury condition, it is not possible to restore the face to its normal symmetry. These deformities can limit the patient's ability to chew, interfere with normal speech, and cause serious emotional and social problems. Malunions of facial bone fractures should be treated by osteotomy to restore normal form and function.

The early complications of bleeding, airway problems, and infection are common to facial fractures in general. Specific to the maxilla is a low incidence of maxillary sinusitis. Air-fluid levels in the sinus associated with unidentified fever should be followed by drainage through a labial sulcus incision.

CEREBROSPINAL FLUID LEAKAGE

When facilities are available, even such problems as a frontal sinus fracture can be repaired at the same time the patient is taken to the operating room for exploration of more serious injuries. CSF rhinorrhea is reported with 25 to 35 percent of Le Fort II and III fractures. Without operative treatment, most CSF leaks close in a few days, and 95 percent close spontaneously within 3 weeks. The value of antibiotics in preventing meningitis has not been demonstrated, although these agents are commonly used.

Le Fort III and nasoethmoid fractures can result in fracture and disruption of the cribriform plate of the ethmoid, leading to a dural tear followed by CSF rhinorrhea. If the patient is supine, the leaked fluid may pass into the nasopharynx and not be detected. CSF otorrhea, mastoid ecchymosis, and lateral scleral ecchymosis can also result from Le Fort III fractures associated with basilar skull fractures.

INTRACRANIAL INJURIES

The patient with displaced mid-facial fractures may also have some degree of intracranial injury. The surgeon treating facial fractures must be competent to make a neurologic assessment. A history of loss of consciousness or amnesia of the traumatic event is indicative of significant intracranial trauma. The examiner must search for evidence of skull fracture and include in the examination anteroposterior and lateral radiographic films of the skull. Subdural hemorrhage may be reflected initially by headaches of varying intensity and a dilated pupil. A neurosurgical consultation is required when there is any indication of intracranial injury, no matter how slight.

LATE COMPLICATIONS

Nonunion

Nonunion is rare and is usually seen with untreated fractures or those with which comminution was severe and fixation was not adequate for the extent of the injury. Treatment consists in exposure of the fracture site, bone grafting, and fixation. Slight mobility of the maxilla, now commonly seen with elective Le Fort I procedures, may be present for months. Eventual firm union can be expected.

Malunion

Untreated fractures or those with inadequate reduction may demonstrate malunion or malocclusion. In one study occlusal disharmony was seen in approximately 20 percent of patients, with approximately 90 percent of these cases corrected by simple means not requiring surgery.

Severe late deformities, such as an elongated face or retruded maxilla, may be corrected with Le Fort osteotomies. When occlusion is satisfactory, onlay bone grafts may correct a nasal or zygomatic deformity. When the upper maxilla is satisfactory, a Le Fort I may be performed to correct malocclusion. A short face resulting from suspension wires used in the presence of severe comminution is difficult to correct electively, and recurrence is common.

Nerve Injury

Anesthesia of the teeth is expected after transverse maxillary fracture. Recovery is usual, and patients should be instructed to inform their dentists, as unnecessary root canal therapy may be instituted during the months before pulp testing returns to normal. Injury to the infraorbital nerve is common, being reported with 40 percent of Le Fort fractures. Persistent infraorbital nerve symptoms are reported in one-half of these patients. Decreased sensation may be permanent and less annoying to the patient over time. Pain may be a significant problem and should be approached through decompression of the infraorbital canal if no relief occurs within 6 to 12 months.

Osteomyelitis

Osteomyelitis is rarely reported after treatment of maxillary fractures. Treatment includes débridement, bone grafting, and fixation.

Lacrimal System

The nasolacrimal duct may be interrupted by the Le Fort II fracture. Le Fort II and III fractures may be associated with injuries of the lacrimal sac. Persistent epiphora is reported in 4 percent of patients. Reconstructive procedures (e.g., dacryocystorhinostomy, Jones tube insertion) may be indicated (see Chapter 17).

Miscellaneous Complications

Anosmia is reported in 2 to 3 percent of patients. Its occurrence is slightly higher in patients undergoing craniotomy for associated cranial injuries. Diplopia is found in approximately one-third of patients with Le Fort II and III fractures. It resolves in 70 percent of patients, with the remainder having persistent diplopia, usually due to entrapment of the lateral oblique muscle. Extraocular muscle surgery is successful in most patients. Chronic maxillary sinusitis is rarely seen.

REFERENCES

1. Knight, J. S., and North, J. K. The classification of malar fractures: An analysis of displacement as a guide to treatment. *Br. J. Plast. Surg.* 13:325, 1961.
2. Yanagisawa, E. Symposium on maxillo-facial trauma III. Pitfalls in the management of zygomatic fractures. *Laryngoscope* 83:527, 1973.
3. Rowe, N. L., and Killey, H. C. *Fractures of the Facial Skeleton* (2nd ed.). London: Livingstone, 1968.
4. Larson, O. D., and Thomsen, M. Zygomatic fractures. I. A simplified classification for practical use. *Scand. J. Plast. Reconstr. Surg.* 12:55, 1978.
5. Dingman, R. O., and Natvig, P. *Surgery of Facial Fractures.* Philadelphia: Saunders, 64:211, 1964.

SUGGESTED READING

Alling, C.C., and Osborn, D. B. *Maxillofacial Trauma.* Philadelphia: Lea & Febiger, 1988.
Foster, C. A., and Sherman, J. E. *Surgery of Facial Bones Fractures.* New York: Churchill Livingstone, 1987.
Rowe, N. L., and Williams, J. L. *Maxillofacial Injuries.* Edinburgh: Churchill Livingstone, 1985.

Commentary on Chapter 15

George C. Sotereanos

Learning is recognition through repetition; and as in every area of training, with greater clinical exposure and experience one becomes more at ease in managing the patient with severe craniofacial injury. The area that may present a problem to the young house staff is recognition of complications that develop owing to either injury or treatment. We, as treating physicians, must be cognizant of anatomy and function. If we remember these basic rules, problems such as global injuries, orbital nerve disorders, bony segmental loss, canthal detachments with and without lacrimal gland and ductal structure dysfunction, dural tears with anatomic extravasation (nasal or laceration), orbital positional asymmetries (dystopia), and speech, hearing, occlusal, masticatory, and swallowing disorders may be addressed accordingly.

Knowledge of anatomic form and function and professional expertise in its restoration are the keys to handling the initial injuries along with all potential sequelae. Finally, a bonafide team approach to management of the acutely traumatized patient with craniofacial injuries lies in the best interest of the patient and the treating physicians. Plastic and maxillofacial surgery has much to gain and to offer our colleagues in ophthalmic and otolaryngologic surgery as well as in neurosurgery. The proper recognition of specialty care practice and proper timing of treatment of injuries negate the potential for developing complications and provide a nucleus of expertise in this small work place called the craniomaxillofacial unit.

Advances in treatment modalities have allowed the facial trauma surgeon to be more aggressive regarding early repair and secondary-stage reconstruction. Mini- and microplating systems are now available for direct reduction of these bony injuries. Development of resorbable implant fixation appliances are not available clinically but have been tested in the laboratory by multiple manufacturers.

16 THE NOSE

Timothy R. Jones

The most prominent feature of the face is the nose. Therefore any abnormality in its size or shape is noticeable. As a result of its prominent position, the nasal bones are vulnerable to injury, making them the most commonly fractured bones of the face. Injury to the nose can produce cosmetic deformity as well as impaired nasal airway function. Prompt recognition and treatment of nasal injuries should minimize the long-term cosmetic and functional deformity.

ANATOMY

The nose is referred to as a nasal pyramid because of its shape. The apex, where the nose attaches to the forehead, is called the nasal root, and the free lower angle is called the nasal tip. The rounded area between the root and the tip is called the nasal dorsum. The base of the nose, where the nostrils open, is formed by the columella in the midline and the alar rims on the lateral sides (Fig. 16-1).

Bony Framework

The skeleton of the nose consists of an upper bony and lower cartilaginous framework bound to the piriform aperture. The nasal bones are thicker and more narrow superiorly and become wider and thinner inferiorly. They articulate with each other in the midline, with the frontal bone superiorly, and with the frontal process of the maxilla posterolaterally.

The upper lateral cartilages attach to the septal cartilage in the midline and to the under surface of the nasal bones superiorly. The lower lateral cartilages form the framework for the columella, tip, and alae. They attach to the upper lateral cartilages superiorly by dense connective tissue. Each lower lateral alar cartilage consists of a medial and a lateral crus. The medial crura provide support for the columella, and the lateral crura provide support for the alae. The medial crura are adherent to each other in the midline and to the anterior inferior edge of the septum by dense connective tissue. The lateral crura extend posterolaterally for a variable distance and are attached to the maxilla (Fig. 16-2).

Soft-Tissue Covering

The nasal skin has variable thickness and is generally thinner in the nasal root and tip areas and thicker in the supratip and over the ala. The skin covering the columella is thin and tightly adherent to the paired medial crura.

365

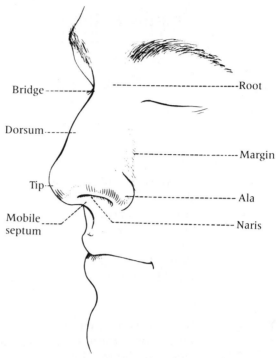

Fig. 16-1. Surface anatomy of the nose. (From W. H. Hollinshead. *The Head and Neck,* 3rd ed. Philadelphia: Harper Medical, 1982. With permission.)

Innervation

Sensation to the nose is provided by the ophthalmic (V_1) and maxillary (V_2) branches of the trigeminal nerve (fifth cranial nerve, CN V) (see Fig. 13-2). The supratrochlear and infratrochlear nerves (CN VI) supply the root, bridge, and lateral sides of the upper nose (see Fig. 16-4 below). The tip is supplied by the external nasal branch of the anterior ethmoidal nerve (CN VI). The remainder of the nose is innervated by the infraorbital nerve (CN VII).

Blood Supply

The nasal root and the bridge receive their primary blood supply from the dorsal nasal arteries. They are terminal branches of the ophthalmic artery and interconnect with the lateral nasal branch of the facial artery or angular artery along the lateral nose (see Fig. 13-1). Branches extending from the superior labial artery provide blood supply to the columella and alae.

Nasal Cavity

The nasal cavity is divided into two triangular chambers by the nasal septum. The entrance into the nasal cavity is referred to as the vestibule and is the only portion of the nasal cavity lined with skin. The remainder of the nasal cavity is covered by a mucous membrane that is tightly adherent to the underlying perichondrium or periosteum. The roof of the nasal cavity is the floor of the anterior cranial

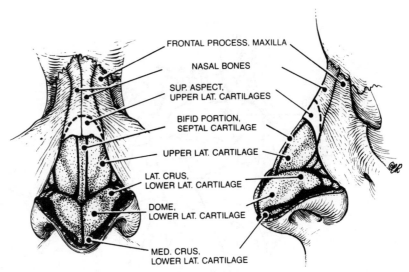

Fig. 16-2. Cartilaginous and bony skeleton of the nose. (From C. A. Foster and J. E. Sherman. *Surgery of Facial Bone Fractures.* New York: Churchill LIvingstone, 1987. With permission.)

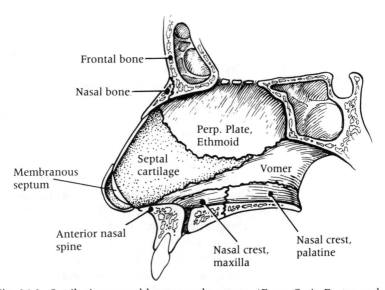

Fig. 16-3. Cartilaginous and bony nasal septum. (From C. A. Foster and J. E. Sherman. *Surgery of Facial Bone Fractures.* New York: Churchill Livingstone, 1987. With permission.)

fossa and is formed by the cribriform plate and the fovea ethmoidalis. The palatine bone forms the nasal floor. The lateral nasal wall is geographic and is composed of several irregular bones that form three or four prominent projections named the turbinates.

The anterior portion of the septum is composed of the quadrilateral cartilage, and the posterior portion of the septum is composed of bone (Fig. 16-3). The perpendicular plate of the ethmoid forms the posterior superior aspect of the bony septum, and the vomer forms

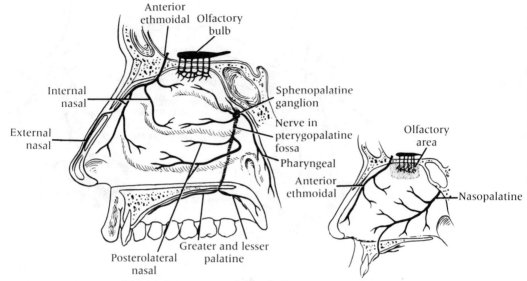

Fig. 16-4. Nerve supply to the lateral wall and septum of the nose. (From C. W. Cummings. *Otolaryngology, Head and Neck Surgery.* St. Louis: Mosby, 1986. With permission.)

the posterior inferior aspect of the septum. The septum articulates inferiorly with the maxillary crest and is joined to the columella anteriorly by connective tissue in the membranous septum.

The septum receives sensory innervation by the nasal palatine nerve and the anterior ethmoidal nerve (Fig. 16-4). The nasal palatine nerve enters the posterior part of the septum and travels anteriorly to the incisive canal where it anastomoses with the greater palatine nerve to innervate the hard palate.

Blood supply to the superior part of the septum is provided by the anterior and posterior ethmoidal arteries, and the posterior septum is supplied by branches of the sphenopalatine artery, which is a branch of the internal maxillary artery. Kiesselbach's, or Little's, area is a portion of the anterior septum where the superior labial artery anastomoses with the sphenopalatine artery to supply the septum. This area accounts for 90 percent of the nosebleeds due to atraumatic causes (Fig. 16-5).

The anatomy of the lateral nasal wall is much more complex than that of the septum. Three turbinates project from the lateral nasal wall into the nasal cavity and function as the major source of humidification of the upper respiratory tract. The superior turbinate is small and difficult to identify, whereas the inferior and middle turbinates are much larger and easier to examine. The nasal lacrimal duct drains into the anterior one-third of the inferior meatus. The ostia of the maxillary sinus, the anterior ethmoidal cells, and the frontal sinus drain into the middle meatus. The posterior ethmoidal cells drain into the superior meatus.

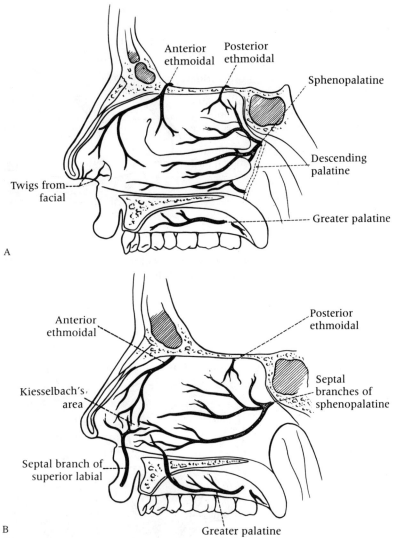

Fig. 16-5. Vascular supply to the lateral wall (*A*) and nasal septum (*B*).
(From W. H. Hollinshead. *The Head and Neck*, 3rd ed. Philadelphia:
Harper Medical, 1982. With permission.)

Paranasal Sinuses

Frontal Sinus
The frontal sinus is an extension of the anterior ethmoidal cells into
the vertical portion of the frontal bone and is separated into
individual cavities by a vertical bony septum. The nasofrontal duct
originates along the posterior medial aspect of the sinus floor and
drains the sinus into the middle meatus underneath the middle
turbinate (Figs. 16-6 and 16-7).

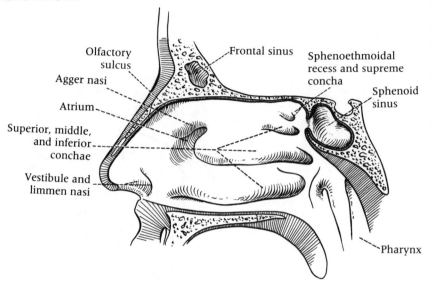

Fig. 16-6. Lateral wall of the nose. (From W. H. Hollinshead. *The Head and Neck,* 3rd ed. Philadelphia: Harper Medical, 1982. With permission.)

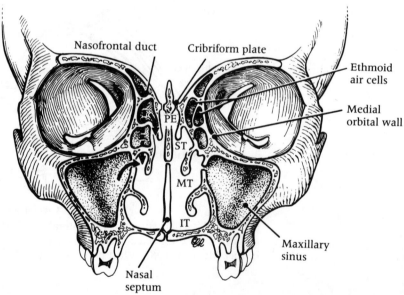

Fig. 16-7. Bony architecture of the nasal cavity and paranasal sinuses (coronal view). (From C. A. Foster and J. E. Sherman. *Surgery of Facial Bone Fractures.* New York: Churchill Livingstone, 1987. With permission.)

Ethmoid Sinus

The ethmoid sinus is composed of numerous air cells divided into two groups: anterior and posterior. The bony walls of the ethmoid sinus are the medial orbital wall laterally, the anterior cranial fossa superiorly, and the lateral nasal wall medially. The anterior ethmoid cells open into the middle meatus and the posterior ethmoid cells into the superior meatus.

Sphenoid Sinus

The sphenoid sinus is the posterior evagination of the nasal cavity. Its border includes the middle cranial fossa and pituitary gland superiorly, the cavernous sinus laterally, the posterior cranial fossa posteriorly, and the pharynx inferiorly. The sphenoid sinus drains above the superior turbinate in the sphenoethmoidal recess.

Maxillary Sinus

The maxillary sinus is enclosed in the maxilla, and its boundaries include the lateral nasal wall medially, the floor of the orbit superiorly, the anterior portion of the maxilla anteriorly, the alveolar and palatine processes of the maxilla inferiorly, and the anterior surface of the pterygopalatine fossa posteriorly. The ostia of the maxillary sinus drains underneath the middle turbinate into the middle meatus.

EVALUATION

A complete history with careful delineation of the mechanism of injury, including the direction and intensity of force, is helpful for predicting the extent of the nasal injury. Assaults, sporting accidents, and falls generally result in isolated nasal fractures, whereas motor vehicle accidents and gunshot wounds are associated with more extensive mid-face injuries that may involve the orbits and maxillae. Other important points to document include a history of previous nasal injury and the presence of pain, nasal obstruction, clear rhinorrhea, or epistaxis.

A complete intra- and extranasal examination of the nose is performed. The external nose is inspected for ecchymosis, edema, lacerations, or bony displacement. Periorbital edema and ecchymoses are identified. The nose is palpated for crepitus, angulation, and mobility of the bony and cartilaginous nasal pyramid.

The intranasal examination, an essential part of the physical examination, is difficult without good lighting, suction, a topical anesthetic, and a topical vasoconstrictor. The nasal mucosa should be inspected for mucosal lacerations, areas of epistaxis, septal hematomas, deformities of the septum, and patency of the airways.

Simple nasal fractures do not require confirmation by conventional radiographic examination, and the diagnosis can be made accurately by careful intra- and extranasal examination. Treatment is based on these clinical findings. If the nasal injury is severe and there is clinical suspicion of a nasoethmoidal fracture, a computed tomography scan should be obtained to better delineate the extent of the injury. Some people advocate routine nasal radiographs for documentation of the injury.

TREATMENT
Epistaxis

Epistaxis resulting from facial injuries can be secondary to nasomucosal lacerations or injury to the ethmoidal and sphenopalatine arteries. Bleeding from simple nasal fractures is usually anterior and due to mucosal lacerations. The epistaxis is typically self-limited or can be controlled by pinching the nostrils against the anterior septum. However, epistaxis associated with nasoethmoidal or midface fractures is associated with injury to the ethmoidal and sphenopalatine arteries and can produce profuse hemorrhage that results not only in significant blood loss but possibly airway compromise. Bleeding is obvious from the anterior nostril, but significant occult loss can occur into the nasopharynx and hypopharynx.

If pressure and ice do not control the epistaxis, intranasal packing is necessary. To localize the source of the bleeding one needs good lighting, suction, a nasal speculum, and a bayonet forceps. The examiner should wear protective gloves and glasses and use topical anesthetics and vasoconstrictors to help locate and control the area of epistaxis. The preferred topical agent is 4% cocaine because it has both properties. Lidocaine 4% and tetracaine HCI 1% are also good topical anesthetic agents to use in the nose. NeoSynephrine 1% can be used as a topical vasoconstrictor if cocaine is not available. The physician planning to use lidocaine with epinephrine must be aware that the concomitant use of topical cocaine can cause a synergistic cardiotoxic effect.

Mucosal lacerations that continue to bleed and are accessible can be controlled with primary chromic suture repair of the laceration. If the laceration is not accessible to repair and the epistaxis needs to be temporarily controlled, hemostatic agents such as surgical gel or foam can be placed over the area, or silver nitrate cautery may be utilized. If these techniques are not successful, an anterior nasal pack should be placed.

An anterior nasal pack is made from a long 0.5 inch ribbon gauze coated with bacitracin ointment. The gauze is placed in the nose in a pleated fashion, starting inferiorly along the nasal floor and packing toward the roof of the nasal cavity. The gauze is placed underneath the inferior and middle turbinates and should be placed with only closed loops posteriorly so that a strand does not fall into the nasal pharynx. There are now commercially available nasal tampons and nasal balloons that serve as an anterior pack (Fig. 16-8). These devices are more easily placed than a nasal pack; in addition, the nasal balloon has an airway in its center that permits airflow through the nostril. The disadvantage of these devices is that they do not allow precise packing of the nasal cavity, and care must be taken to avoid pressure necrosis, especially along the alar rim.

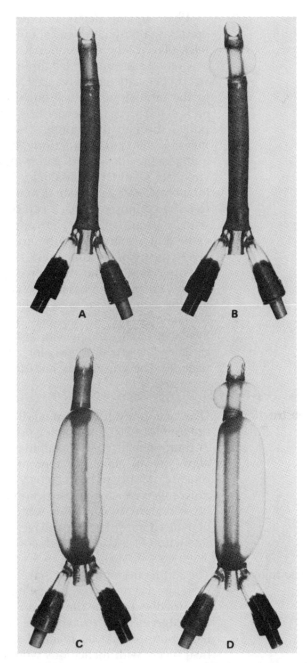

Fig. 16-8. Nasal balloon for epistaxis. *A.* Uninflated. *B.* Posterior balloon inflated. *C.* Anterior balloon inflated. *D.* Both balloons inflated. (From N. L. Rowe and J. L. Williams. *Maxillofacial Injuries.* Edinburgh: Churchill Livingstone, 1986. With permission.)

When an adequately placed anterior pack fails to control the epistaxis, a posterior bleed should be assumed and a posterior nasal pack placed. The conventional posterior pack is comprised of two separate 0 silk sutures tied around a dental gauze roll. A 23 French red rubber catheter is advanced along the floor of the nose, visualized in the oropharynx, and brought out through the mouth. The free ends of the 0 silk sutures are tied to the end of the catheter previously pulled through the mouth. The catheter protruding through the nostril is then pulled anteriorly, bringing the sutures out of the nose and placing the dental gauze snugly against the posterior nasal choanae. An anterior nasal pack is then applied, and the silk sutures are placed over a separate dental gauze roll (Fig. 16-9). An alternative type of posterior pack can be fashioned from a Foley catheter with a 30-ml balloon. The catheter tip is trimmed and the Foley catheter advanced along the floor of the nose until the tip is seen below the uvula. Normal saline is used to inflate the balloon, and the proximal end of the catheter is pulled until the balloon is snug against the posterior nasal choanae. An anterior nasal pack is placed, and the catheter is secured to the nostril with a C-clamp. Care must be taken to prevent necrosis of the alar rim. The commercially available nasal balloons can also be used as a posterior pack. The catheter has separate ports for an anterior balloon and a posterior balloon. The advantages and disadvantages have been previously discussed.

Nasal Obstruction

Obstruction resulting from nasal trauma can be caused by injury to the osteocartilaginous framework or the mucosal lining of the nose. A thorough intranasal examination using topical vasoconstrictors allow one to make the appropriate diagnosis. Obstruction due to mucosal injury can be treated by systemic decongestants and topical mucosal constrictors. Obstruction due to a displaced framework can be secondary to a fractured septum, severely displaced nasal bones, or avulsed upper lateral cartilages with resulting nasal valve collapse. Reduction of the framework corrects the obstruction.

Soft Tissue Injury

The soft tissues of the nose have a tremendous vascular supply, and therefore even severe injuries may heal unnoticeably. Lacerations that involve the alar rim should be carefully reapproximated at the free edge in order to avoid the noticeable "notch." Full-thickness lacerations should be repaired in layers. Partial-thickness injuries heal nicely with meticulous wound closure using 6-0 nylon. Often the cartilage and mucosa can be reapproximated in a single layer with chromic sutures, and the skin is repaired with a separate skin closure. If it is necessary to repair the injury in three layers, the mucosa is approximated first with 5-0 chromic catgut, the cartilage with chromic catgut or 6-0 clear nylon, and the skin with fine 6-0 nylon sutures.

Avulsion injuries of the nasal alae should be repaired primarily with fine sutures. Like the ear, the avulsed tissue has a good chance

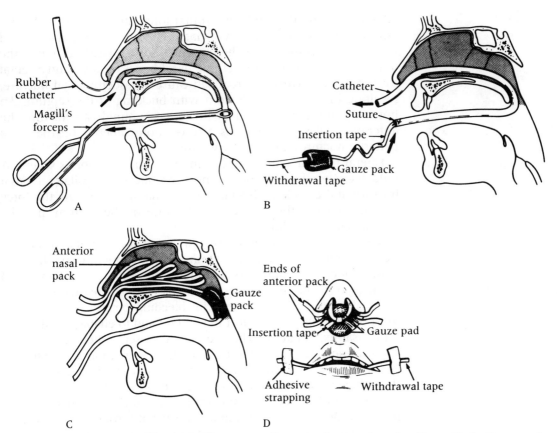

Rubber
catheter

Magill's
forceps

A

Catheter

Suture

Insertion tape

Gauze pack

Withdrawal tape

B

Anterior
nasal
pack

Gauze
pack

C

Ends of
anterior pack

Insertion tape

Gauze pad

Adhesive
strapping

Withdrawal tape

D

Fig. 16-9. Placement of a posterior nasal pack. (From N. L. Rowe and J. L. Williams. *Maxillofacial Injuries.* Edinburgh: Churchill Livingstone, 1986. With permission.)

of surviving even if there is just a small pedicle of skin attached. A completely avulsed segment of the nostril may be replaced as a free graft if it is less than 2 cm in length. Injuries with full-thickness skin loss may need skin grafting or local flaps. Full-thickness skin grafts from the retroauricular, preauricular, or supraclavicular areas can be used.

Nasal Fractures

Nasal bones are the most commonly fractured facial bones. Treatment of these fractures starts with a thorough intranasal and external examination. Signs of nasal fractures include edema, intranasal and external lacerations, displacement of the nose, angulation of the nasal pyramid, crepitus, epistaxis, and cerebrospinal fluid rhinorrhea. With time, edema and ecchymosis progress, making accurate physical examination more difficult. Symptoms associated with nasal fractures include pain, epistaxis, and nasal obstruction. It is important to determine the mobility of the nasal pyramid in order to distinguish a recent injury from an old injury.

Nasal fractures can be classified into two categories: frontal and lateral (Fig. 16-10). Moderate frontal force causes fracture of nasal bones at their caudal ends. Associated fracture and displacement of the septum is common, as the septum absorbs a large portion of the impact. With a greater impact, the nasal bones collapse and a septal fracture results. Greater forces can cause a nasoethmoidal fracture, resulting in a flat, wide dorsum with buckling of the septum. An impact to the lower aspect of the nasal pyramid can fracture the anterior nasal spine, whereas a force more superior on the nasal pyramid fractures the maxillary buttress.

Lateral nasal fractures are common and usually not as severe. A mild blow to the side of the nose produces an ipsilateral nasal fracture and associated buckling of the nasal septum. As the force becomes greater there may be a fracture of the septum and the contralateral nasal bone.

Radiographs of the nose are not mandatory for diagnosing or treating simple nasal fractures. Immediate treatment of nasal septal injuries includes control of epistaxis, prevention of edema, and drainage of septal hematomas. Epistaxis with isolated nasal injuries is usually self-limiting. When the bleeding persists, the epistaxis must be controlled to comfort the patient and to enable an adequate intranasal examination. The presence of a septal hematoma mandates immediate evacuation by aspiration or incision and drainage. It can be performed after adequate topical anesthesia of the septum. If further anesthesia is needed, the septum is injected with 1% lidocaine with 1:100,000 epinephrine. An incision is made at the inferior aspect of the hematoma and carried through the mucoperichondrium down to the septal cartilage. The hematoma is evacuated and the incision left open. The mucoperichondrial flap is pressed against the cartilage with nasal packing and septal splints; and the septum is reexamined within 24 hours. Prophylactic antiobiotics against *Staphylococcus* should be used.

Once the intranasal problems have been addressed, the external problems are treated. Simple lacerations commonly occur with nasal fractures and are usually located over the area of the fracture. They are treated as one would treat any acute laceration — with irrigation, débridement, and primary closure. If the nasal fracture is to be reduced acutely, the laceration is closed after the nasal bones are reduced. When nasal reduction is to be delayed, the nasal laceration should be closed within the first 12 hours. Prophylactic antibiotics against *Staphylococcus* should be used for 5 to 7 days.

The timing of the treatment of the nasal fractures depends on the amount of edema and extent of injury. Immediate closed reduction can be performed in the emergency room if there is minimal edema and minimal injury to the septum. The ideal candidate for immediate reduction is the patient who sustained a lateral blow to the nose that resulted in an ipsilateral, medially displaced nasal bone fracture without septal fracture. Delayed treatment of nasal fractures may be best in patients with extensive nasal edema, comminuted nasal fractures, or septal fracture. When the treatment of the nasal fracture

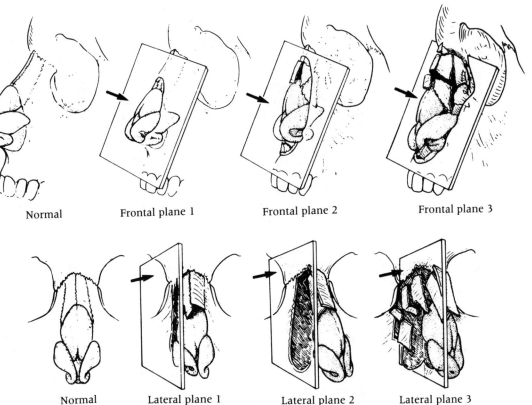

Normal   Frontal plane 1   Frontal plane 2   Frontal plane 3

Normal   Lateral plane 1   Lateral plane 2   Lateral plane 3

Fig. 16-10. Nasal fracture patterns. (From C. W. Cummings. *Otolaryngology, Head and Neck Surgery.* St. Louis: Mosby, 1986. With permission.)

is delayed, it should be performed within 7 days in a child and 10 days in an adult. During this interval the patient may benefit from the use of systemic and topical nasal decongestants, prophylactic antibiotics, and saline nasal spray.

When treating septal injuries, attention must be given to both the nasal bones and the septum if a good long-term cosmetic and functional result is desired. Most nasoseptal fractures can be treated by a closed technique. General anesthesia is used in children and young teenagers. Older teenagers and adults usually tolerate local anesthesia well.

The nose can be adequately anesthetized using a combination of topical and injectable anesthetic agents. First the nasal cavity is anesthetized topically with cotton pledgets moistened with either 4% cocaine, 4% topical lidocaine, or 1% tetracaine. If cocaine is not used, 1% NeoSynephrine should be added as a topical mucosal constrictor. Three cotton pledgets are placed in each nasal cavity: (1) along the floor of the nose, adjacent to the inferior turbinate; (2) against the middle turbinate, being sure to reach the sphenopalatine ganglion at the posterior extent of the turbinate; and (3) high in the

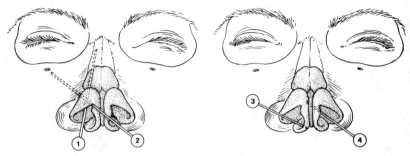

Fig. 16-11. Technique of local anesthesia for the nose. (From C. W. Cummings. *Otolaryngology, Head and Neck Surgery.* St. Louis: Mosby, 1986. With permission.)

nasal cavity. After waiting 5 to 7 minutes, 1% lidocaine with 1:200,000 epinephrine is injected submucosally along the septum, the inferior turbinate, and the posterior aspect of the middle turbinate.

After anesthetizing the nasal cavity, the external nose is anesthetized with 1% lidocaine with 1:200,000 epinephrine (Fig. 16-11). This process includes injections through the nasal radix to anesthetize the external nasal branches (infratrochlear nerve), along the lateral nasal pyramid to anesthetize the infraorbital nerve contributions, and at the base of the columella to block the contributions of the greater palatine nerve. When using topical cocaine and injectables with epinephrine, strict adherence to the recommended doses should be observed and cardiac monitoring performed. When the procedure is performed under general anesthesia, topical and injectable vasoconstrictors are still essential.

When treating nose injuries, attention must be given to both nasal bones and septum if good cosmetic and functional results are to be obtained. Minimally displaced nasoseptal fractures can be treated by closed techniques. The closed reduction of the nasal fracture is addressed first. A medially displaced fracture can be reduced with flat elevator or Ballinger elevator by lifting the bone upward and laterally. More control can be provided by using a Walsham forceps and grasping the nasal bone directly. A laterally displaced fracture can be reduced medially with the operator's thumb or with the Walsham forceps. Once the nasal fracture is reduced, the septum can usually be closed reduced with the Asch forceps. The forceps are placed on both sides of the septum and traction applied in a superior anterior direction (Figs. 16-12 and 16-13).

Occasionally open reduction is indicated when the fractures are immobile and cannot be reduced by closed techniques. It is performed with an intracartilaginous incision and elevation of the skin without elevating the periosteum. A small osteotome is tapped into the fracture line, and the fracture is gently mobilized. If reduction of the nasal pyramid is desired, open reduction should be delayed for 6 months after the injury to stabilize the nasal pyramid. Severely

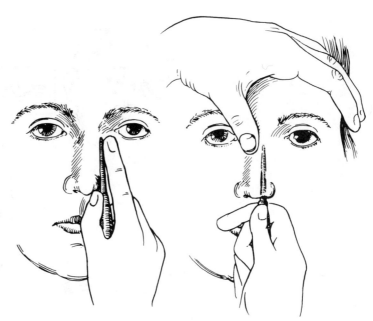

Fig. 16-12. Reduction of a medially displaced nasal fracture. (From C. W. Cummings. *Otolaryngology, Head and Neck Surgery.* St. Louis: Mosby, 1986. With permission.)

comminuted nasal fractures associated with nasoethmoidal fractures require open reduction and internal fixation. In addition, bone grafting of the orbital walls and nasal dorsum is often needed. Exposure through existing lacerations, a bicoronal approach, or an "open sky" incision can be utilized.

The inability to reduce the septum by closed techniques is an indication for an open septoplasty, which should be performed at the time the nasal fracture is reduced. A limited cartilage resection is performed by removing overlapping cartilage segments in horizontal and vertical strips. Extensive submucosal resection of the cartilage is avoided if possible.

The proper use of internal and external splinting is a valuable component of nasal/septal fracture treatment. Intranasal packing with 0.5-inch ribbon gauze covered with bacitracin ointment should be used sparingly to control epistaxis. Overpacking widens the nose, and the packs should be removed in 1 to 2 days.

Intranasal septal splints are valuable for treating septal injuries. They are placed on both sides of the septum and secured with transseptal mattress sutures. Their major contribution is to stabilize the septum, but they also serve to prevent septal hematomas and nasal synechiae. Minimal airway obstruction is created, and the patients tolerate their presence for as long as 10 days postoperatively.

External nasal splints are made of plaster of paris, aluminum, and plastic materials. They protect the reduction of the nasal pyramid but cannot stabilize an unstable reduction. If a stable reduction cannot be obtained, a transnasal external splint or open reduction is

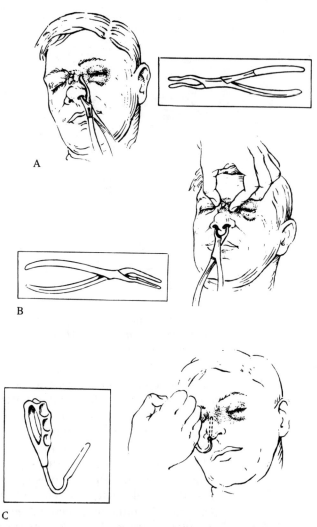

Fig. 16-13. Reduction of complex nasal fractures. *A.* Walsham forceps used to disimpact and reconstruct nasal pyramid. *B.* Asch forceps used to disimpact and replce nasal septum in midline. *C.* Salinger reduction instrument used to further shape and contour nasal pyramid and reduce fractures of nasal tip. (From R. C. Schultz. *Facial Injuries,* 3rd ed. Chicago: Year Book, 1988. With permission.)

necessary. Once the edema subsides in 5 to 7 days, the external splint no longer fits and it should be replaced by a new splint.

Treatment of nasal injuries in children is different from that in adults. First, children do not cooperate for an intranasal examination, and general anesthesia is usually required. Second, children are more apt to develop septal hematomas and incomplete (greenstick) nasal bone fractures. Third, fractures heal more rapidly in children, and so these nasal injuries should be addressed within 5 to 7 days of the injury. Most displaced septal fractures can be treated adequately with closed techniques; if unsuccessful, however, limited open septoplasty should be performed to obtain an open nasal airway. Nasal bone fractures can likewise almost always be treated with closed reduction; it is best to avoid open reduction, if possible, until the age of 15 to 16.

Young children are particularly intolerant to nasal obstruction. Septal splints can be used; and if nasal packing is needed, soft tubing with gauze packing around it is usually better tolerated.

COMPLICATIONS

Nasal synechiae can result from unprotected mucosal injuries involving the medial and lateral sides of the nasal cavity. The use of septal splints keeps the injured mucosal linings divided, allowing them to epithelialize separately.

An unrecognized septal hematoma can lead to loss of the cartilaginous septum with a resulting saddle nose deformity, retracted columella, and widened nasal base. The external nasal deformities can be prevented by reconstructing the septum at the time of injury once the infection is under control.

Septal injuries are responsible for most posttraumatic functional and cosmetic problems. The convolutions and spurs of the septum often result after septal injuries, even when they are not present on the day of injury. The fibrosis that occurs with healing can produce osseous and cartilaginous overgrowth resulting in subsequent nasal airway obstruction. If the internal nasal deformity is severe, it can produce an external nasal deformity as well (i.e., twisted nose). Many of these problems can be prevented by adequate treatment of the septum at the time of the initial injury.

Hematoma of the nasal dorsum is uncommon and is produced by tearing of the upper lateral cartilage from the nasal bones. It can be treated by intra- or extranasal evacuation of the hematoma and prophylactic antibiotics.

Commentary on Chapter 16

Dennis J. Hurwitz

The early diagnosis of displaced nasal fracture can be difficult. It is important to determine the force of injury. (Did the patient hear the crack of broken bones?) Displaced nasal bones lacerate nasal mucosa and cause profuse nasal bleeding; therefore the absence of epistaxis is significant. Also, many patients experience anosmia. The patient may have noticed an immediate posttraumatic nasal deformity before swelling obscured it, interfering with the physician's evaluation. Preinjury facial photographs are helpful, as is a history of prior nasal trauma or rhinoplasty. The physical examination should specifically search for deficient projection, saddling of the nose, distortion of the pyramid, deviation of the septum, and retraction of the columella. Blood clots are removed by cotton swabs or suction. Skin and mucosal lacerations, as well as hematomas and septal dislocations, are noted.

In addition to routine nasal radiographs, Waters views demonstrate the dorsal bony pyramid and the lateral walls of the nose. Further radiographic studies of the face, including computed tomography scans, are ordered as indicated. Although nasal radiographs are rarely medically necessary, they do serve medicolegal and insurance purposes.

If there is limited nasal swelling, immediate reduction of the fracture should be attempted. Moderate swelling does not permit precise palpation of the nasal bones, so realignment cannot be assessed.

Nasal fractures are reduced by closed technique unless there are extensive lacerations or the closed reduction is unsatisfactory. In those cases, an open approach is indicated. Topical anesthesia, usually in the form of 4% cocaine, and limited amounts of local infiltration with epinephrine and lidocaine are important. Sedation is helpful. For the very young or uncooperative patient, general anesthesia is required.

Proper reduction of nasal bone fractures requires an appreciation of the bone displacement and anticipation of the required manipulation. Depressed bone must be elevated with a bimanual maneuver using an instrument within the nasal passageway and palpation along the dorsum. Premeasurement of the length of the inserting instrument on the dorsum of the nose is helpful. The bones are pulled out of their displaced position by steady pressure and are overreduced so they can be manipulated into proper position. Use only as much force as is necessary, thereby avoiding further tissue injury. The opposite hand is used to mold the bones into position. Thus the depression is corrected first, and lateralization is done second. For comminuted fractures, special forceps may be necessary. Once the nasal bones are in position, the septal position must be checked. Asch forceps can help elevate the dorsum and disimpact the displaced septum. When all is in place, hematomas are drained through small incisions. Multiple nasal bone commamution or an unstable septum requires special attention to splinting. Intranasal polyurethane splints and transnasal wiring over splints may be required.

A common adverse result following reduction of nasal fractures is the persistence of a small mid-dorsal hump due to the tearing of the upper lateral cartilages from the septum or nasal bones with the result of minute hematoma formation. Subsequent fibrosis and osteophyte deposition forms a mild deformity. Another common problem is persistence of a depressed fragment that appears to be aligned at the completion of a nasal reduction but is unstable and loses position as the swelling subsides. Finally, persistent lack of nasal projection may be due to telescoping injuries into the orbitoethmoidal complex that require craniofacial exposure for reduction.

Unrealistic expectations, particularly of young women, should be anticipated. The postreduction state may not match the preinjury appearance. Imperfections are expected and require a formal rhinoplasty to correct.

17 SOFT-TISSUE INJURIES OF THE EARS, EYELIDS, FACIAL NERVES, AND PAROTID DUCTS

Mark S. Granick

The repair of soft tissue injuries of the face requires strict adherence to the general principles of wound management. A thorough comprehension of the regional anatomy is necessary to describe the location and extent of the injury. Needless to say, a facial nerve injury, for instance, can be repaired only if it is first detected.

An accurate assessment must be conducted of the wound and injured tissues by direct examination. Prior to injecting local anesthetics, nerve function must be evaluated. Patients with wounds that require extensive exploration and repair must obviously be taken to the operating room. It is generally best to be well prepared and to know preoperatively if any major structures have been injured. If possible, local anesthetics can be injected into the area of the wound after the initial neurologic and gross examinations. This procedure allows painless but thorough cleansing of the wound and more specific evaluation of the injury.

EAR

Anatomy

This anatomic discussion is limited to the external ear and skin overlying the mastoid process. It must be remembered that there is an external auditory canal that extends from the pinna to the tympanic membrane and the temporal bone. The external ear consists primarily of a cartilage framework supporting a thin layer of enveloping skin (Fig. 17-1). The prominent landmarks on the external ear include the helical rim, which surrounds the superior and posterior portions of the ear. The antihelix is the large fold that runs longitudinally through the center of the ear and splits superiorly into a posterior and anterior crus. The antihelix blends into a prominence inferiorly known as the antitragus, below which sits the ear lobule. Anteriorly, the tragus defines the anterior extent of the ear and is present just anterior to the orifice of the external auditory canal. Enveloped within the antihelix is a depression known as the concha. The medial surface of the ear is relatively smooth and lacks the well defined fold seen on the lateral surface. Fortunately, in patients who have injured one ear, the opposite ear is available as an

385

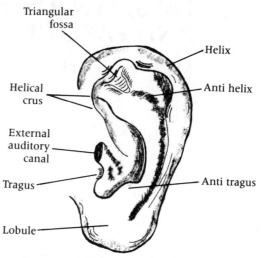

Fig. 17-1. External ear anatomy.

anatomic model. When attempting to identify and repair landmarks on the injured ear, reference can be made to the opposite side for purposes of orientation.

Evaluation

The physical examination of an injured ear requires that the ear be thoroughly cleaned and the extent of the injury carefully assessed and categorized. Of prime importance is the vascularity of the remaining segments of the ear and whether cartilage is involved in the injury. Whenever an injury occurs to the external portions of the ear, a physical examination must rule out involvement of any of the middle or inner ear structures as well. Such examination can be performed quickly and accurately with a few simple tests. The first is obviously to look in the external auditory canal with an otoscope and evaluate the canal and tympanic membrane. The presence of a hemotympanum suggests the possibility of a temporal bone fracture and requires that the patient undergo formal audiometric testing and radiographic evaluation. This regimen includes air and bone conduction hearing tests and a computed tomography (CT) scan of the temporal bones. A gross hearing test can be performed by determining if the patient can hear the ticking of a watch or the rubbing of two dry fingertips held adjacent to his ear. The results can be compared with those from the normal side. If available, the Rhinne and Weber tuning fork tests can determine if a conductive hearing loss is present.

The nature of the wound and timing of the injury clearly dictate the treatment of the defect. If the wound is secondary to a bite, particularly a human bite, the patient should be placed on antibiotics and, if any evidence of cellulitis exists, admitted to the hospital for intravenous antibiotics. If cartilage is involved in a human bite wound, the exposed cartilage should be débrided from the wound prior to wound closure and the patient admitted for intravenous antibiotic therapy. If only soft tissue is involved by a bite, the wound edges can be débrided and the wound irrigated and closed using skin sutures only. The patient should be sent home on oral antibiotics and checked in 24 hours. With grossly contaminated or dirty wounds or wounds that have been left open for a period of time, it is best not to attempt closure in the emergency room setting. Wounds that are older than 18 hours should simply not be closed for fear of developing postoperative wound infection. They can be allowed to heal secondarily and revised at a later date. Another option is to perform a delayed primary closure after the wound has been observed and appears to be free of infection. Hence there is clearly a considerable degree of judgment the surgeon must exercise when determining which wounds are suitable for closure in the emergency room setting.

Operative Techniques

Simple lacerations can be treated as they would be at any other site. Skin sutures are all that are necessary on the ear. On the medial surface of the ear, which is generally not easily seen, the skin can be closed with chromic catgut.

On the lateral surface a 5-0 monofilament suture is appropriate. The contours of the ear provide excellent guides for the surgeon as the wound edges are aligned prior to closure. It is a good idea to suture the key landmarks first to be sure that subsequent repair is anatomically correct. A vertical mattress suture should be used along the helical rim to approximate the edge and prevent notching.

Any hematoma noted below the skin of the external ear *must be drained.* If a hematoma is left undrained it can become secondarily infected and lead to a disfiguring "cauliflower" ear deformity. This injury is seen frequently in wrestlers but may accompany any sort of blunt trauma to the ear. An auricular hematoma is easily drained with a small incision overlying the fluid, drainage of the blood, and application of a compressive dressing over the ear fashioned like a mastoid dressing. The ear is then reevaluated in 24 to 48 hours; if any blood has reaccumulated, it should be drained and a Penrose drain placed in the defect. Another compressive dressing is then applied. A compressive ear dressing is simple and effective if properly applied. In my experience, patients are most comfortable if the first layer of the dressing is packed into all the contours of the external ear prior to placing a bulky compressive wad on top of it: A 5 × 9 inch sheet of Xeroform is cut into 2 cm wide strips, which are then packed into the lateral ear crevices. A 4 × 4 inch pad is then opened and tucked behind the medial surface. A wad of fluffed gauze is placed over the ear, and the head is wrapped with a 3-inch Kling and a 3-inch Ace bandage. The opposite ear is left free of the dressing. The outer layer must be taped well, or it may fall off.

Complex lacerations of the external ear include skin and cartilage. For small cartilaginous defects, skin approximation may be all that is necessary to restore the auricular contour. When the cartilage laceration is extensive, it may be necessary to repair the cartilage as a separate layer. The cartilage and perichondrium should be closed in one layer and the skin in a separate layer. When closing cartilage, simple sutures using Dexon or Maxon should be placed with the knots on the medial side so they are not palpable or visible from the lateral surface. A compressive dressing is placed around the ear postoperatively, and the ear is checked in 48 hours to be sure that no hematoma has accumulated. When segments of the ear have been avulsed, the best way to manage the acute wound is to achieve wound closure, with reconstruction being performed at some later time if necessary.

When large segments of the ear have been avulsed, they can be repaired in any of a number of fashions. The amputated segment can be dermabraded, reattached to the remaining portion of the ear, and then covered with a temporoparietal fascial flap, a temporalis fascia "fan flap," or a subgaleal fascial flap; or it can simply be buried under the scalp. When the ear is buried it needs to be released in approximately 2 weeks and skin-grafted. When an ear has been fully amputated, microvascular reimplantation can sometimes be performed. Alternatively, the cartilage framework can be exposed, after which the cartilage is replanted as a nonvascularized graft and covered with a thin vascularized tissue flap and skin-grafted. None of these more elaborate reconstructions can be performed in an emergency room setting, and all require the expertise of a specialist. There are numerous other local flaps available to repair or conceal segmental defects of the ear.

There are several complications unique to ear surgery of which the physician should be aware. Foremost is infection of the cartilage (*chondritis*). This problem is a medical emergency because it can result in severe permanent deformity of the ear if not aggressively treated.

Another complication that occurs frequently is *stricture* of the external auditory canal. Stricture that occurs as a consequence of a circumferential laceration is seen along the soft-tissue portion of the external canal. This situation is one instance where local skin flaps are useful adjuncts for closure of an acute wound. If a straight circumferential excision exists around the external auditory canal, the repair should include one or two Z-plasties to break up the line of potential cicatrix and prevent stenosis.

The next problem frequently seen in ears is *notching* along the rim of the ear. It can be minimized by meticulous skin closure.

The final complication, particularly around the ears, is *keloid* formation. Keloids are difficult to manage. Patients must be warned about their possibility, particularly if there is a history of keloid formation. The best preventive measure for keloid formation is to have a surgically clean wound and use meticulous technique during wound closure. If the patient appears to be developing a thickening of the scar during the early postoperative period, steroid injections

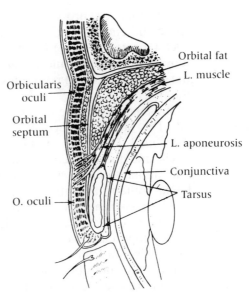

Fig. 17-2. Eyelid anatomy. The filaments of the levator expansion penetrate the orbital septum and orbicularis oris to insert into the pretarsal dermis, forming a palpebral fold. (From K. J. Lee. Comprehensive Surgical Atlases in Otolaryngology and Head and Neck Surgery. In D. D. Dedo (ed.), *The Atlas of Aesthetic Facial Surgery.* New York: Grune and Stratton, 1983. With permission.)

and local pressure can help to prevent it from developing further. Careful follow-up is important for these patients.

EYELIDS
Anatomy

Eyelid anatomy is complex (Fig. 17-2). A detailed knowledge of the anatomy of the eyelids is necessary if an attempt is made to repair complicated injuries. A basic understanding is important for all physicians who treat and evaluate lacerations in the region of the eyelid.

The upper eyelid consists of a layer of skin overlying the orbicularis muscle, which is found immediately below it. The inner margin of the eyelid, which is applied against the orbit, is lined with the conjunctiva. Sandwiched between the conjunctiva and the skin muscle unit on the outer surface is a layer consisting of a strip of cartilage known as the tarsal plate along the inferior border and a complex of muscles above it that are responsible for eyelid elevation. The levator muscle attaches to the external surface of the tarsus. This muscle is the primary elevator of the eyelid. When the levator insertion to the tarsus is disrupted, ptosis is the result. Just deep to the levator muscle is Müller's muscle, which is a thin muscle that is usually injured only with extensive injuries to the eyelid. Superior to the level of the tarsal plate is the orbital septum, which extends off the levator aponeurosis. It forms the anterior border of the orbital fat space and encloses the fat surrounding the orbit. The border of the eyelid contains hair follicles and glands associated with eyelid lubrication along its inferior surface. There is a faint gray line along the eyelid border that represents the attachment of the tarsal plate to the mucosa.

The anatomy of the lower lid is comparable to that of the upper lid. The tarsal cartilage of the lower lid, however, is less well developed. The tissue comparable to the levator muscle is primarily fascial and does not serve a major function as it does in the upper lid. The orbital septum, which emanates from the capsulopalpebral fascia, contains the orbital fat pad in the lower portion of the eyelid. The outer skin muscle layer, the eyelid border, and the conjunctival lining are comparable to those in the upper lid. The lacrimal system is also important. It consists of the lacrimal gland, which is located superiorly and laterally in the upper lid generally under the protection of the supraorbital ridge. The other components of the lacrimal system are the orifice and ducts, which drain tears from the eye. They are located at the medial margins of the upper and lower eyelids. The ducts extend from the orifices and travel around the medial canthal ligament into the lacrimal sac, which then drains into the nasal lacrimal duct and the nose. The only other comment with regard to eyelid anatomy concerns the medial and lateral canthi. In both areas a strong ligament is present that attaches to bone and supports the position of the eyelids.

Evaluation

Physical examination of the eye begins with a vision test. This test is easily performed with a standard chart in all but the most severely injured patients, for whom a hand-held eye chart can be used. Occasionally, when only gross vision can be checked, it can be done by counting fingers.

The next stage of evaluation is the ophthalmoscopic check of the orbit. Pupillary reflexes are examined. The cornea is examined for abrasions, the anterior chamber for hyphema, the iris for tears, the vitreous for hemorrhage, and the retina for a host of potential problems. If any abnormalities are noted during the orbital examination, an opthalmologist should be consulted.

For suspected corneal injuries a fluorescein test is helpful. A moistened fluorescein paper strip is touched against the eyelid margin, and the patient is asked to blink. A Wood's lamp is then held to the eye. Corneal abrasions stain positive with fluorescein.

Extraocular muscle function is then evaluated. The eyelid position and function are compared to those of the noninjured side. The lids are checked for ptosis (injury of the levator mechanism), epiphora (lacrimal duct injury), and alteration of the palpebral angle (canthal disruption).

The facial bones surrounding the eye are examined for tenderness, irregularities, and abnormal position relative to the noninjured side.

Facial bone and orbital radiographs can be obtained if there are any questions about the integrity of these structures.

Finally, when the important but easily overlooked portions of the examination are complete, the laceration can be fully evaluated. Its size, location, and depth are assessed. Simple lacerations involving skin and orbicularis muscle can be easily evaluated. More penetrating injuries may need to be fully evaluated in the operating room, as they may require the use of anesthesia, loupe magnification, and specialized instruments.

Operative Technique

Simple Lacerations

Simple lacerations of the eyelid skin can be repaired with local anesthesia (lidocaine with epinephrine) in the emergency room setting. Remember that meticulous hemostasis is mandatory when handling any periorbital wound. Hematoma around the eye creates a potential for loss of vision. It is unnecessary to use buried sutures for simple laceration repair. Simple or running subcutaneous pull-out sutures are sufficient in most instances. A thin monofilament synthetic suture such as nylon or Prolene, 5-0 or 6-0, should be used. The sutures are removed in 3 to 5 days. Eyelid skin has a tendency to develop epithelial cysts along the suture tracts. Consequently, subcutaneous pull-out sutures are preferred if technically possible during the repair.

Complex Lacerations

Eyelid Margin Repair. A full-thickness laceration of the eyelid margin requires precise alignment of the tissue to obtain a good outcome. A lid margin notch or step-off results if the lacerated lid margin is not perfectly repaired. These deformities can be noticeable even if they are only 1 to 2 mm.

The best way to start is to line up the gray line of the margin, which corresponds with the attachment line of the tarsus (Fig. 17-3). This landmark is carefully brought together with a 5-0 buried chromic catgut simple suture, being certain to evert the edges. After the gray line is brought together, the remaining skin defect is closed with 6-0 nylon or Prolene, and the conjunctiva is closed with buried 6-0 chromic catgut sutures.

Lacrimal System Repair. The lacrimal puncta are located on the medial borders of the upper and lower lid margins. The lacrimal ducts extend for 1 to 2 mm perpendicular to the lid margin. They then turn medially and course under the medial canthal ligament. Evaluation of the lacrimal system, when it is potentially involved in the eyelid laceration, consists in passing a lacrimal probe gently through the canaliculus and ductal system described above (Fig. 17-4). If the probe does not easily pass into the lacrimal sac, a lacrimal duct tear is presumed. These ducts are so fragile that direct repair is not feasible. It is necessary to place a lacrimal stent, which can be done

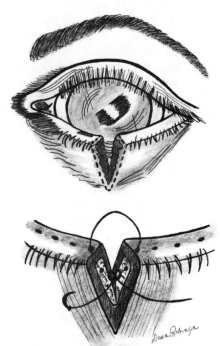

Fig. 17-3. Eyelid margin repair. The gray line is repaired with a buried chromic catgut suture.

under local or general anesthesia. This stent consists of a thin Silastic tube swedged onto a metal lacrimal probe. The probe is passed through the opening of the lacrimal duct along the pathway of the duct into the sac and through the sac into the nose. This procedure can be performed relatively atraumatically in an intact duct. When a duct is destroyed or lacerated, the open end of the duct is sought with loupe magnification in the injured tissues and cannulated with the lacrimal stent probe. If the distal end of the duct cannot be located, a new opening can be made into the lacrimal sac with the probe. Once the probes are passed through both the upper and lower ducts into the nasal area via the nasal lacrimal orifice, the Silastic tube is tied together to form a complete circle, which is then cut off and left in the nasal cavity for later removal. The stents are left in place for 6 months and are then removed in the office.

Upper Lid Repair. A laceration through the skin and orbicularis muscle requires only skin closure in most cases. If skin is avulsed, this wound can usually be closed primarily. Total lid avulsion requires complicated flap reconstruction, which obviously requires general anesthesia and a trip to the operating room.

In situations where the laceration extends through the orbicularis muscle, the levator aponeurosis and its attachment to the tarsal plate must be carefully inspected (Fig. 17-5). An unrepaired tear or

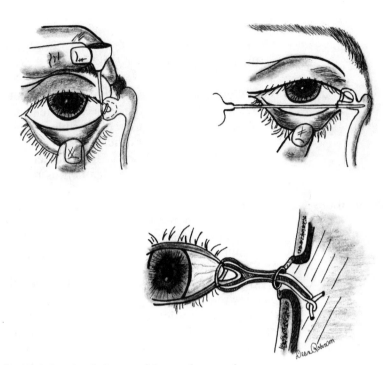

Fig. 17-4. Lacrimal duct probing and stent placement.

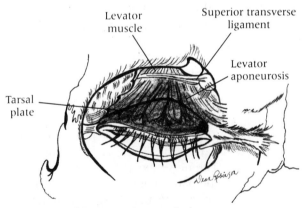

Fig. 17-5. Levator attachment to the tarsal plate.

avulsion of the levator apparatus results in a ptosis deformity. If the levator system requires repair, a 5-0 Maxon, Vicryl, or permanent suture is needed. Levator repairs should be done under local anesthesia so that voluntary lid excursion can be checked and compared to that on the uninjured side.

Lower Lid Repair. Once again injuries to the skin and orbicularis muscle require only skin repair. Buried sutures in the deep lower lid structures can lead to tethering and an annoying postoperative entropion or ectropion. Ectropion can also result from primarily closing a skin defect resulting from a skin avulsion. Any avulsed or missing skin on the lower lid should be repaired using a full-thickness graft of upper lid skin.

Canthal Ligament Repair. The medial and lateral canthal ligaments are densely attached to the adjacent bone (Fig. 17-6). Any displacement of the canthi suggests a possible facial fracture. The patient is carefully assessed for other clinical signs of fracture, and appropriate radiographs and CT scans are obtained (see Chapter 13). Complete laceration of the canthal ligament is rare.

Complications

Eyelid margin *notching* is a noticeable deformity. The scars should be allowed time to soften; then, in an operating room, the notch should be excised and the margin properly realigned.

Entropion and *ectropion* can occur after repair of almost any lower lid laceration. During the early phase of scar maturation, taping the lower lid up and laterally and massaging the lid in that same direction can often resolve the problem. If these deformities persist, they may require revision 3 to 6 months later.

Ptosis of the upper lid is usually due to edema during the early postoperative period. After the edema subsides, persistent ptosis suggests an inadequate levator repair. The upper lid should be reexplored and the aponeurosis reattached to the tarsus.

The final complication distinctive to eyelid injuries is *epiphora* (drainage of tears down the cheek). It indicates a failure of the lacrimal system to function. This late complication can usually be avoided by repairing the lacrimal system as noted above. If it is noted as a late complication of eyelid repair, an elective secondary repair of the lacrimal system must be undertaken.

CHEEKS
Anatomy

The facial nerve is responsible for most of the muscles of facial expression. There is no peripheral sensory component to this nerve. The nerve exists from the skull at the stylomastoid foramen deep to the parotid gland below the ear. It then travels superoanteriorly and enters the parotid gland, where it divides into multiple branches (Fig. 17-7). The nerve emerges from the gland at the level of the fascia of the facial muscles and spreads out through the face to innervate the muscles of expression. Five major branches of the facial nerve have been described: (1) the temporal nerve, which innervates the muscles of the forehead; (2) the zygomatic nerve, innervating the eyelid muscles; (3) the buccal nerve, innervating the facial expressive muscles of the central cheek; (4) the marginal mandibular nerve, which innervates the depressor muscles of the lower lip; and (5) the cervical branch, which innervates the platysma. There is, however, much variability in the anatomic pattern and distribution of these nerves. The temporal nerve frequently emerges from the parotid substance just anterior to the

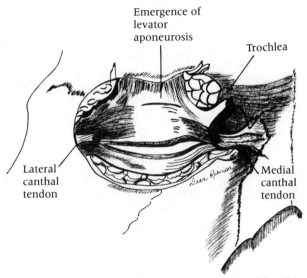

Fig. 17-6. Canthal ligament attachment to the periorbital facial bones.

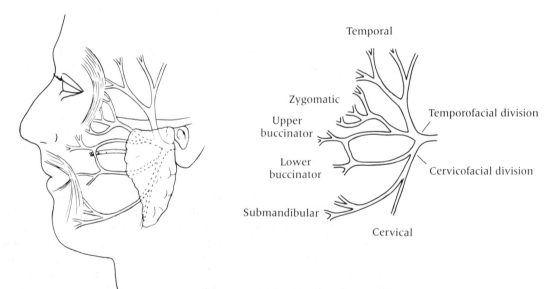

Fig. 17-7. Facial nerve anatomy. (From C. E. Silver. *Atlas of Head and Neck Surgery.* New York: Churchill Livingstone, 1986. With permission.)

superficial temporal vascular pedicle. It then travels on the muscle fascia and is immediately subcutaneous in the area over the zygoma, following a pathway between the tragus and a point 1.5 cm above the lateral aspect of the eyebrow. The zygomatic branch emerges from the parotid gland just at the anterior extension of the superior border of the gland below the zygoma and travels up toward the orbicularis muscles of the eye. The buccal branch frequently emerges from the gland adjacent to the parotid duct and fans out into the face overlying the masseter muscle. The marginal mandibular branch emerges inferiorly from the parotid gland, travels deep to the platysma muscle, crosses over the facial vein complex, and follows a path above the submandibular gland approximately 1 to 2 cm below the lower border of the mandible. It then travels upward at a level anterior to the submandibular gland to innervate the depressor muscles of the lower lip. The cervical branch of the nerve travels in a directly inferior fashion just below the parotid gland into the platysma muscle.

Parotid Gland and Duct
The parotid gland fills the cheek from the area below the zygoma anterior to the ear and lateral to the masseter muscle (Fig. 17-8). It extends slightly below the jaw anterior to the sternomastoid muscle of the neck. The gland contains the facial nerve. The portion of the parotid lateral to the nerve is artifically designated the superficial lobe, although the gland is actually a continuous structure. The parotid duct emerges from the superior anterior border of the superficial lobe of the parotid gland, travels over the masseter muscle, and pierces the buccinator muscle to enter the mouth. The orifice to the parotid duct is present opposite the second maxillary molar on the adjacent cheek (Fig. 17-9).

Evaluation

Evaluation of the facial nerve and parotid duct is easy. When injuries to these structures are missed, it is usually because the structures are not specifically examined during the evaluation of the wound. Any laceration over the masseter area of the cheek must include testing of the facial nerve and evaluation of parotid duct function. Facial nerve testing is simply accomplished by testing the muscle function in different regions of the face. Be sure to examine these muscle groups *prior* to injecting the wound with anesthetic, as lidocaine can block the facial nerve. The temporal branch is responsible for motion of the muscles of the forehead and can be examined by asking the patient to raise the eyebrows. The zygomatic branch is responsible for eyelid closure and can be tested by having the patient close the eyelids tightly. The buccal branch is responsible for creating the nasolabial fold, and absence of the nasolabial fold or mid-facial motion indicates injury to this branch. The marginal mandibular branch innervates the depressor muscles of the lower lip. Injury to this branch causes the lower lip to become elevated and immobile.

Parotid duct function can be assessed by observing the orifice of the duct intraorally on the buccal mucosa opposite the second maxillary molar. When the gland is gently compressed, clear saliva should be seen emanating from the duct orifice. The duct can also be directly cannulated in the operating room to locate the level of injury to the duct. It is unwise to inject surgical dyes such as methylene blue because this material stains the tissues once it escapes from the duct.

Surgical Management

Emergency room management of cheek lacerations requires that a thorough examination be conducted first. If the wound involves only skin and subcutaneous tissue, it can be closed in the emergency

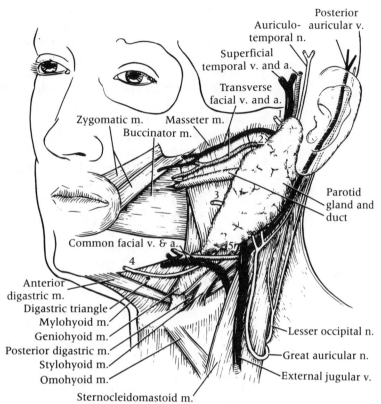

Fig. 17-8. Parotid gland and the facial nerve and its relationship to the surrounding structures. (From D. D. DeWeese et al. *Otolarygology — Head and Neck Surgery.* St. Louis: Mosby, 1988. With permission.)

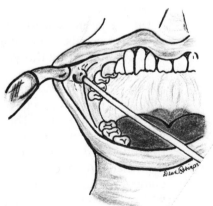

Fig. 17-9. Placement of a probe in Stenson's duct (second upper molar) to rule out parotid duct injury.

room in the usual fashion. Macerated edges must be trimmed. The wound edges are then aligned, and simple buried 4-0 or 5-0 polyglycolic acid sutures can be used to approximate the edges. Buried sutures are used sparingly, as they may become a nidus for infection in contaminated wounds. The skin is then closed with 5-0 or 6-0 monofilament nylon or similar sutures, taking care to evert the wound edges. These stitches need to be removed in 4 to 5 days to prevent cross-marking.

If deeper structures are involved in a cheek laceration and the examination is normal, the wound is anesthetized, irrigated with saline, and carefully inspected. The patient should undergo operative exploration for any extensive deep wounds or if there is any question of significant injury. The timing of operative intervention is not critical with nerve injuries. The skin can be closed and the wound reopened electively in the operating room. Facial nerve contusions can result in a facial palsy (Fig. 17-10), with recovery of function usually within 1 to 2 weeks. If the nerve is clearly severed at the onset, it is best to proceed with neurorrhaphy as soon as the patient is stable. Stensen's duct lacerations should be repaired soon after the injury to prevent a sialocele, salivary fistula, and secondary infection. If the repair cannot be done immediately, it is best to close the skin and leave any buccal lacerations open until the patient can be taken to surgery.

Any injury to the facial nerve requires microsurgical repair and should not be attempted in the emergency room setting. The laceration on the face can be extended into a standard parotidectomy incision if necessary. Frequently, to locate the ends of the nerve, it is necessary to perform a superficial parotidectomy. The key to successful nerve repair is adequate exposure. It is important to carefully trace the anatomy of the nerves in surrounding tissue to avoid unwanted injury to adjacent branches.

During facial neurorrhaphy it is obviously critical to identify the distal nerve ends, which may be difficult. A nerve stimulator can be of assistance during this part of the surgery, but only if the surgeon reminds the anesthesiologist to avoid using long-acting paralytic agents. One of the advantages of repairing the nerve soon after the injury is that for 4 to 5 days following the laceration the distal nerve end can be stimulated. This option is unavailable during late repairs because distal nerve function degenerates quickly. As the neurorrhaphy proceeds, the appropriate nerve ends are identified and freshened. A microanastomosis with 9-0 microvascular nylon epineural sutures is performed, attempting to align the fascicles without tension. For late repairs there may be tension at the planned neurorrhaphy site. In that setting or when a segment of the nerve has been avulsed or crushed, a nerve graft using the great auricular nerve as the donor is preferred.

Operative repair of parotid duct injuries provides a surgeon with three options. First, the ends of the lacerated duct can be directly sutured under magnification with 7-0 nylon, Prolene, or Vicryl. This

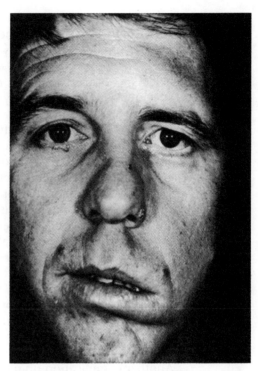

Fig. 17-10. Patient with a complete right facial nerve palsy. Note the loss of forehead wrinkling, increased palpebral fissure, flattening of the nasolabial fold, and drooping of the lateral portion of the mouth. (From H. Anderl. The head and neck. In J. M. Converse (ed.), *Reconstructive Plastic Surgery,* 2nd ed. Philadelphia: Saunders, 1977. With permission.)

method necessitates placement of a Silastic stent for a period of time postoperatively. The next best option after duct repair is repositioning, which involves transposing the cut end of Stensen's duct on the parotid side into the oral cavity via a perforation in the oral mucosa, which is created posterior to the normal orifice. The duct is then sutured with 4-0 chromic catgut or 5-0 Vicryl directly to the oral mucosa. A large fistula must be created, or it will stenose. The final and least desirable option is ligation of the parotid duct. This method, however, leads to immediate swelling and pain in the parotid gland for a period of several days postligation, after which the gland ceases to function and atrophies. Soft-tissue closure of the facial wound can be performed after any of these repairs is completed.

Complications

There are several unique complications that can occur after surgical repair of the facial nerve or parotid duct. Obviously, *paralysis* of the muscles innervated by the facial nerve is a direct result of the injury. Young children tend to recover almost complete function of these muscles after the repair, and young adults recover most of it. Middle-age individuals recover significantly less, and older people recover minimal function after repair of the nerve. Patients are always advised that full return of function is unlikely. There may be a significant delay between the time of repair and the end results, sometimes a period of months to more than a year. There are two nerve branches that, if injured, lead to the most significant functional problems associated with the facial paralysis. First is a zygomatic branch injury, leading to paralysis of the orbicularis oculi muscle and deficient eyelid closure.

Corneal injuries can result from exposure keratitis and can be treated symptomatically with taping, patching, and ophthalmic ointment. Another option is to perform a temporary lateral tarsorrhaphy until eyelid function returns.

The long-term management of *deficient eyelid closure* consists in many approaches. Gold weights can be used to provide gravity assist during eyelid closure. The levator muscle and Müller's muscle continue to function after facial nerve injury and provide adequate eyelid opening. Small wire springs can also be used to assist eyelid closure, as can a variety of fascial slings.

Late correction of *paralysis of the marginal mandibular branch of the facial nerve* is best performed by transfer of the anterior belly of the digastric muscle, which is innervated by the trigeminal nerve. A variety of masking procedures can be performed to hide this deformity by revising the lower lip margin.

Another complication unique to the parotid gland is formation of a collection of *salivary secretions* below the skin. Sialoceles look and act like seromas. They usually resolve with direct pressure and limitation of stimulation to the production of salivary flow. Salivary fistula is a comparable lesion. Instead of accumulating below the skin, the salivary fluid drains out through an opening in the skin. Salivary fistulas generally resolve with local wound care and by decreasing salivary output. Surgical intervention is rarely necessary for either of these complications.

Another unique syndrome associated with parotid duct and facial nerve injuries is the possible development of *Frye's syndrome*. This syndrome occurs when the skin overlying the parotid muscle is elevated and the parotid tissue is violated. After healing has occurred, frequently a year or more after surgery, the skin develops the disconcerting function of sweating or erythema production during periods of salivary stimulation. This phenomenon is due to abnormal connections between the parasympathetic stimulators of salivary flow and the sweat glands of the overlying skin. Virtually all patients who have had parotidectomy report some degree of Frye's syndrome if questioned carefully. It fortunately improves over a period of time. Rarely is it a significant enough problem to warrant surgical intervention.

SUMMARY

Management of injuries to the important structures of the face requires attention to the details of proper wound management. The wounds must be properly cleaned and assessed and the injured structures carefully identified. Injury to any of the major structures requires repair in an operating room setting. Minor lacerations of the face, even in highly visible areas, can generally be repaired in an emergency room setting. Perhaps the most important aspect of evaluating these injuries is to avoid overlooking an injury to a potentially repairable and important structure, such as the facial nerve or the parotid duct.

Commentary on Chapter 17

H. Wolfgang Losken

Dr. Granick suggested that individuals with human bites of the ear must be given intravenous antibiotics and be admitted to the hospital. I agree that the wound must be irrigated, débrided, and sutured but believe that the patient can then safely be given antibiotics orally and discharged home.

Dressings on the ear are important in that they provide pressure and so prevent hematoma. Bacitracin ointment is applied to the wound, with Telfa and paper tape molded to the ear to give good support. I agree that it is essential to check the wound in 24 hours.

For treatment of a hematoma of the ear, the hematoma is drained and a monofilament nylon suture inserted through all the layers of the ear. The suture is inserted through the Xeroform dressing on each side of the ear, which provides good support and keeps the skin on each side firmly adherent to the cartilage. This method significantly reduces the incidence of recurrent hematoma formation. If the hematoma has been present for longer than 24 hours, the contents may thrombose, which makes it impossible to aspirate the hematoma adequately and so results in a permanent deformity of the ear. This problem should be treated in the operating room. The hematoma may need to be formally opened and curreted and irrigated. The ear could then be packed with cotton gauze soaked in saline, which can be well molded into the crevices of the ear.

If a patient has a history of keloid formation, the skin edges should be injected with triamcinolone. It is important to inject intradermally only. If cortisone is injected subcutaneously, fat necrosis results. The steroid injection may need to be repeated 3 weeks later if it appears that a hypertrophic scar is forming.

The edge of the eyelid should be sutured with a soft suture such as 6-0 Nurolon, which is a multifilament nylon suture that is soft and nonirritating to the cornea; it is less reactive than silk. With a full-thickness laceration of the eyelid, the tarsal plate must be repaired. It is sutured with 6-0 chromic catgut suture inserted through the tarsal plate and conjunctiva, with the knot on the exterior surface. The suture is tied only after the eyelid margin has been meticulously approximated.

If the skin laceration is recent (less than 6 hours since the injury), clean cut, and 90 degress from the skin surface, suture without débridement is possible. All other wounds must be débrided. It is of concern that excessive débridement may distort important landmarks. If a nevus was present on the same site, a small amount of skin can be excised without fear of distortion; and with débridement it is seldom necessary to remove more than 1 mm from each side.

With severe lacerations, important landmarks must be maintained to ensure that the correct areas are sutured together. If necessary, temporary tacking sutures are inserted, and the rest of the wound is then débrided.

Suturing lacerations under local anesthesia is a painless procedure if a few basic rules are followed. The patient must be reassured that every endeavor will be embarked on to repair the laceration with the least amount of discomfort possible. A peaceful environment without excessive noise helps the patient to relax. Nursing staff are instructed never to say the words "needle," "syringe," "knife," or "blade." Sedation is sometimes of assistance when suturing lacerations, although not every child requires it.

Cleaning the skin is started some distance from the wound to obtain the confidence of the patient. Local anesthetic is sprayed on the wound surface, anesthetizing the wound and making needle insertion painless. The needle is advanced slowly. Never advance the needle and inject anesthetic at the same time. Give small amounts and wait for it to become effective before injecting greater quantities. Taking a slightly longer time with the infiltration could convert the experience from an unpleasant one to one that is bearable.

IV LOWER EXTREMITY

18 ACUTE CARE OF LOWER EXTREMITY TRAUMA

Michael J. White

The management of lower extremity trauma begins with a comprehensive evaluation of the entire patient and his or her injuries. The emphasis on airway, breathing, and circulation followed by primary and secondary surveys, as espoused by the Advanced Trauma and Life Support (ATLS) course, appropriately prioritizes this care so as to preserve life and function. Emergency care of the injured lower extremity begins with the cessation of life-threatening hemorrhage and temporary stabilization of fractures to prevent further injury. Definitive care of the lower extremity includes characterization of the injury, determination of salvageability, and definitive reconstruction encompassing revascularization, fracture stabilization, soft tissue coverage, and the special considerations of reinnervation and restoration of muscle function.

The goal of restoring a painless, sensate, functioning limb for locomotion may not be attainable or appropriate for every patient. Considerable judgment and skill must be exercised to provide the most satisfactory result with the least morbidity.

PERTINENT ANATOMY

Lower extremity salvage and reconstruction demand a detailed knowledge of the appropriate anatomy and physiology. An in-depth discussion of the pertinent anatomy is beyond the scope of this chapter; however, a brief review of the appropriate pertinent soft-tissue anatomy is presented.

Thigh

The quadriceps muscles comprise the rectus femoris and the vastus medialis, intermedius, and lateralis. They originate primarily from the pelvis and femur and insert into the anterior tibial tubercle by way of the patellar tendon and its associated ligaments. They are innervated by the femoral nerve and receive their blood supply from the lateral femoral circumflex artery and its associated branches or directly from muscular branches of the profunda femoris. They are principally responsible for extending the leg or flexing the thigh (Fig. 18-1).

The gracilis, semitendinosis, and sartorius muscles originate from

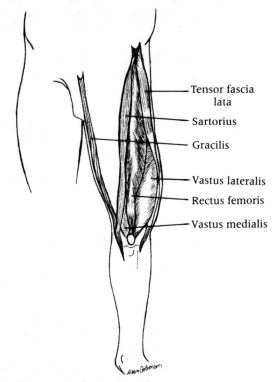

Fig. 18-1. Anterior thigh, regional anatomy.

three separate locations but insert commonly into the pes anserinus on the medial surface of the upper tibia. The nerve supply to the sartorius is segmental from the femoral nerve as is its blood supply from the femoral artery. The gracilis is innervated by the anterior branch of the obturator nerve. The principal blood supply is from the medial femoral circumflex artery and the muscular branches of the profunda femoris. The semitendinosis is innervated by the sciatic nerve and derives its blood supply from the perforating branches of the profunda femoris and popliteal arteries (Fig. 18-2).

The semimembranosis and biceps femoris in conjunction with the semitendinosis make up the hamstring musculature. This posterior group of muscles inserts on the posterior aspect of the leg both medially and laterally, and they are the principal flexors of the leg. They are innervated by the sciatic nerve and receive their blood supply from perforating branches of the profunda femoris and the muscular branches of the popliteal (Fig. 18-3).

The adductors of the thigh are innervated by the obturator nerve. They are supplied by the muscular branches of the profunda femoris artery as well as the obturator artery (see Fig. 18-2).

The musculature of the leg can be divided into four compartments with distinct anatomic boundaries. The anterior compartment comprises the tibialis anterior, extensor hallucis longus, extensor digito-

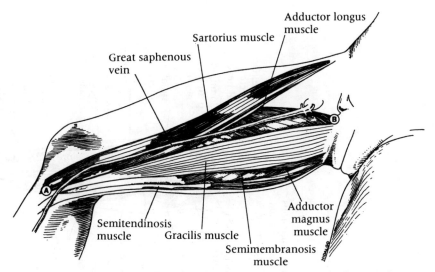

Fig. 18-2. Medial thigh, regional anatomy. (From W. W. Shaw and D. A. Hildalgo. *Microsurgery in Trauma.* Mt. Kisco, NY: Futura, 1987. With permission.)

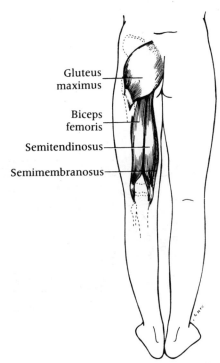

Fig. 18-3. Posterior thigh, regional anatomy. (From S. J. Mathes and F. Nahai. *Clinical Atlas of Muscle and Musculocutaneous Flaps.* St. Louis: Mosby, 1979. With permission.)

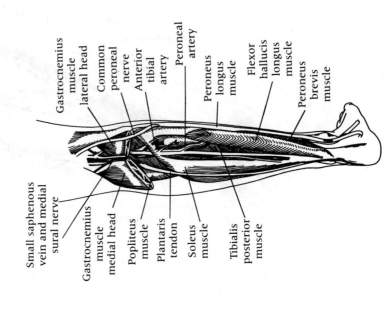

Fig. 18-5. Posterior leg, regional anatomy. (From W. W. Shaw and D. A. Hildalgo. *Microsurgery in Trauma.* Mt. Kisco, NY: Futura, 1987. With permission.)

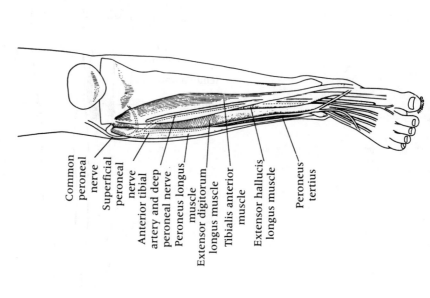

Fig. 18-4. Anterior leg, regional anatomy. (From W. W. Shaw and D. A. Hildalgo. *Microsurgery in Trauma.* Mt. Kisco, NY: Futura, 1987. With permission.)

rum longus, and peroneus tertius muscles. They are each supplied by the deep peroneal nerve and receive their blood supply from the muscular branches of the anterior tibial artery.

The lateral compartment comprises the peroneus longus and peroneus brevis muscles, which plantar flex and evert the foot. These muscles are both supplied by the superficial peroneal nerve with an arterial supply from the anterior tibial and peroneal vessels (Fig. 18-4).

The superficial posterior compartment of the leg comprises the gastrocnemius, soleus, plantaris, and popliteus muscles. These muscles are innervated by the tibial nerve. The blood supply to the gastrocnemius muscle is from the sural branches of the popliteal. Similarly, the plantaris receives its blood supply from the sural branches of the popliteal. The popliteus receives its blood supply from branches of the popliteal artery. The soleus receives blood supply from the posterior tibial, peroneal, and popliteal arteries.

The deep posterior compartment includes the flexor hallucis longus, flexor digitorum longus, and tibialis posterior muscles. These are innervated by the tibial nerve and supplied by the branches of the posterior tibial or peroneal arteries (Fig. 18-5).

Foot

The soft-tissue anatomy of the dorsal foot includes the skin and subcutaneous tissue, which immediately cover an extensive venous network overlying the superficial and deep peroneal nerves. This layer also includes the dorsalis pedis artery and its branches. The dorsal musculature of the foot includes the extensor hallucis brevis, extensor digitorum brevis, and dorsal interossei muscles, which are supplied by the deep peroneal nerve and dorsalis pedis artery, with the exception of the interossei, which are innervated by the lateral plantar nerve. The muscles are covered by the tendons of the extensor digitorum longus and extensor hallucis longus (Fig. 18-6).

The muscles of the plantar surface of the foot can be divided into four levels. The first level underneath the skin and plantar fascia also encompasses the medial and lateral plantar arteries and associated plantar nerves. This first muscular layer comprises the abductor hallucis brevis, flexor digitorum brevis, and abductor digiti minimi. The second plantar level consists of the quadratus plantae and the lumbricals. The third muscular plantar space includes the flexor hallucis brevis, adductor, hallucis, and flexor digiti minimi brevis. The fourth level contains the dorsal and plantar interossei.

Vascular Anatomy

The external iliac artery descends underneath the inguinal ligament, giving rise to the common femoral artery, which soon bifurcates giving off the profunda femoris branch and continues as the superficial femoral artery. Vessels of particular importance to the reconstructive surgeon include the lateral femoral circumflex artery from the profunda femoris artery, supplying the quadriceps musculature and the tensor fascia lata. The medial femoral circumflex branch from the profunda femoris is the principal blood supply to the

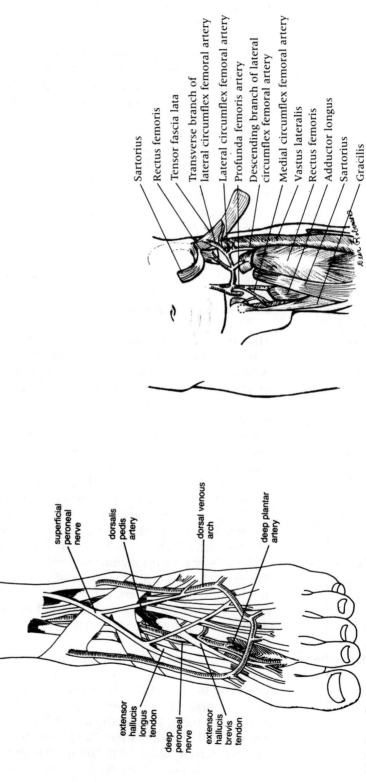

Sartorius
Rectus femoris
Tensor fascia lata
Transverse branch of
lateral circumflex femoral artery
Lateral circumflex femoral artery
Profunda femoris artery
Descending branch of lateral
circumflex femoral artery
Medial circumflex femoral artery
Vastus lateralis
Rectus femoris
Adductor longus
Sartorius
Gracilis

Fig. 18-7. Blood supply of the anterior thigh. (Modified from S. J. Mathes and F. Nahai. *Clinical Atlas of Muscle and Musculocutaneous Flaps.* St. Louis: Mosby, 1979.)

superficial
peroneal
nerve
dorsalis
pedis
artery
dorsal venous
arch
deep plantar
artery
extensor
hallucis
longus
tendon
deep
peroneal
nerve
extensor
hallucis
brevis
tendon

Fig. 18-6. Dorsal aspect of the foot, regional anatomy. (From W. W. Shaw and D. A. Hildalgo. *Microsurgery in Trauma.* Mt. Kisco, NY: Futura, 1987. With permission.)

gracilis, which is also a useful muscle during lower extremity reconstruction (Fig. 18-7).

As the femoral artery descends to the popliteal space and becomes the popliteal artery, several important anastomotic communications arise, that is, the superior and inferior geniculates. In addition, the sural arteries form the principal blood supply of the medial and lateral heads of the gastrocnemius. This extensive collateral network may provide satisfactory vascular supply to the lower extremity in the event of an isolated popliteal injury, maintaining viability while reconstruction can be accomplished. As the popliteal artery descends from the popliteal fossa, the anterior tibial artery is given off and enters the anterior compartment over the proximal edge of the interosseus membrane. The tibial-peroneal trunk descends, giving rise to the peroneal and posterior tibial arteries. The posterior tibial artery continues to the foot from behind the medial malleolus, dividing underneath the flexor retinaculum into the medial and lateral plantar vessels, which are important contributors to the foot and useful as axial vessels for flap reconstruction. The anterior tibial artery descends within the anterior compartment between the tibialis anterior and extensor muscles to exit on the dorsum of the foot underneath the extensor retinaculum. The dorsalis pedis is a continuation of the anterior tibial artery and supplies the intrinsic extensors of the foot before giving off the deep plantar vessel, which communicates with the plantar vessels. The metatarsal extensions of the dorsalis pedis form the basis of multiple free flaps, including the first web space, great toe transfer, second toe transfer, and so on (Fig. 18-5).

Venous return from the lower extremity can be divided into superficial and deep systems. Although there is a multitude of superficial branches, appropriate understanding of the superficial anatomy is important because of its significant role as graft material for arterial and venous reconstruction, free tissue transfer, and the proximity of the greater and lesser saphenous veins to the saphenous and sural nerves, respectively. The deep system accompanies the arterial supply and coalesces to form the popliteal vein.

Nervous Anatomy

The nervous anatomy of the lower extremity is particularly important in helping to assess salvageability of the lower extremity. Restoration or preservation of cutaneous sensibility of the foot is a prerequisite for successful reconstruction. The cutaneous innervation of the foot is demonstrated in Figure 18-8. The motor innervation has been described previously.

EVALUATION

Initial evaluation of an injury requires a detailed and pertinent history and physical examination. Although life-saving measures demand immediate attention, a pertinent history can often be obtained simultaneously from family members, emergency personnel, and transport personnel. The important aspects that relate to lower extremity trauma are depicted in Table 18-1. Documenting the

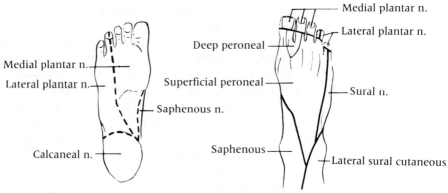

Fig. 18-8. Cutaneous innervation of the foot.

nature of the injury, including the time since injury and the mechanism of injury, provides invaluable information as to the possibilities for reconstruction. Airway status, the presence of hypotension or significant blood loss, and loss of consciousness are parameters that not only place lower limb salvage in perspective but also suggest the degree to which the clinical evaluation will be accurate or complete. For example, the conscious, cooperative patient who can participate in the history and physical examination process may be able to provide diagnostic tip-offs to the complete injury that are unavailable with the comatose or uncooperative patient. Similarly, medical problems such as coronary artery disease, pulmonary disease, and peripheral vascular disease directly affect diagnostic and therapeutic decision-making.

Information related to the treatment rendered at the scene should be obtained to assist in understanding the mechanisms of injury. Such information might include a difficult extrication from a motor vehicle, a long contamination time, or exsanguinating hemorrhage that required tourniquet application or direct ligation of a bleeding vessel. These bits of information contribute to a more complete understanding of the severity of the injury.

Physical examination of the lower extremity is part of the secondary survey and is outlined in Table 18-2. The lower extremity must be examined with knowledge of the patient's level of consciousness and vital signs. Evaluation of the vascular status of the lower extremity includes the presence or absence of pulses, capillary refill, and the appropriate color in a normotensive patient. Similarly, neurologic evaluation requires a detailed examination of defined motor and sensory nerve distributions. Orthopedic injuries must be documented by satisfactory radiographic evaluation based on a thorough physical examination. Soft-tissue injuries not only must be

Table 18-1 Components of the history

Nature of the injury
    Time, date, location
       Mechanism of injury
           Penetrating versus blunt
           Degree of energy transmitted
           Degree of crush injury
           Degree of contamination
       First aid rendered
           Time and location of initial intervention
           Type of treatment rendered (at the scene, en route, at other hospitals)
           Treatment rendered to the amputated part
Patient information
    Extent of injury
        Airway status
        Hypotension
        Blood loss
        Loss of consciousness
    Extent of lower extremity injury
        Pain
        Paresthesia/anesthesia
        Loss of function
    Complete preinjury medical history

Table 18-2. Physical examination of the lower extremity

Level of consciousness
Vital signs
Vascular status
    Color
    Capillary refill
    Pulses (palpation vs. Doppler examination)
Neurologic status
    Sensation in defined nerve distribution
    Motor ability
Orthopedic status
    Obvious deformity
    Tenderness
Soft-tissue injury
    Ecchymosis or contusion
    Laceration or avulsion
        Proximity to major neurovascular bundle
        Exposure of bone, tendon, neurovascular bundle

---

documented as to type and location but must be placed in the context of associated injury (e.g., an open fracture or major neurovascular injury). Soft-tissue injury in proximity to a major neurovascular bundle must be evaluated thoroughly, and it often requires surgical exploration or arteriographic assessment. Similarly, soft-tissue injury in proximity to a major fracture must be investigated to exclude continuity with the fracture site itself.

Laboratory Evaluation

Laboratory tests do not often reflect lower extremity trauma directly; however, several tests may be helpful and certainly are an indicated part of the overall evaluation of the injured patient. Blood loss and the adequacy of resuscitation can be roughly monitored by hemoglobin and electrolyte analyses, which are used in conjunction with the patient's vital signs and urinary output. On the other hand, a severe crush or electrical injury to the lower extremity may produce significant myoglobinuria requiring alkalinization of the urine to prevent renal tubular injury; therefore serum myoglobin levels should be evaluated.

Radiologic Evaluation

Patients who have experienced any lower extremity trauma must be evaluated radiographically to identify fractures. Certain high risk injuries, such as posterior knee dislocations, associated with a high incidence of popliteal artery injury or open wounds in close proximity to major neurovascular structures should be considered for arteriography. Surgical exploration with or without arteriography is often the most appropriate intervention so as not to miss potentially dangerous vascular injuries [1].

CLASSIFICATION OF LOWER EXTREMITY INJURIES

Obtaining a careful history and performing an accurate physical examination allows the examiner to classify lower extremity trauma so as to predict salvageability and, more importantly, the quality of the salvaged limb. The classification systems are based on mechanism of injury, viability of the extremity, and functional assessment of the injured extremity.

Mechanism of Injury

Understanding the mechanism of injury cannot be overstated. Types of injuries may be classified (1) as penetrating versus blunt, (2) as high energy versus low energy, (3) by the degree of crush injury, and (4) by the degree of contamination.

Viability

Viability of an extremity may be compromised by an arterial, venous, or crush injury. The length of ischemia is crucial for determining outcome and therefore is a vital component of any classification system.

Viability of the extremity may also be compromised by a *compartment syndrome*. Compartment syndromes not infrequently occur in the leg where four defined anatomic compartments are confined by stout investing fascia and bone. The diagnosis of compartment syndrome is made on the basis of: (1) an appropriate history for significant lower extremity injury; (2) subjective complaints of pain out of proportion to the injury; (3) hypesthesia or paresthesia in defined nerve distributions and the physical findings of a painful, swollen extremity with exquisite tenderness on passive motion; (4) decreased sensation to examination; or (5) diminution or absence of distal pulses. Adjunctive measures such as measuring compartment pressures by any number of published techniques (e.g., Whitesides' method or Wick catheter) may be helpful in the comatose patient or the patient who is unable to cooperate with the evaluation. Brumback and Blick [2] recommended that pressures measuring more than 30 mm Hg be considered pathologic and an indication for compartment fasciotomy in an extremity with significant injury.

Once a compartment syndrome is diagnosed, immediate fasciotomy is indicated, which can be accompanied by any number of techniques. In the traumatized patient the double incision technique of Mubarek and Owen [3] is recommended because of the completeness with which all four compartments can be decompressed. Total fibulectomy is not recommended because of its potential use during subsequent reconstruction and the added stability it gives the lower extremity, particularly one that is traumatized. Similarly, minimal incision fasciotomies provide limited exposure and increase the risk of damaging vital structures such as the common peroneal nerve. The double incision technique of fasciotomy is shown in Figure 18-9.

Functional Assessment

Classification systems of lower extremity injury also account for the functional losses of the extremity, including weight-bearing, neuromuscular function, and soft-tissue protection. Skeletal stability must be ascertained as to both the integrity of the bones and the ligamentous structures to preserve fully articulated joints. Fractures are classified as open or closed by site, displacement, angulation, and degree of comminution and contamination. High energy wounds of the lower extremity usually result in fractures that place the greatest demands on the orthopedic and reconstructive surgeon.

Adequate débridement of the fracture site, stabilization of the bone, and adequate coverage with vascularized tissue are the principal ingredients of successful limb salvage. Because open fractures with soft-tissue injury represent the most challenging types of reconstruction, several classification systems have been devised to study them and predict outcome. Categorization of lower extremity fractures allows accurate comparison of fractures and treatment outcome.

Gustillo and Anderson [4] first classified open fractures of the lower extremity in 1976. This classification system was based on the nature of the fracture as well as soft-tissue injury. Subsequent classification systems have sought to further identify those subgroups of open fractures with varying prognoses based on the nature of the fracture, soft-tissue injury, and neurovascular status of the extremity [5–9].

Gustillo and Chapman's [5] modification of the original description in 1983 is perhaps the most widely recognized and utilized classification system (Table 18-3). Mears and Stone [9] sought to subdivide type III fractures by further defining the zone of injury. Swartz and Mears [10] in 1985 classified lower extremity wounds on the basis of their reconstructive requirements rather than the nature of the injury itself.

On the basis of these classification systems, prognostic information

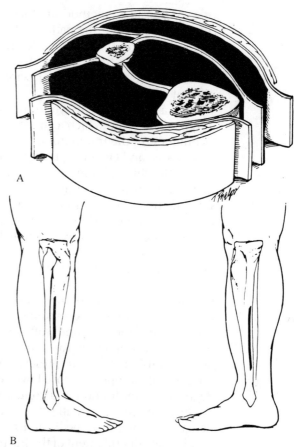

Fig. 18-9. Double incision technique for fasciotomy of the leg.
A. Cross-sectional diagram depicting the medial and lateral incisions and the release of the myofascial compartments. B. Anatomic location of the medial and lateral skin incisions; note that the medial incision is more distal than the mid-calf lateral incision. (From R. J. Bumback and S. S. Blick. Lower Extremity Salvage and Reconstruction. In M. J. Yaremchuk, A. R. Burgess, and R. J. Bumback (eds.), *Compartment syndrome*. New York: Elsevier, 1989. With permission.)

can be obtained that, when considered in conjunction with the patient's overall evaluation, leads to a determination of salvageability.

DETERMINATION OF SALVAGEABILITY

Caring for patients with an extensively traumatized lower extremity (e.g., type III$_c$ open fracture) requires that salvageability be determined. This multifactorial decision-making process must determine not only if the limb *can* be salvaged but if it *should* be.

The importance of this decision was lucidly pointed out by Bondurant et al. [11]. In their study 263 patients with grade III open tibial fractures were studied of whom 43 ultimately underwent

Table 18-3. Classification of lower extremity open fractures[a]

Grade	Gustillo and Chapman [5]	Mears and Stone [9]	Swartz and Mears [10]
I	Open fracture with clean wound < 1 cm long	Perforation from within; minimal soft-tissue injury; indirect, low energy absorption	Soft tissue Clean Infected
II	Soft tissue wound > 1 cm but without extensive soft-tissue damage, flaps, avulsions	Perforation from without; moderate soft-tissue injury; direct, moderate energy absorption	Soft tissue and bone (< 8 cm) Clean Infected
III	Wounds with extensive soft-tissue laceration or flaps, or wounds of high-energy trauma but with adequate soft tissue to cover the fractured bone	Laceration or avulsion; severe soft-tissue injury; direct high energy absorption	Massive soft tissue and bone Clean Infected
	Wounds with extensive soft-tissue injury or loss with periosteal stripping and bone exposure		Bone only Clean Infected
	Open fractures associated with arterial injuries requiring repair		

[a]This classification system is based on reconstructive requirements rather than a description of the fracture and associated soft-tissue injury.

amputation. Of the 43 patients, 14 (32.6%) underwent primary amputation. this group averaged 22.3 days of hospitalization, 1.6 surgical procedures on the affected extremity, and $28,964 in hospital costs. The 29 patients who underwent attempts at salvage with delayed amputation had an average of 53.4 days of hospitalization, 6.9 surgical procedures, and $53,462 in hospital costs. Six of these patients (20.7%) developed sepsis secondary to their involved lower extremity and died, whereas no patient in the primary amputation group developed sepsis or died. These findings underscore the importance of making an accurate determination of salvageability early in the course of treatment. Such a determination, however, is not easy to make and requires astute clinical judgment. Salvageability depends on both patient factors and factors related to the injury itself.

Patient factors to be considered include the underlying medical condition of the patient and the degree of traumatic injury suffered. Consideration must be given to the occupational and personal aspects of the patient. The status of the ipsilateral foot and opposite

extremity also influence the decision to salvage a severely traumatized limb.

Certain questions relate to the injured extremity: Can the bony
stability be restored? Can vascularity be restored? *Protective sensation
must be restorable if the reconstruction is to provide any advantage over
amputation and a prosthesis.* The goal of limb salvage remains one of
restoring a stable, sensate limb for locomotion. The extent to which
reconstruction cannot meet this condition alters the risk/benefit ratio
in favor of amputation.

Lange [12] has analyzed the decision-making process of whether
to reconstruct or amputate a traumatized limb. Reviewing some
series of type III_c tibial fractures, he pointed out the "prolonged
hospitalization, requirement for multiple operations, high infection
rate, high failure rate, increased mortality rate, prolonged disability
time, high rate of significant functional sequelae, psychological
attachment to the limb, socioeconomic disability, psychosocial disability, and medical-legal considerations" attendant to attempted
limb salvage. In his own series of type III fractures, Lange [13]
correlated the worse prognosis for salvage with crush injury, segmental fractures, and revascularization delays of longer than 6
hours. In this series, 9 of 17 salvage attempts (53%) underwent
amputation. Similar series reported by Caudle and Stern [14] and
Lancaster et al. [15] confirmed the low salvageability rate of type III_c
tibial fractures, with amputation rates of 78 percent and 87 percent,
respectively.

These studies suggest that lower extremity reconstruction and
salvageability is a highly individualized and demanding process.
Multiple variables and clinical experience must be considered.

**LOWER EXTREMITY
RECONSTRUCTION**

Reconstruction begins with appropriate first aid at the scene and
during transport. Cessation of life-threatening hemorrhage, stabilization of the fracture, adequate resuscitation, and prevention of
edema and contamination are the basic tenets.

Treatment in the emergency department, in addition to evaluation
of the injury, includes adequate resuscitation, intravenous antibiotics, tetanus prophylaxis, and appropriate use of radiologic studies
including arteriography.

The operative strategy for limb salvage should include neurovascular exploration followed by fracture stabilization and definitive
revascularization of the extremity. This process must be carefully
orchestrated between the orthopedic, vascular, and reconstructive
surgeons so as not to compromise each discipline's procedure. From
the plastic surgical perspective, this cooperation may be essential to
providing optimum reconstruction. For example, should the orthopedic surgeon find it necessary to use an external fixator for a tibial
fracture, placement of the external fixator pins in an anterior
position provides optimum access to both the medial and lateral

aspects of the leg without directly compromising local muscles, skin, or flaps. Similar cooperation is required between the vascular and orthopedic surgeons for injuries requiring limb salvage. If limb ischemia has not been prolonged, fracture stabilization is usually accomplished first so that the length of neurovascular disruption can be accurately appreciated and the vascular reconstruction is not disrupted during manipulation of the fracture fragments. For limbs with relatively prolonged ischemia, temporary shunts or definitive revascularization with careful monitoring of the repairs during fracture fixation permit expeditious reperfusion of the limbs prior to fracture fixation. Soft-tissue débridement is performed, and appropriate dressings are chosen. The patient is monitored to confirm satisfactory perfusion of the limb and to delineate progressive soft tissue injury. The wound is observed and débrided as necessary until the soft tissues are stable. Serial bacterial cultures may assist in this determination. Definitive soft-tissue coverage can be planned at this time. Bony reconstruction is usually performed secondarily if necessary.

Timing of Reconstruction

The timing of soft tissue reconstruction for open lower extremity fractures has been studied relative to the incidence of complications such as infection, delayed nonunion, and subsequent amputation. In 1986 Godina [16], reviewing a personal series of 532 extremity reconstructions, concluded that acute soft-tissue reconstruction within the first 72 hours after injury was critical to obtaining superior results. This finding was supported by an extremely low infection rate (1.5%) and a flap failure rate of 0.75 percent in the early coverage group.

Byrd et al. [7] similarly concluded that acute soft-tissue coverage was crucial for maintaining a low complication rate. In their series of 54 open tibial fractures requiring flap coverage, 27 patients had acute (within the first 6 days) soft-tissue coverage, with an 18 percent complication rate compared to a 50 percent complication rate for the 20 patients whose fractures were closed during the subacute period (1–6 weeks). A similarly high complication rate (40%) was found in the seven patients who underwent delayed reconstruction during the chronic period (after 6 weeks). These two studies [7, 16] would lead the reconstructive surgeon to believe that acute soft-tissue coverage is mandatory for obtaining satisfactory results after lower extremity trauma.

Yaremchuk [17], on the other hand, subscribed to a more pragmatic approach for the multiply injured patient. As he pointed out when reviewing the Maryland Institute for Emergency Medical Services Systems Shock Trauma Center experience, most patients treated at that facility for lower extremity trauma also had other systems injured, requiring additional care. Moreover, the zone of injury was often difficult to discern during the first 3 to 4 days after the injury. Serial débridement of their multiply injured patients with lower extremity trauma was performed every 48 to 72 hours until the wound was deemed ready for definitive soft-tissue closure. Flap coverage was usually performed within the first 7 to 10 days after injury; however, even longer delays of up to 3 to 4 weeks did not appear to be detrimental to the ultimate outcome. In a series of nearly 100 patients treated in this manner, nine flaps were lost with a 10 percent acute infection rate. This approach of serial débridement to a clinically clean and stable wound followed by soft-tissue coverage appears to be most appropriate for the multiply injured patient, although arguably with a slightly higher complication rate. Unnecessary delays in soft tissue coverage are to be avoided, but timing must also take into consideration the patient's other injuries and condition.

Débridement of the Wound

Serial wound débridements are performed to accomplish total excision of all nonviable tissue while preserving such vital structures as nerve, tendon, and periosteum. It is best accomplished by serial observation and operative intervention as necessary. Sharp débridement under regional or general anesthesia is most effective in removing all nonviable tissue. We have also found the jet lavage irrigating system to be of benefit in further cleansing the wound.

Adjunctive Measures

In a large series of over 1,100 fractures, Patzakis and colleagues [18] demonstrated the efficacy of prophylactic antibiotics. In the group receiving a parenteral cephalosporin and an aminoglycoside, the infection rate was 4.5 percent compared to a 24.0 percent incidence of infection in those patients who did not receive prophylactic antibiotics.

Antibiotic therapy should be culture-specific once these results have been obtained. For this reason, the wound is cultured initially at the time of the first débridement with follow-up cultures as necessary.

At complex fracture sites, antibiotic delivery may be enhanced by the use of antibiotic-impregnated beads placed within the wound. These methyl methacrylate beads have been shown to leach relatively high doses of antibiotics locally without systemic absorption [19].

Choice of Flaps for Reconstruction

Thigh

Extensive soft tissue reconstruction of the thigh is seldom indicated because of the relative abundance of muscle mass covering the femur. Often muscles can be moved locally to provide sufficient coverage for any bony defect. Thigh flaps frequently used for coverage of the thigh, groin, or pelvis include the tensor fascia lata, vastus lateralis, biceps femoris, rectus femoris, and gracilis muscle flaps. These flaps can also be raised as myocutaneous flaps. In addition, fasciocutaneous flaps can be elevated, such as the inferior gluteal thigh flap, for local transposition. For the most part, however, adequate soft-tissue coverage can usually be obtained by local transfers combined with skin grafts.

Table 18-4. Choice of flaps for lower extremity coverage

Flap	Description	Disadvantages	Comments
Knee and proximal third			
Medial gastrocnemius	Medial head of gastrocnemius based on sural artery Robust muscle belly with wide arch of rotation for medial and anterior aspect of upper leg and knee		Workhorse of soft-tissue reconstruction in the proximal third of the leg
Lateral gastrocnemius	Lateral head based on sural artery for lateral aspect of knee and proximal leg	Limited length due to shorter muscle belly and rotation over proximal head of fibula	Seldom reaches much beyond midline but useful for lateral defects; common peroneal nerve must be protected
Others Soleus	Posterior tibial and peroneal artery supply	Limited to distal proximal third	Although principally used for middle third coverage, this muscle has sufficient arc of rotation to cover defects in the lowest portion of the proximal third
Tibialis anterior	Bipedicled mobilization of muscle, allowing coverage of small anterior defects	Limited usefulness; function should not be sacrificed	
Fasciocutaneous flaps (e.g., saphenous, posterior calf)	Useful for covering surface wounds without significant depth	Requires limited zone of injury to ensure perfusion of flap; requires skin graft of donor defect	
Middle third Soleus	Broad origin, tapered insertion, based on posterior tibial and peroneal arteries	More difficult dissection; arc of rotation limited by number of preserved perforators	Workhorse of middle third defects

Table 18-4. (continued)

Flap	Description	Disadvantages	Comments
Hemisoleus	Smaller than soleus but increased arc of rotation		
Gastrocnemius myocutaneous	Fasciocutaneous extensions based on medial or lateral head; can extend to within 5 cm of medial malleolus for medial gastrocnemius or 10 cm from the malleolus for lateral gastrocnemius	Requires skin graft of significant posterior donor defect	Excellent choice for long anterior middle third defects
Others Flexor digitorum longus Tibialis anterior Extensor hallucis longus Flexor hallucis longus			Limited usefulness due to small size of coverage and consideration of functional deficits
Distal third Free flap	Allows coverage of any size defect with great versatility	Requires microsurgical expertise and longer operative time	Workhorse of distal third reconstruction; flap selection based on size, depth, and type of defect, length of pedicle rquired to reach vessels outside the zone of injury, and external cover requirements
Soleus	See Middle Third		Soleus is often sufficiently long to cover small distal third defects

Table 18-4. (continued)

Flap	Description	Disadvantages	Comments
Extensor digitorum brevis	Small island muscle flap based on dorsalis pedis	Small size, sacrifices dorsalis pedis	Versatile flap despite its small size; useful for medial and lateral malleolar defects
Reversed peroneal island flap	Island fasciocutaneous flap based on retrograde peroneal arterial flow	Requires normal arterial anatomy and limited zone of injury; more extensive dissection required	
Others Flexor mallucis longus Flexor digitorum longus Tibialis anterior Abductor hallucis Peroneus brevis Peroneus tertius	Local advancement or transposition of these flaps may cover small defects in the distal third	Requires limited zone of injury and small defect	Functional deficits must be considered; the author has found these flaps to be of limited usefulness for major lower extremity injury

Leg

Significant soft-tissue avulsions and defects in the leg can be particularly challenging because of the decreasing muscle mass and increasing density of neurovascular, tendinous, and bony structures as one approaches the ankle and foot. The leg is typically divided into three reconstructive areas: proximal, middle, and distal one-thirds. Customary muscle flap choices for each of these anatomic locations can be seen in Table 18-4. In simplest terms, the proximal one-third is the usual domain of the gastrocnemius muscle. The middle one-third is most frequently covered by the soleus muscle flap, and the distal one-third not infrequently requires free tissue tranfer (Fig. 18-10). Several excellent textbooks are available for review of each of these flaps, including anatomic dissections [20–22].

In addition to the muscle flaps described in Table 18-4, the reconstructive surgeon must be cognizant of other modalities that may be appropriate for smaller defects. They include local random pattern flaps from noninjured sites, fasciocutaneous flaps described for the lower extremity, and tissue expansion for wounds that do not need immediate coverage.

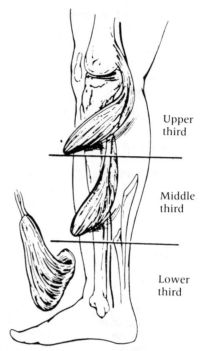

Fig. 18-10. Soft-tissue coverage for the leg. Upper third: gastrocnemius muscle. Middle third: soleus muscle. Lower third: free tissue transfer. (From R. J. Brumback and S. S. Blick. Compartment syndrome. In M. J. Yaremchuck, A. R. Burgess, and R. J. Brumback (Eds.), *Lower Extremity Salvage and Reconstruction.* New York: Elsevier, 1989. With permission.)

Table 18-5. Classification of foot injuries

Type	Description
I	Limited soft-tissue injury
II	Major soft-tissue loss with or without distal amputation
III	Major soft-tissue loss with an open fracture of the ankle, calcaneus, or distal leg

Source: D. A. Hildalgo and W. W. Shaw. Reconstruction of foot injuries. *Clin. Plast. Surg.* 13:664, 1986. With permission.

Foot

Hildalgo and Shaw have classified foot injuries into types I, II, and III, corresponding to the extent of soft-tissue loss and associated injury (Table 18-5). In an excellent review of foot anatomy and reconstruction [23], these authors provided an intelligent choice of options based on injury type and location (Table 18-6).

Table 18-6. Reconstructive options by location and injury type

Site	Type I	Type II	Type III
Weight-bearing heel and mid-plantar area	PPSP flap Myocutaneous fasciocutaneous flap FDB muscle flap Skin graft	Muscle free flap Skin free flap Ipsilateral gluteal or thigh flap (children)	Muscle free flap Amputation
Distal plantar area	Toe flap Skin graft	Muscle free flap Skin free flap Ipsilateral gluteal or thigh flap (children)	Muscle free flap Amputation
Dorsum	Skin graft Fascial free flap	Fascial free flap Skin free flap	Muscle free flap Fascial or skin free flap
Malleolus	EDB muscle flap Fascial free flap Muscle free flap Dorsalis pedis flap Abductor muscle (below malleolus)	Fascial free flap Muscle or skin free flap	Muscle free flap Fascial or skin free flap
Posterior (non-weight-bearing) heel, Achilles tendon	Lateral calcaneal artery flap EDB muscle flap; abductor/FDB muscle flap Fascial free flap Dorsalis pedis/first webspace flap Skin graft	Muscle free flap Skin free flap Ipsilateral gluteal or thigh flap (children)	Muscle free flap Amputation

PPSP = proximal plantar subcutaneous plexus; FDB = flexor digitorum brevis; EDB = extensor digitorum brevis.
Source: D. A. Hildalgo and W. W. Shaw, Reconstruction of foot injuries. *Clin. Plast. Surg.* 13:672, 1986. With permission.

REPLANTATION

Although successful lower extremity replantation has been accomplished, the efficacy of this extensive procedure is often limited. Frequently lower extremity amputations are avulsive in nature, comprising significant areas of crush injury that require unacceptable shortening of the extremity. In addition, the likelihood of restoring plantar sensation is so limited that careful consideration must be given to any lower extremity replantation. Shaw [24], reviewing 100 traumatic lower extremity amputations, attempted only 29 replantations of which 12 survived. He suggested six indications/prerequisites for lower extremity replantation: (1) a medically stable patient; (2) débridement of less than 3 inches of bone; (3) bilateral amputations; (4) adequate soft tissue and potential for nerve restoration; (5) a well motivated patient; and (6) the patient is a child.

Acknowledgment. The author thanks Margie Gazda for her invaluable assistance in preparing the manuscript.

REFERENCES

1. Richardson, J. D., Vitale, G. C., and Flint, L. M. Penetrating arterial trauma: analysis of missed vascular injuries. *Arch. Surg.* 122:678, 1987.
2. Brumback, R. F., and Blick, S. S. Compartment syndrome. In M. J. Yaremchuk, A. R. Burgess, and R. F. Brumback (eds.), *Lower Extremity Salvage and Reconstruction.* New York: Elsevier, 1989.
3. Mubarek, S. J., and Owen, C. A. Double incision fasciotomy of the leg for decompression in compartment syndromes. *J. Bone Joint Surg.* [*Am.*] 59:184, 1977.
4. Gustillo, R. B., and Anderson, J. T. Prevention of infection in the treatment of 1,025 open fractures of long bones. *J. Bone Joint Surg.* [*Am.*] 58:453, 1976.
5. Gustillo, R. B., and Chapman, M. W. Management of type III open fractures. In *Orthopedic Surgery Viewpoints 1983.* Indianapolis: Eli Lilly, 1983.
6. Johner, R., and Wruhs, O. Classification of tibial shaft fractures in correlation with results after rigid internal fixation. *Clin. Orthop.* 178:7, 1983.
7. Byrd, H. S., Cierny, G., III, and Tebbetts, J. B. The management of open tibial fractures with associated soft tissue loss: external pin fixation with early flap coverage. *Plast. Reconstruct. Surg.* 68:73, 1981.
8. Tscherne, H., and Gotzen, L. (eds.), *Fractures with Soft Tissue Injury.* Berlin: Springer-Verlag, 1984.
9. Mears, D. C., and Stone, J. P. The management of open fractures. *Orthop. Surg.* 3:247, 1988.
10. Swartz, W. M., and Mears, D. C. The role of free tissue transfers in lower extremity reconstruction. *Plast. Reconstruct. Surg.* 76:364, 1985.
11. Bondurant, F. J., et al. The medical and economic impact of severely injured lower extremities. *J. Trauma* 28:1270, 1988.
12. Lange, H. Limb reconstruction versus amputation decision making in massive lower extremity trauma. *Clin. Orthop.* 243:92, 1989.
13. Lange, H., et al. Open tibial fractures with associated vascular injuries: prognosis for limb salvage. *J. Trauma* 25:203, 1985.
14. Caudle, R. T., and Stern, P. J. Severe open fractures of the tibia. *J. Bone Joint Surg.* [*Am.*] 69:801, 1987.
15. Lancaster, S. J., Honwitz, M., and Alonso, J. Open tibial fractures: management and results. *South. Med. J.* 79:39, 1986.
16. Godina, M. Early microsurgical reconstruction of complex trauma of the extremities. *Plast. Reconstruct. Surg.* 78:285, 1986.
17. Yaremchuk, M. J. Flap reconstruction of the open tibial fracture. In M. J. Yaremchuk, A. R. Burgess, and R. F. Brumback (eds.), *Lower Extremity Salvage and Reconstruction.* New York: Elsevier, 1989.
18. Patzakis, M. J., Wilkins, J., and Moore, T. M. Use of antibiotics in open tibial fractures. *Clin. Orthop.* 178:31, 1983.
19. Seligson, D. Antibiotic-impregnated beads in orthopedic infectious problems. *J. Ky. Med. Assoc.* 82:25, 1984.

20. McGraw, J. B., and Arnold, P. B. *McGraw and Arnold's Atlas of Muscle and Musculocutaneous Flaps.* Norfolk: Hampton Press, 1986.
21. Mathes, S. J., and Nahai, F. *Clinical Atlas of Muscle and Musculocutaneous Flaps.* St. Louis: Mosby, 1979.
22. Mathes, S. J., and Nahai, F. *Clinical Applications for Muscle and Musculocutaneous Flaps.* St. Louis: Mosby, 1982. Pp. 532–584.
23. Hildalgo, D. A., and Shaw, W. W. Reconstruction of foot injuries. *Clin. Plast. Surg.* 13:664, 1986.
24. Shaw, W. W. Microvascular surgery. In H. Haimovici (ed.), *Vascular Surgery: Principles and Techniques,* 2nd ed. Norwalk, CT: Appleton-Century-Crofts, 1984. Pp. 289–309.

Commentary on Chapter 18

William M. Swartz

The plastic surgeon's role in acute lower extremity trauma is an important and sometimes decisive one. The successful long-term result with a severe lower extremity injury depends on the coordinated efforts of general surgeons, orthopedic surgeons, and plastic surgeons, with their input starting at the beginning of the patient's care. The first decisions are ultimately the most important and should center around (1) whether to salvage the extremity and (2) the development of a sound surgical plan with a reasonable chance for successful completion in a timely manner. The ultimate test of success is whether the patient is able to return to functional ambulation and a productive role in society. A young patient, for instance, may be condemned to a lifetime of dependence on a prosthetic device, and the elderly patient may find it significantly difficult to deal with a prosthetic device, particularly when getting up in the middle of the night. In both cases, then, it would be desirable to preserve the lower leg if possible.

Modern techniques of extremity reconstruction, including microsurgical free tissue transfers and leg lengthening by the Ilizarov method, have changed the outcome of severe injuries. With this point in mind, the decision to salvage the leg should encompass technical, social, and economic factors, which vary among patients. In general, if it is predicted that one can achieve full weight-bearing and painless ambulation within 18 months and that the number of procedures required to achieve this end is predictable, salvage may be considered. In descending order of importance, the factors that militate limb salvage are as follows.

1. *Patient's psychosocial environment.* The patient must be able to deal effectively with an 18- to 24-month program of surgical interventions and rehabilitation with the likelihood that independent ambulation and return to work is possible.

2. *The presence of sensibility in the distal leg and foot.* Transection of the posterior tibial or popliteal nerves lead to severe difficulty achieving successful ambulation despite nerve repairs. Not only does loss of sensation lead to breakdown of the weight-bearing surface of

the foot, but loss of sensibility has secondary effects including chronic pain and paresthesias.

3. *Technical feasibility of soft-tissue and bone restoration.* Severe lower extremity injuries generally require soft-tissue replacement, often with microvascular free-tissue transfers. Primary wound closure within the first 5 to 7 days of injury in general permits rapid progression to wound healing and bone union provided large segments of bone have not been completely devascularized. In the latter category, secondary bone reconstruction and the ability to achieve bone union with full weight-bearing is the ultimate problem of extremity salvage.

4. *Bone reconstruction.* Provided primary soft-tissue wound healing is feasible, early plans for bone reconstruction must take into account the nature of the injury and the time required for restoration. For short segmental defects of less than 6 cm or for anterior cortical defects where a posterior cortex is intact, delayed cortical cancellous grafting has proved efficacious in restoring the bone column. An important adjunct is the presence of an intact fibula, which adds stability to the grafted tibia as it is being solidified. For larger defects, of more than 6 cm, three techniques of bone restoration have been employed. Each has its proponents, and each claims a reasonable degree of success. They are (1) cortical cancellous bone grafting underneath vascularized muscle flaps; (2) free vascularized bone grafts from the contralateral fibula; and (3) bone lengthening techniques using the Ilizarov method. Although there are no controlled studies to date that compare these three methods, it is becoming apparent that each has a significant role to play in individual patients. Of singular importance, however, is the provision for healthy soft tissue, the elimination of necrotic bone sequestra, and a reconstruction plan that provides continual progress toward the goal of complete weight-bearing by 18 to 24 months after the injury.

Our approach to the acute care of severe lower extremity injuries is as follows.

1. The circulatory status is restored and limb length is preserved by temporary bone stabilization. In most circumstances, it requires an external fixator device.

2. All devitalized tissue is débrided, including bone fragments that do not have secure periosteal attachments to the wound bed. Muscle that does not bleed readily or contract upon stimulation should be débrided at this first setting. Transected blood vessels in the wound should be marked for possible use as donor vessels in delayed primary wound closure.

3. Temporary wound coverage should be provided during the interval between successive débridements; it may include occlusive dressings with bacitracin ointment, which is our first preference, or biologic dressings such as amniotic membrane or lyophilized pig

skin. Exposed vital structures including blood vessels and nerves should be covered by mobilization of local tissues or acute primary free tissue transfer where indicated.

4. Definitive soft-tissue coverage should be provided as soon as technically feasible. The requirement here is a biologically clean wound, which may be ascertained by the use of quantitative wound cultures and rapid slide techniques. Immediate free tissue transfers should be considered when the vital structures of essential blood vessels and nerves cannot be covered by local tissues during the interval between débridements. Within 5 to 7 days definitive wound coverage should be provided. For the proximal and middle thirds of the tibial region, soleus and gastrocnemius muscle flaps are the procedures of choice. For the distal one-third and below the ankle, free tissue transfers are the most reliable procedures.

5. Secondary management of the bone defects must be effected. Whereas the orthopedic surgeon frequently becomes responsible for the osseus defect, the plastic surgeon has a significant role to play in the provision of well vascularized soft tissue preceding bone reconstruction and potentially the provision for vascularized bone grafts where indicated. Additional methods at the orthopedist's disposal include fibula tibia bypass grafting, cortical cancellous bone grafting for segmental defects, and bone lengthening techniques for closure of defects.

In this organized, coordinated fashion, predictable salvage after severe lower extremity injury can be realized. Prolonged, unsuccessful outcomes can be avoided by properly assessing the patient's potential for rehabilitation and use of the surgeon's ability to provide timely, effective care.

V GENERAL INFORMATION

19 DRESSINGS AND SPLINTS

Mark D. Liang

There are several specific purposes of dressings: (1) immobilization of the injured part; (2) protection of the area from further trauma; and (3) keeping the area clean or in a dry or wet state. In addition, a good dressing should be secure and neat (dressings are often the only evidence of one's work initially seen by the patient and the family) and should be tailored to fit the particular area.

SKIN WOUNDS

The choice of dressing materials and techniques is important not only for achieving the above purposes; it may play a significant role in the biologic process of wound healing itself. Occlusive dressings may affect healing by keeping tissues moist and preventing the buildup of crust, both of which facilitate epithelialization and collagen synthesis.

Sutured Wound

The first layer in contact with the freshly sutured wound should be a porous, finely meshed gauze with or without a moisturing agent (fine mesh gauze, Xeroform, Adaptic) that is cut to cover the laceration and sutures. It is then followed by a couple of layers of coarse gauze to absorb any blood or serum. This gauze is also trimmed so it is not bulky. One of the most useful ways of securing these two layers, especially on the face and trunk, is to first apply a thin layer of benzoin or Mastisol on the skin. This step allows better adherence of the tape to the skin and may provide some measure of protection for the skin. Tape (0.5 inch paper tape) is then applied in multiple layers to fashion a "cocoon dressing" (Fig. 19-1). These five to ten layers of tape essentially splint the skin surrounding the laceration, thereby decreasing motion at the suture line and providing protection against minor trauma to the wound.

Steri-strips placed directly over skin sutures (subcuticular sutures are the exception) are not advocated. These adherent strips can be uncomfortable to take off and can cause trauma to relatively fresh wounds when removed. Moreover, without several layers of gauze adjacent to the wound there is a tendency to retain blood and serum under these strips.

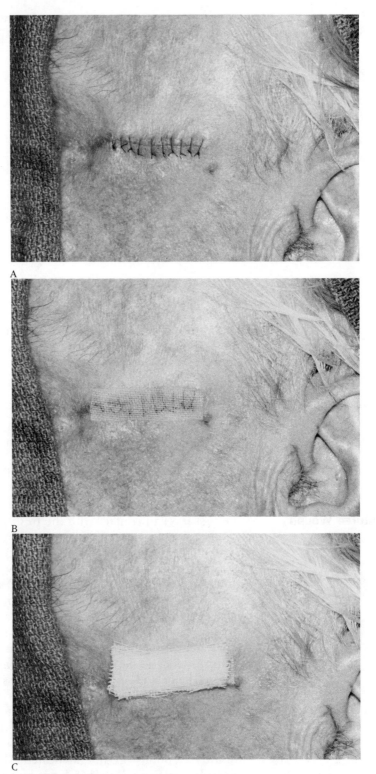

Fig. 19-1. A., B., and C. "Cocoon Dressing" is created by multiple layers of ½ inch paper tape applied over a coarse gauze dressing in order to immobilize the underlying skin and suture line.

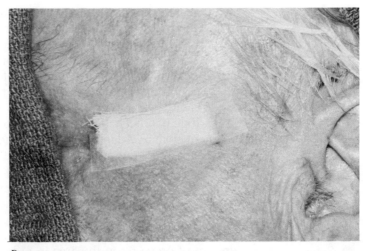

D

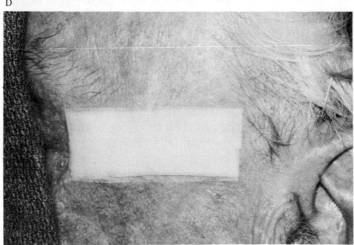

E

Fig. 19-1. D., E. "Cocoon Dressing" is created by multiple layers of ½ inch paper tape applied over a coarse gauze dressing in order to immobilize the underlying skin and suture line.

Dressing tape is removed as gently as possible by pulling the tape either toward the laceration or along the length of the laceration in order to not create excessive tension on the wound. The surrounding skin is gently stabilized by the physician's hand. An adhesive solvent such as Freon, Stripease, or Unisolve may facilitate removal of adherent tape.

Open Wounds: Abrasions and Burns

Abrasions and minor burns are often best treated on an outpatient basis. These wounds are treated by one of two methods: open or closed. Open therapy is usually used for selected wounds of the head, neck, and perineum, where maceration can be a problem and where dressings might be difficult to keep in place. Occasionally, abrasions and burns of the hands are treated open in order to facilitate movement of the joints. A thin layer of topical antibiotic ointment may be applied daily. One of the disadvantages is that there is often an increased tendency to drying and crusting.

The most common approach to abrasions/burns is the use of closed occlusive dressings composed of several dressing materials, each providing a specific function. The first layer, which is in direct contact with the wound, should be a nonadherent porous mesh gauze that has been lightly impregnated with a petroleum-based ointment such as Adaptic. The gauze should be porous enough that it does not allow ingrowth of new tissue but coarse enough to allow weeping of wound exudate. Covering it should be a layer of fluffed, coarse gauze that helps absorb wound exudate and provides a layer of padding to protect the wound from mechanical trauma.

These layers can be held in place by a gentle wrap of slightly elastic gauze, such as Kling or Kerlix. Care must be taken not to apply large amount of pressure on the area in order to prevent further damage to the wound by constricting the blood flow. Dressings can be changed on a daily basis if no topical antibiotic therapy is used. If a topical antibiotic such as Silvadene is utilized, a twice-a-day dressing is in order to maintain the antibiotic effect.

Synthetic dressings such as Opsite provide a more modern solution to treating open wounds. These products consist of a plastic film that is permeable to oxygen and water vapor while being impermeable to liquids. The advantages of these dressings include pain relief, ability to continually visualize the wound, and maintaining the wound in a moist environment. Alternative synthetic dressings for abrasions are Duoderm and Biobrane. In the future there may be dressings impregnated with antibiotics, growth factors, and so on for continued delivery directly to the healing wound.

DRESSINGS OF SPECIFIC AREAS

Head and Neck

As mentioned above, small dressings about the face are best accomplished with a small "cocoon dressing." Large wounds about the forehead, posterior cheek, and submental and submandibular regions can be dressed with a pressure dressing (Barton bandage). Wounds can be dressed with the same fine mesh gauze and coarse gauze as noted above and then wrapped with a Kling gauze as shown in Figure 19-2. This bandage should be wrapped firmly with a C-shaped dressing placed behind the ear. It can be made by folding a 4 × 4 inch gauze and cutting a semicircle out of it.

Eyes

Repaired lacerations around the eyelids may be treated by applying ointment to the eyes and eyelashes and over the lacerations. A standard eye pad (which consists of two layers of fine mesh gauze separated by cotton padding) may be moistened slightly and placed over the closed eyelids. This pad may be taped with 0.5-inch paper tape, or a 3-inch Kling may be wrapped circumferentially around the

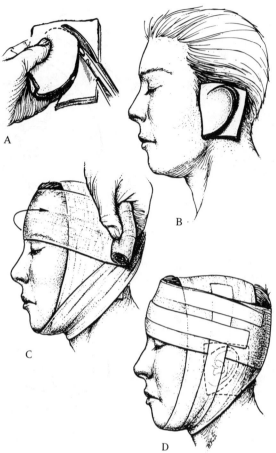

Fig. 19-2. The "Barton Bandage" is a useful pressure dressing of the head and neck region. The ear is cushioned with a C shaped gauze posteriorly. (From R. C. Schultz, *Facial Injuries*, 3rd ed. Chicago: Year Book, 1988. With permission.)

head to secure the eye patch. A slight amount of compression may be achieved by this technique.

Nose

Nasal trauma is often associated with fractures to the fragile nasal bones. A useful nasal splint is a plaster of paris cast that is used to stabilize nasal fractures; it helps to minimize swelling while protecting the nose from further trauma. Usually five or six thicknesses of quick-drying plaster of paris can be cut into a shape as shown in Figure 19-3. Customizing the height and width of the splint is essential for each patient. This splint may be placed over intact nasal skin or over a light gauze bandage if there has been a laceration or abrasion of the skin of the nose.

Lukewarm water is used to wet the splints. Hot water should be avoided if the plaster is to be in direct contact with the skin because the drying of plaster is an exothermic reaction and may produce excessive heat if hot water is utilized. The plaster is then molded about

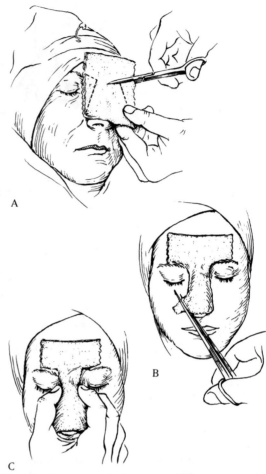

Fig. 19-3. Nasal splints made of plaster of Paris are very useful in treating nasal fractures. A. Cutting plaster splint to measure. B. Trimming splint to nasal contour while still wet. C. Accurate shaping with fingers before plaster sets. (From R. C. Schultz, *Facial Injuries,* 3rd ed. Chicago: Year Book, 1988. With permission.)

the nose and forehead and held in place with paper tape. Care must be taken to trim the plaster in the gabellar region in order not to irritate the sensitive eyelid skin or interfere with the patient's vision.

Hands and Arms
Lacerations or abrasions about the hands and fingers should be treated with a nonadherent gauze such as Adaptic or Xeroform. When bandaging the hand it is important to keep dry gauze between the fingers to decrease sweating and maceration. It is also important to splint the hand in the correct position. Almost all hand and wrist lacerations should be splinted in order to (1) minimize swelling, (2) decrease motion at the suture line, and (3) place the hand in a position that is most beneficial to decrease stiffness and maximize rehabilitation.

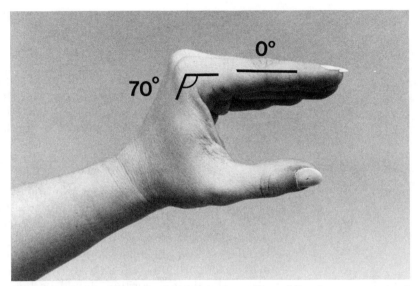

Fig. 19-4. The position of safety keeps the collateral ligaments at maximal length and facilitates rehabilitation postoperatively.

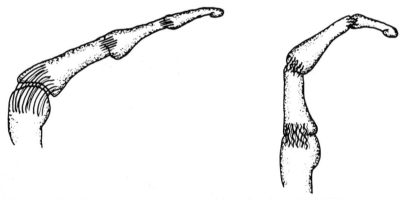

Fig. 19-5. The ligaments are at maximal length when the MCP joints are flexed and the PIP joints are straight.

There are basically two positions for hand splinting: the position of safety and the position of function. Most hand lacerations seen in the emergency room should be splinted in the position of safety (Fig. 19-4). The wrist in the safety position is neutral relative to supination and pronation and in 15 to 30 degrees of extension. The metacarpophalangeal (MCP) joints are flexed 70 to 90 degrees and the interphalangeal joints 0 to 10 degrees. This position keeps the collateral ligaments of the fingers at maximal stretch (Fig. 19-5). The collateral ligaments of the interphalangeal joints are straight when the fingers are straight. However, those over the MCP joints drape more dorsally, putting them at maximal stretch with the joint at 90 degrees. If the thumb is not injured, the splint should be molded away from the hypothenar eminence in order to allow freedom of motion of all three joints of the thumb. If the thumb is to be incorporated into the splint, it should be placed in position where the web space is maximally stretched to prevent web space contracture (Fig. 19-4).

Splints for the hand may be fashioned from either plaster of paris or fiber glass. These splints can be placed on the volar or dorsal aspect. For most hand problems a volar (palmar) splint can be created from the proximal forearm to the fingertips. An adequate padding of Webril over the skin is recommended, with the splint being held in place by a 2- or 3-inch Ace wrap.

Lower Extremity

The lower leg, ankle, and foot can and should be splinted when lacerations occur in this region or when a sprain is present. Splints should be made of 15 to 20 layers of 5-inch plaster or fiber glass after padding the extremity with adequate amounts of Webril. Care must be taken to keep the ankle at 90 degrees to prevent shortening of the achilles tendon. A 4- or 6-inch Ace wrap is used to hold the splint in place. The desired position should be held until the plaster dries adequately.

Commentary on Chapter 19

Ross Musgrave

It is my belief, in agreement with Dr. Liang, that personal preference is the rule rather than the exception for wound dressings (as well as for wound care). Many physicians/surgeons use the dressing as a physical and psychological barrier to protect the emotional sensitivities of both the patient and the family, to say nothing of the patient's coworkers.

Americans in particular who are now in their mid to late thirties and younger have been essentially brain-washed by the Mickey Mouse or Flintstone "bandaids," which they have been led to believe by commericals on kiddies' television to be a "cure-all" for every "boo-boo." Even toddlers not yet toilet-trained are led to believe that mommy's kiss plus the magic "bandaid" promote healing and somehow ensure a miraculous cure. There is a certain amount of personal conviction that "out of sight, out of mind" is the safer course, particularly in children and adolescents, to say nothing of squeamish adults. Sometimes even the neatest row of precisely placed fine nylon sutures (worthy of being projected on a large screen) appear "yukky" to a sizable segment of the population. What I am trying to emphasize is that protection of the area is both a physical and a psychological protection. If there is some adjacent ecchymosis, it too is "masked" by the dressing.

The neatness of the dressing cannot be overemphasized. Prior to the Federal Trade Commission's ruling on the permissibility of advertising by physicians, the dressing or splint and its neatness — the only visible initial evidence of the proficiency of the surgeon — served as a subliminal advertisement.

I cannot recommend too highly the "cocoon dressing" described by Dr. Liang. It is efficient in that in addition to providing the elements of protection and coverage, it provides *splinting*. (Sometimes I use several layers of cloth tape over the laminated layers of paper tape in cocoon dressings.)

Steri-strips can be of considerable value in the right patient at the right place and for the right purpose. They are particularly good for children and work well if a subcuticular or subcutaneous suture has been used as a buried suture. *Note:* Something must be said here about the removal of Steri-strips. Each end of the Steri-strip should be taken off and gently pulled toward the middle, as the physician or nurse who pulls only in one direction after the half-way point is disrupting the wound by distracting the coapted edges.

As for slightly elastic gauze, such as Kling or Kerlix, care indeed must be taken not to apply it with undue pressure. If too much pressure is used, further damage to the wound (by constriction of blood flow) may occur. Therefore in many instances the slightly crimped gauze (e.g., Kling or Kerlix) is preferable to using an Ace elastic bandage.

Dressings around the eye, particularly after suturing, should be lightly applied and changed perhaps as often as every 6 hours. An alternative method, if a cooperative patient is involved, is to use cold saline compresses; sometimes these 4 × 4 inch sterile gauze dressings are placed in a custard cup of saline that sits in a larger basin of ice. The compresses are changed at least every 30 minutes or every hour, sometimes by the patient or family. An ophthalmic ointment frequently used is either bacitracin or a polysporin-polymyxin ointment. (Care must be taken that the patient has no history of allergies to any of these medications.)

An alternative to the plaster of paris nasal splint is one of the easily molded and trimmed lightweight aluminum splints padded with a thin felt layer. To obviate the sharp edges of such a trimmed splint, a "piping" of 0.25 inch adhesive tape — 0.5-inch adhesive tape split down the middle — can be used, applied in two pieces from 12 to 6 o'clock and 6 to 12 o'clock on the splint. I hasten to add that these metal splints can be spread further apart if the physician believes there is too much pressure being exerted. Conversely, this type of splint can provide slightly more pressure by merely squeezing the lateral sides together between thumb and forefinger.

Dressings for the hands and arms frequently can be simplified if the emergency room has available a "universal splint," which comes in a lightweight metal and can be wrapped with a Kling or Kerlix gauze before placing the hand and forearm in place with the wrist bent slightly up. A smaller size can be used for older children and young adolescents. This splint is not available for small children. Most splints should extend to the proximal forearm, care being taken not to impinge on the antecubital space. If an Ace bandage is used over plaster of paris, it can become moist; then, when the cotton material in it shrinks, the bandage may exert too much pressure. For this reason the Ace wrap may have to be removed and reapplied somewhat more loosely after it has been allowed to dry.

The same precaution should be observed with an Ace bandage over wet plaster of paris when used for lower extremity splinting. If the knee is involved in the splint or casting, foresight or forethought should be used when deciding on the amount of knee flexion that can be tolerated so the patient can ambulate with crutches and get in and out of automobile seats.

In summary, something should be said about dressings in general:

First, cleanliness is next to godliness. Second, immobilization, although at first cumbersome, can pay dividends in the immediate suture line area as well as in the adjacent soft-tissue structures. Third, when dealing with extremities, elevation of the injured or sutured part on a pillow after the dressing has been applied does aid in the healing. Fourth, when upper extremity trauma or surgery is more than trivial, a properly applied sling should be used without question. Frequently the sling is of psychological value: Particularly in children and adolescents, it is a reminder that the wound is going to heal better if it is not only protected but immobilized. Thus the sling may have the same psychological "warning" value as the colorful bandaids noted in the first portion of this commentary.

20 LOCAL ANESTHESIA AND SEDATION FOR THE PEDIATRIC PATIENT

Holly W. Davis
Bruce W. Rosenthal
Angela M. Tangredi

Assessment and treatment of pediatric patients with wounds that require plastic surgical repair often pose special challenges. Failing to understand our helpful intent and the need for their cooperation, and tending to perceive attempts at examination and treatment as an attack, many young patients not only are uncooperative but indeed often are frankly combative. Optimal wound closure is impossible and the situation potentially hazardous when the surgeon is dealing with a flailing, screaming child and an operative field that is a perpetually moving target. Thus physical restraint or administration of some form of sedation often becomes necessary.

The decision to sedate a child must never be taken lightly or considered routine. The potential risks must be weighed against possible benefits, tailoring the approach to the needs of each individual child. Furthermore, the surgeon must have reasonable expectations as to what can be achieved safely by the use of sedation in the outpatient setting and must bear in mind that currently there is no one ideal method. The size of the wound, its complexity, the probable severity and duration of pain when administering the local anesthetic, and the likely duration of the procedure should be considered.

The surgeon must also recognize that there are many situations in which problems that could be managed easily in the emergency department with an adult patient require closure under general anesthesia in the operating room when the patient is a child. It is also important to appreciate that one's manner of approach, use of reassurance, and collaboration with parents may enhance cooperation and obviate the need for sedation, especially with older children. Hence before discussing types and methods of administering topical and local anesthetics and sedative agents, we address methods of approaching patients and parents, emphasizing relevant developmental stages and methods of reassurance and distraction.

APPROACH TO PATIENTS AND PARENTS

The accident that precipitates a trip to the emergency department with a wound requiring plastic surgical repair is typically an unexpected and frightening experience for a child. A warm, supportive,

447

calm, unhurried approach, beginning with the triage nurse and extending to the plastic surgeon, can help set the stage for a more optimal assessment and treatment experience.

One should gently attempt to engage and get to know the child. When the children are verbal, find out their version of what happened, empathizing in age-appropriate terms with how "scary" that must have been and conveying that we are going to do our best to help them get better. A small investment of time in finding out about the patient's home, brothers and sisters, best friends, favorite stories, activities, and heroes can pay off handsomely as assessment and treatment proceed. At each step in the examination and during the procedure, the physician should explain in simple, nonthreatening terms what he or she is about to do, making reassuring comments as appropriate. It is also of utmost importance to be honest with a child; saying something will not hurt when it usually will results in complete loss of trust and a marked reduction in cooperativeness. One should avoid highly charged terms such as "pain" and "needle," using "hurt," "ouch," or "pinch" instead — and bring this point up only shortly before the painful stimulus in order to avoid a long period of anticipation [1,2].

An understanding of a few highly relevant developmental phases, their associated behavioral characteristics, and measures designed to reduce their impact is often helpful. The first of these phases, *stranger anxiety* (manifest by fearfulness and crying at the sight of an unfamiliar face) tends to develop at 5 to 6 months of age and may last until age 3 or 4. To avoid triggering this reaction, the physician should attempt to avoid making eye contact with older infants and toddlers for more than a few seconds at a time. Keeping a parent's face in the child's line of sight as much as possible and having the parent talk to the patient to maintain his or her attention as one does the examination and even as one performs the procedure are also helpful.

Separation anxiety begins at around 1 year of age and lasts until age 5 or 6. During this phase children become frightened often to the point of panic when separated from their parents. Hence the parent should be supported and encouraged to stay with the child *at all times*. Only when parents are so anxious that they cannot be reassured and their anxiety is adding to that of the patient should they be asked to leave.

Negativism is a trait typical of children between 15 to 18 months and 3 years of age; it is characterized by stubbornness and a tendency to say "no" to everything. It is therefore wise to avoid questions with yes/no answers and approach such patients with a warm, yet firm, quietly confident manner. Children of this age group often are more cooperative for examination maneuvers when their parents are shown the movement first and then ask the child to imitate it.

Fear of loss of body integrity with injury and of loss of emotional control begins during the late preschool years, peaks at age 5 to 6, and then resurfaces during adolescence. Here reassurance that they will be okay and that their injury can be repaired is of great importance. Furthermore, giving them suggestions regarding things they can do to help and praise for doing so are well received. Adolescents need considerable reassurance regarding long-term outcome, as they often anticipate the worst in terms of handicap and disfigurement.

At all ages, most children are distractible. Throughout infancy, sucking is of great import and comfort, whether on a nipple or a pacifier; often, when allowed to suck, the infant is oblivious to the examination unless it is painful. Toddlers and preschoolers love funny noises, stuffed animals, and puppets. Older preschoolers usually can be distracted by stories read or told during procedures. Young school-age children frequently can be engaged in conversation or even fantasy about favorite characters, heroes, and activities [1,2]. If available, videotaped cartoons are powerful distractions.

A few other techniques have proved useful in part as distractors and in part because they make the situation seem less threatening. When possible, the examination is performed with the patient seated on the parent's lap (Fig. 20-1A). The threat of the gloved hand can be lessened by making a balloon out of a rubber glove, drawing a face on it and giving it to the patient to hold while examination proceeds. Letting the child help hold nonthreatening instruments such as lights and tongue blades and making a game of looking in dental mirrors or blowing out examining lights can make the examination seem much less threatening (Fig. 20-1B&C).

School-age and adolescent patients who are not unduly anxious may be amenable to relaxation techniques. These techniques include having the children take slow, deep breaths in and out; having them try to make their arms and legs limp like Raggedy Ann, first gently shaking them; or having them close their eyes and imagine or pretend to be in their favorite place doing their favorite thing. Some children are adept at these exercises, but often in the acute care setting such measures fail; rather, they tend to be more successful for children with chronic problems requiring repetitive procedures where patients are given repeated instruction and practice in these techniques [1,2].

Attending to the concerns and needs of parents is highly important, as the parents are understandably anxious and often struggling with feelings of guilt stemming from their perceived failure (however real or unreal) to prevent the inciting accident. Furthermore, in cases of wounds necessitating the skills of a plastic surgeon, the parents have concerns that their child may be permanently disfigured or handicapped. Here too warmth, empathy, supportive explanations, and reassurance as assessment and treatment proceed are of great help, as parents can serve as invaluable assistants when carefully supported. They can demonstrate movements needed for the examination, having their child follow their lead, and can perform palpation. When confident in and reassured by the physician, they are

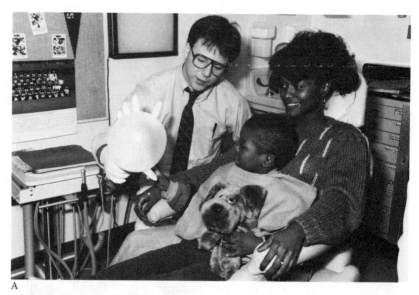

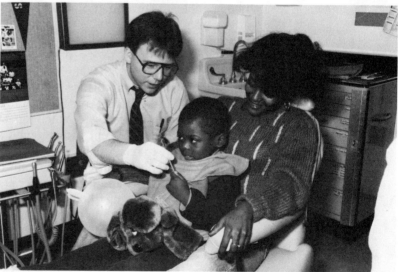

Fig. 20-1. Methods of distraction and anxiety reduction during examination. *A.* The patient is seated on his mother's lap. Having been introduced to a puppet, which he now holds, he is given a rubber glove blown up into a balloon to reduce fear of the gloved hand. *B.* Before starting the intraoral examination the patient is introduced to the dental mirror and is allowed to look at himself in it.

often able to calm the child and maximize his or her cooperation. Enlisting their assistance often reduces parental feelings of helplessness, which further allays anxiety. Finally, during an era in which informed consent is a necessity, one should be careful to explain about risks and possible complications in a manner that does not add to parental anxiety, and it should be done out of earshot of the patient.

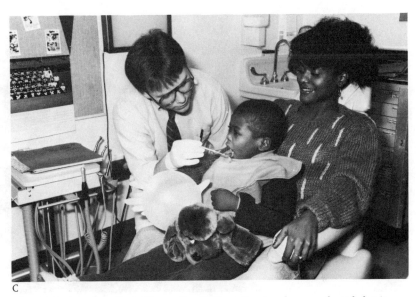

C

Fig. 20-1. (continued) C. The patient's fears having been reduced, he is
now able to cooperate with the examination.

Although attention to the above may take extra time at the outset,
it can save much time and wear and tear on patient, parents, and
personnel in the long run. In many cases it obviates the need for
sedation, especially in older preschoolers and young school-age
children with relatively small wounds.

USE OF RESTRAINT   There are numerous instances in which there is need for physical
restraint when performing plastic surgical procedures in the emer-
gency department setting, for example, the young child with a small
laceration requiring only a few sutures for closure and children who
have other injuries, concurrent bronchospasm, or some underlying
condition that contraindicates use of sedation. Even when sedation
has been administered, restraint is often required during the period
of infiltration of the local anesthetic agent because the depth of
sedation feasible in the emergency department does not ablate pain.

When the period of restraint is likely to be brief and the patient has
not manifested agitation during the examination, restraint is generally best applied in the form of firm holding by an assisting nurse. In
situations necessitating longer periods of restraint, a papoose board
(Fig. 20-2) is often helpful. Although it does not obviate the need for
a restraining nurse, it does reduce the amount of force and strength
required to keep the patient still. The papoose board must be used
with caution, however. Its chest bands make observation of respiratory effort difficult, if not impossible, and probably produce some
decrease in ventilation. Furthermore, the patient is supine and
absolutely flat, creating some element of risk if vomiting should
occur, and at times making it difficult to prevent aspiration of blood

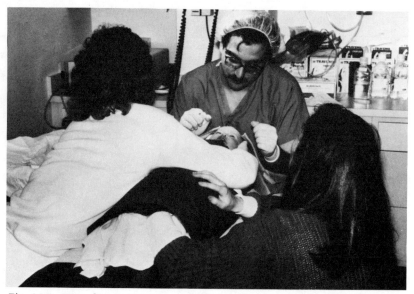

Fig. 20-2. Use of restraint. This toddler has been placed in a papoose device. The assisting nurse is helping to fully immobilize the patient's head. The child's mother remains to provide reassurance and comfort.

and irrigating solutions when large through-and-through oral or cheek lacerations are being repaired. Often when the patient has been sedated, he or she can be released from the papoose after the local anesthetic agent has been administered if the child is given 5 to 10 minutes to relax and become calm.

When restraint is required, the concept should be introduced and the need for helping the child to hold still explained before any effort is made to hold the patient down or strap him or her onto the papoose board. This phase is best done in a gentle, firm manner, using phrasing such as "It's going to be real important for you to keep very still while we fix your cut. The nurse is going to give you a big, long hug to help hold you still," or "To help you hold still, we're going to wrap you up nice and snug in this papoose which sort of gives you a big, long hug."

LOCAL ANESTHESIA
Agents

Most plastic surgical repairs done in the emergency department require use of a local anesthetic. These agents act on neuronal membranes to prevent depolarization, thereby blocking nerve conduction of painful impulses. Procaine, chlorprocaine, and tetracaine are esters of paraaminobenzoic acid, whereas lidocaine, mepivacaine, bupivacaine, and etidocaine are amides. Allergic reactions are uncommon with the esters and exceedingly rare with the amides. Procaine and chlorprocaine are of low potency and act for a short period of time; lidocaine and mepivacaine are of intermediate potency and duration; and tetracaine, bupivacaine, and etidocaine

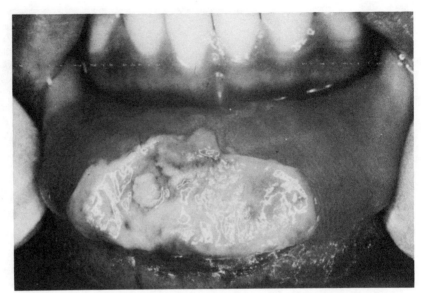

Fig. 20-3. Severe lip ulceration caused by chewing following use of a long-acting local anesthetic. (From B. J. Zitelli and H. W. Davis (eds.), *Atlas of Pediatric Physical Diagnosis.* St. Louis: Gower Medical, 1987. With permission.)

are of high potency and have a long duration of action. Of these agents, lidocaine has gained relative popularity because of the rarity of allergic reactions, its relatively rapid onset of action, and its duration of action of 9- to 200 minutes [3,4]. Longer-acting agents are rarely needed for the types of repair done in the emergency department and can in fact result in complications when used for wounds involving the lips or mouth, because with prolonged anesthesia children often produce significant ulcers by chewing on the anesthetized mucosa (Fig. 20-3).

Technique of Administration

Except for small superficial abrasions, lidocaine must be injected rather than administered topically. Its administration is therefore painful and likely to ablate the cooperation of the young patient. Preparation of the suture tray and drawing up of the local anesthetic agent should be done quietly and out of the child's line of vision to prevent unnecessary fear and anticipation [1]. Use of proper equipment and careful technique can reduce the pain of injection, although it cannot eliminate it. Syringes equipped with thumb rings facilitate control, and use of a long, thin needle (27 gauge, 1.5 inch) minimizes the number of entry sticks (Fig. 20-4).

The skin is stretched taut to facilitate penetration, and the needle is introduced through the wound margin (at the level of the dermis or dermal subcutaneous junction) rather than through intact skin. There is some evidence that use of counterirritation by scratching the skin ahead of the point may reduce pain perception; furthermore, injection of the proximal portion of the wound first may produce

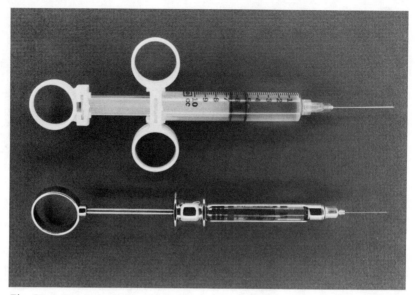

Fig. 20-4. Equipment for enhancing control during administration of local anesthetic. *Top.* Disposable syringe with thumb and finger rings attached to a 27-gauge 1.5-inch needle. *Bottom.* Dental cartridge syringe with thumb ring and a 28-gauge needle.

some blocking effect as the needle is advanced distally. Finally, injecting at a slow rate while gradually moving the needle prevents overdistension of the tissue which, in and of itself, is painful [3]. It must be noted that although slow injection reduces pain it does prolong the period of pain, and this point must be weighed against the patient's ability to tolerate a longer period of injection.

Studies have shown that addition of sodium bicarbonate to lidocaine in a ratio that buffers it to a pH of 7.4 significantly reduces pain on injection [5,6]. It probably stems from the fact that buffering shifts the cation/base ratio of this weak base resulting in better diffusion and more rapid onset of action. One part sodium bicarbonate (1 mEq per milliliter) is added to ten parts lidocaine just before injection, as the addition of base markedly shortens the shelf life of the anesthetic.

Complications

As with any pharmacologic agent, use of local anesthetics carries a risk of toxicity, as a result of either inadvertent intravascular injection or overdose. Initial signs of toxicity stem from action on the central nervous system. Lightheadedness and restlessness often accompanied by perioral parasthesias, diplopia, and tinnitis may progress to twitching, tremors, and seizures. High serum levels produce arrhythmias, circulatory collapse, respiratory depression, and loss of consciousness [3,7]. Intravenous diazepam (0.1–0.3 mg per kilogram) administered at the first sign of toxicity can curb the severity of toxic reactions [1]. Intravascular injections can be avoided by moving the needle as one injects the anesthetic slowly or by frequently aspirating back during the injection.

Overdose is considerably more likely in the small pediatric patient with an extensive wound; therefore the *maximum dosage should always be calculated prior to administration*. The maximum dose is 3 to 5 mg per kilogram, which should be reduced by 20 to 25 percent in infants and toddlers [3]. Injectable lidocaine comes in three concentrations: 0.5% (0.5 mg per milliliter), 1% (10 mg per milliliter), and 2% (20 mg per milliliter). Given the fact that the effect of each concentration is the same and that only duration of action (and not analgesic efficacy) increases with increasing concentrations, the 0.5% and 1% solutions are generally safer to use [3]. Addition of epinephrine reduces bleeding and systemic absorption by producing local vasoconstriction and increases duration of anesthetic action and the maximum dose to 7 mg per kilogram [3,8]. Epinephrine does, however, increase the intensity of pain felt on injection. Because local vasoconstriction produces some degree of ischemia of wound margins, epinephrine can be used only in well vascularized areas (e.g., face, neck, and scalp), and its use is contraindicated for infection-prone wounds (animal bites, dirt-contaminated wounds) and at anatomic sites supplied by end-arteries (fingers, toes, nose, ears, penis) [3,9,10].

Note: Prior to deciding on repair in the emergency department the physician must (1) assess wound size, depth, and extent; (2) estimate the likely amount of lidocaine needed; and (3) compare it with the maximum dose allowable. If the dose required approaches or exceeds the maximum, repair under general anesthesia is advisable. The importance of making and double-checking this calculation cannot be overstressed.

One final point merits emphasis: The physician should wait 5 to 10 minutes after administration of the local anesthetic to give the agent time to take effect and then check its efficacy by testing the patient's response to pinprick. This wait also gives the pediatric patient time to calm down; and the use of stories, puppets, videotapes, or conversation during this period may help reduce fear such that good cooperation is achieved.

Jet Injector

Because injections, no matter how skillfully performed, are to some extent painful, and because so many children have needle phobias, a number of alternative devices and agents have been developed, one of them being the jet injector (Fig. 20-5). This apparatus is a spring-loaded piston device that can deliver a 0.5 to 2.0 ml of local anesthetic with a pressure of 2000 psi, penetrating to a depth of up to 1.5 cm [1,3]. The injector is relatively expensive, and some models produce a loud noise that can be frightening. Administration does cause a brief stinging sensation. Use of an injector frequently produces bruises, and if not held steady, at the appropriate angle, or with the proper amount of light pressure, can even cause lacerations [3]. Given the problem of the moving pediatric target, we have found it of limited usefulness.

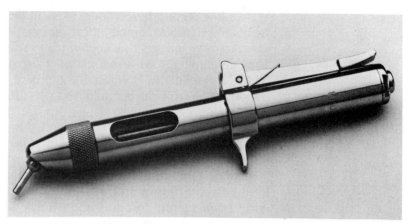

Fig. 20-5. Jet injector. (Courtesy of Mada Equipment Co., Inc.)

**TOPICAL
ANESTHESIA**

Because topical administration of local anesthetic agents avoids the pain of injection, there has been considerable interest in their use in pediatrics. Being well absorbed from mucous membranes, they are widely used to anesthetize the cornea for ophthalmologic evaluation, nasal mucosa for otolaryngologic procedures, and oral mucosa in dentistry prior to injection of local anesthetic agents (Table 20-1). All such agents approved for mucosal application are of low concentration to reduce risk of toxicity, the only exception being benzocaine, which is poorly soluble in water and thus slowly absorbed [3].

Unfortunately, topical agents have a number of limitations in managing nonmucosal wounds. Most diffuse poorly into the wound margins of lacerations; hence anesthesia is usually incomplete. When applied to extensive areas of abraded or burned skin, significant systemic absorption can occur resulting in seizures, respiratory arrest, and even cardiovascular collapse. Hence these agents should be used with caution when managing such wounds, and the dose must be carefully calculated to ensure that it does not approach or exceed the maximum (Table 20-1) [3,11–13].

TAC

A relatively new agent, TAC, has shown promise of efficacy in clinical trials when applied to selected wounds. TAC is a solution consisting of tetracaine (0.5%), epinephrine (adrenaline, 1:2000), and cocaine (11.8%) in normal saline. The tetracaine and cocaine act as local anesthetics, and the vasoconstrictor activity of the cocaine and epinephrine combine to concentrate the anesthesia at the wound site, reducing systemic absorption. Studies have demonstrated complete anesthesia in 80 percent of patients with facial or scalp lacerations, which compares favorably with the results obtained with injected lidocaine [3,14,15]. Efficacy is considerably lower when TAC is applied to less well vascularized areas. Its use has been favorably accepted by patients, especially the toddler, preschool, and early school age populations.

TAC is applied in the following manner. A few drops are placed in

Table 20-1. Topical anesthetics

Site of application	Agent	
	Generic name	Proprietary name
Cornea	Proparacaine 0.5%	Alcaine, Ophthaine
	Tetracaine 0.5%	Pontocaine
Nasal mucosa	Benzalkonium chloride 0.5%/cetyl dimethyl ethyl ammonium bromide 0.005%	Cetacaine 0.5% spray
	Cocaine 2%	Hurricaine
	Benzocaine spray 20%	
Oral mucosa	Benzocaine gel 20%	Hurricaine
	Ethyl aminobenzoate	Topex
	Viscous lidocaine 2%	
Abraded skin	Lidocaine solution 4%	Xylocaine
	Lidocaine ointment 2%	Xylocaine
Lacerated skin	Tetracaine 0.5%/ epinephrine 1:2000/ cocaine 11.8% in normal saline	TAC

the wound, and then approximately 1 ml per centimeter of laceration is dripped onto a 2 × 2 inch gauze pad or a cotton ball, which is pressed over the laceration by one of the parents for 10 to 15 minutes (Fig. 20-6). The parent should wear a rubber glove as some absorption can occur through intact skin. When the gauze is removed, blanching should be seen along the wound margins (Fig. 20-7). If the latter is incomplete, an extra 0.25 ml per centimeter can be applied for another 5 to 10 minutes.

Although its efficacy is good, TAC does have limited application. Because of its intense vasoconstrictor activity, it cannot be used on areas with terminal arterial circulation (e.g., fingers, toes, ears, nose, and penis). Furthermore, its use is inadvisable for infection-prone wounds (e.g., lacerations from animal bites, those contaminated by dirt, or those with devitalized wound edges), as the ischemia it produces increases the risk of infection [16]. Its use is thus probably best restricted to clean lacerations of the face, scalp, and neck where the rich blood supply counteracts the risk of wound margin ischemia.

Care must also be taken to prevent toxicity, which can manifest as tense wide-eyed staring, euphoria, restlessness and irritability, seizures, hypertension, tachyarrhythmias, and even death [3,14,15,17,18]. Although some institutions use up to 5 to 10 ml, we have tried to limit dosage to 3 to 5 ml, as higher doses have resulted in toxicity. Significant systemic absorption can occur and cause severe reactions if the drug is applied to mucous membranes, abrasions, or burns.

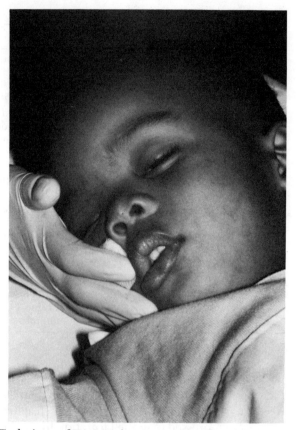

Fig. 20-6. Technique of TAC application. A few drops of TAC have been dripped into the wound and the rest onto a 2 × 2 inch gauze pad, which is pressed over the laceration by the child's parent.

Hence its use is contraindicated for lesions of these types. Even when applied to nonmucosal lacerations, the patient must be positioned so as to eliminate the possibility of any of the solution trickling into the eye, ear, or mouth. Finally, application of TAC necessitates that the child sit or lie relatively still for 10 to 15 minutes, and some toddlers find this state intolerable despite attempts at distraction.

REGIONAL BLOCK ANESTHESIA

Although a complete discussion of regional block anesthesia is beyond the scope of this chapter, a few comments are in order. Administration of regional blocks can be less painful than local injections, especially for wounds involving the palm of the hand and large lip lacerations. Local tissue distension and distortion at the wound site, further tissue trauma, and possible local tissue toxicity are avoided as well. However, their use necessitates a clear knowledge of anatomy and skilled technique, which requires considerable practice. The patient must be placed in a comfortable position such that landmarks are readily visible. The dose should be calculated

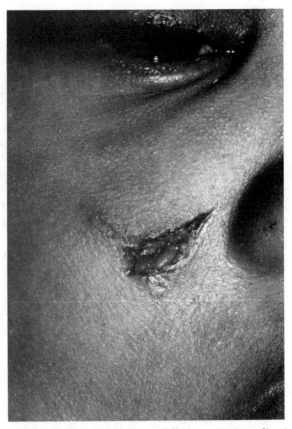

Fig. 20-7. Blanching of wound margins following TAC application is best seen along the inferior wound edge.

prior to the procedure and compared with the maximum allowable, given the patient's weight. The solution is then warmed to body temperature, and a small wheal is raised in the overlying skin. After this step the operator waits a few minutes to ensue its effect. The needle is then advanced while the anesthetic is slowly injected with frequent aspiration, avoiding undue movement of the needle and trying to elicit parasthesias as the needle is advanced [1, 3, 19–21]. Although feasible in school-age children and adolescents, identifying the presence of parasthesias and minimizing movement of the needle can be impossible in younger children. Complications include inadequate anesthesia, overdosage, or intravascular injection with resultant toxicity, as well as intraneural injection, which can result in persistent paresthesias [3, 19–21].

SEDATION

Use of sedation when handling selected pediatric plastic surgical cases in the emergency department has a number of advantages. It can reduce anxiety and pain for the patients, making the experience considerably less frightening for them and their families. Subsequent follow-up for suture removal is then faced with much less apprehension, as are any future visits to the emergency department or doctor's office. Long-term problems with nightmares and adverse behavioral side effects are often prevented as well [22]. Good pain and anxiety control can enable the patient to cooperate more fully with the plastic surgeon for the examination; and having a calm, quiet patient makes planning and approaching repair immeasurably easier. It often substantially reduces the time required for actual wound closure, and quality of repair is enhanced when the patient is quiet and the field thereby motionless.

Thus in many cases use of sedation has advantages that far outweigh the risks. To ensure optimal or proper use, one must be aware of the indications for sedation and of the various agents available: their properties, onset and duration of action, and potential complications. Furthermore, the emergency department must have the staff and equipment necessary, not only for administration of the sedative selected but also for monitoring the patient and for handling potential complications.

Two major levels of sedation — "conscious" and deep [23] — are described in the literature; the former term is somewhat misleading, however, in that optimal sedation, of necessity, results in some degree of alteration in level of consciousness. As the same agents are used to produce both levels, they differ primarily in dosage used and the degree of the resulting depressed level of consciousness. Somewhat more recently, the use of dissociative sedation has received attention and gained advocates for use in the emergency setting [24].

Conscious sedation is defined by the American Academy of Pediatrics as producing "a minimally depressed level of consciousness that retains the patient's ability to maintain a patent airway independently and continuously (e.g., protective reflexes remain intact), and respond appropriately to physical stimulation and/or verbal command. . . . The drugs and techniques used should carry a margin of safety wide enough to render unintended loss of consciousness unlikely" [23]. Vital signs are not altered, although physical stress is reduced. Anxiety is relieved, and pain is reduced but not ablated. In fact, attempts to ablate pain result in deep sedation or even general anesthesia [24].

Deep sedation is defined as "a controlled state of unconsciousness from which the patient is not easily aroused, which may be accompanied by partial or complete loss of protective reflexes, including the ability to maintain a patent airway independently and respond purposely to physical stimulation or verbal command" [23]. Pain is nearly ablated — but at the expense of loss of protective reflexes.

As noted above, many of the regimens used can produce either level of sedation, depending on the dose administered. Regardless of level, cardiorespiratory monitoring and continuous pulse oximetry should be standard. Furthermore, oxygen and airway equipment must be readily available (Fig. 20-8). In fact, delivery of supplemen-

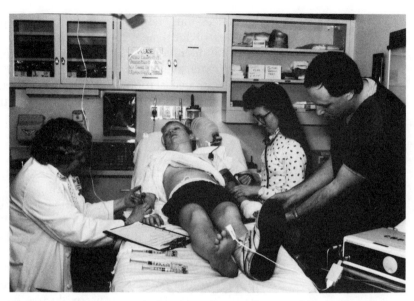

Fig. 20-8. Monitoring and airway equipment for conscious intravenous sedation. The patient lies supine on the stretcher with the head slightly elevated. A rolled towel has been placed under his neck to facilitate airway patency, and he is receiving low-flow oxygen via nasal prongs. His chest has been exposed to facilitate observation of respiratory effort. The patient is being monitored with a cardiorespiratory monitor and a pulse oximeter. The appropriate-size bag and mask are attached to the oxygen outlet and are ready for use. Naloxone has been drawn up and is readily available if needed.

tal oxygen during the period of sedation is probably advisable to prevent hypoxia 2,25]. Both levels require a second physician or an anesthetist familiar with sedative agents, skilled in their administration, and fully capable of airway maintenance and of handling adverse effects. Deep sedation requires yet a third person to assist.

Dissociative sedation is touted as retaining the benefits of consciousness while providing profound analgesia. The patient enters a trance-like state characterized by mind-body separation, dreaming, and some degree of catalepsy, yet remains responsive and obedient to verbal command with intact protective reflexes. Amnesia is also characteristic [24]. Achievement of a dissociative state, in contrast to general anesthesia, is dose-dependent, however, and not totally predictable [26].

Note: For reasons of safety and practicality, "conscious sedation" is the only acceptable level in the emergency department setting.

Patient Selection

Children with small wounds requiring only a few sutures for closure generally should not be considered for sedation. Likewise, children who are receptive to verbal reassurance and able to be calm for examination are unlikely to require sedation. Conversely, patients with extensive and complex or large, heavily contaminated wounds that necessitate lengthy irrigation and repair or in which large volumes of local anesthesia are needed should be considered for closure under general anesthesia. The same pertains to children having extensive abrasions with embedded dirt or tar that necessitates prolonged scrubbing. Conscious sedation is not adequate in these cases because it does not ablate pain; thus when it is relied on for such extensive wounds, the patient experiences protracted and unnecessary suffering.

Sedative Agents

As noted above, the goal of conscious sedation is to reduce anxiety and minimize the pain endured during a procedure, thereby making the experience less traumatic for the patient, enhancing cooperation, and facilitating the task of surgical repair. A wide variety of agents have been used for this purpose, either singly or in combination. Narcotic analgesics have been mainstays for pain control, and benzodiazepines, barbiturates, phenothiazines, antihistamines, and chloral hydrate have seen application as sedatives because of their anxiolytic properties. Nitrous oxide has dual effects, whereas ketamine acts primarily as a dissociative agent. Before discussing specific regimens, a brief discussion of the properties of these agents is warranted, as they become important in selection of the best method of sedation for the individual patient.

Narcotic Analgesics

The narcotics or opiates are a group of drugs structurally related to morphine sulfate. Their major action is to provide potent analgesia. Of these agents, *morphine,* a naturally occurring opium alkaloid, and two synthetic agents, *meperidine* (Demerol) and *fentanyl* (Sublimaze), have seen the widest application in producing sedation. When administered intravenously, fentanyl has a rapid onset (3–5 minutes) and short duration of action (20–60 minutes), and meperidine has a delayed onset (15–20 minutes) with a relatively long duration of action (2–4 hours); morphine is intermediate (onset in approximately 7–10 minutes and duration of 30 minutes to 4 hours). In therapeutic (pain-relieving) doses, these agents can produce excellent analgesia, which tends to be accompanied by a mild degree of euphoria without oversedation. They also have the advantage of being readily reversible by *naloxone* (Narcan) [27–29].

The therapeutic dose varies up to tenfold among patients and is not related to age, sex, weight, or surface area; thus the standard dosage range cited in textbooks is inadequate for some patients and excessive for others [30–32]. Furthermore, these agents have steep dose response curves such that at a given serum level a small increment in dose can make the difference between severe pain and little or no pain [30,33]. Hence dosage should be titrated to the individual patient needs if pain control is to be optimized without oversedation, which necessitates intravenous administration [2,26, 27,34,35]. Although narcotic analgesics are available in preparations for intramuscular injection, this route makes titration impossible, and absorption is highly variable, making over- or undersedation likely.

Complications

Potential adverse side effects of these agents must be considered before their use [2,26–29,34,35]. All three can produce respiratory depression with resultant CO_2 retention, which results in cerebral vasodilation and increased intracranial pressure, contraindicating their use in patients with any possibility of increased intracranial pressure. Respiratory depression is dose-related; its risk is minimized with careful intravenous titration, and it is reversible with naloxone. Respiratory depression is more likely to occur in patients who have recently ingested alcohol or depressant medications and in those with underlying pulmonary disease (asthma, bronchopulmonary dysplasia, pneumonitis). Hence these situations are also relative contraindications. As effective analgesia is produced by doses lower than those required to achieve good sedation, and as the latter are more likely to cause respiratory depression, the opiates are rarely used alone for sedation [2].

Morphine and meperidine can cause histamine release, resulting in urticaria at the injection site (not a true allergic reaction), bronchoconstriction, and vasodilation. These effects can pose significant problems for patients currently having bronchospasm, those with uncorrected hypovolemia, and those with severe cardiac disease. Nausea and vomiting are seen in some patients, although this side effect is reduced by recumbency. Meperidine can produce prolonged and unsettling excitatory central nervous system side effects in a small percentage of patients, consisting of nervousness, agitation, disorientation, hallucinations, tremors, and even seizures.

Fentanyl does not cause histamine release and thus has fewer adverse cardiovascular effects. Although respiratory depression does occur with use of fentanyl in sedative doses (most commonly within 5 minutes of injection), *slow administration and careful titration usually prevent it;* and in *most* cases, patients respond to stimulation and the command to take deep breaths and so do not require assisted ventilation or naloxone, although a small percentage have required ventilatory support and reversal [36]. Delayed respiratory depression can also occur [37]. Fentanyl has another disadvantage in that it typically causes intense facial pruritus with an irresistible urge to scratch, which can interfere with repair of facial lacerations. We have also seen paradoxical excitation in toddlers following fentanyl administration. When given in high doses (much higher than those recommended for sedation), fentanyl can cause severe muscular rigidity, making respiratory support and ventilation difficult if not impossible. This phenomenon is also reversible by naloxone.

Benzodiazepines

The benzodiazepines have good anxiolytic and sedative properties and the added benefits of producing mild muscle relaxation and partial, sometimes total, amnesia [2,38,39]. Benzodiazepines do not have analgesic properties; rather, they blunt the reaction to pain.

Diazepam

Diazepam (Valium), the member used most often, can be administered orally (although onset of effect is slow and difficult to predict [26]) or intravenously. Intramuscular injection is prohibitively painful, and absorption by this route is erratic. Intravenous infusion is also somewhat painful, although less so, and onset of action begins within 1 to 2 minutes [2,26].

Midazolam

Midazolam (Versed) is the newest of these agents to be used for conscious sedation. More water-soluble than diazepam, it can be given intramuscularly as well as intravenously. Intranasal administration is also showing great promise [2,40–43]. Although possessed of a much shorter half-life than diazepam, because of its water solubility, it takes twice as long to achieve clinical effect; thus great patience and care must be exercised during intravenous titration to prevent overdosage. Rate of recovery is similar for both following intravenous use, being 30 to 60 minutes [44].

Note: Experience with use of midazolam in children is thus far limited and still investigational in many institutions; dosage guidelines and safety are not yet clearly established.

Complications

The major adverse side effects of the benzodiazepines are central nervous system depression, respiratory depression, and occasionally a mild decrease in blood pressure [38,39,45]. Paradoxically, increased anxiety has been reported with midazolam [46]. There is some evidence that benzodiazepines may decrease cerebral blood flow and oxygen metabolism; hence they should be used with caution following head injury. They also have the disadvantage of their effects not being reversible, although an antagonist (flumazenil) has been developed and is currently undergoing testing [47].

Barbiturates

The barbiturates are sedative/hypnotic agents that cause drowsiness without significant respiratory or cardiovascular depression when administered in sedative doses rather than hypnotic doses. They offer flexibility in that they can be administered by intravenous, intramuscular, oral, or rectal routes. Like the benzodiazepines, they have no analgesic properties; and in fact they appear to have antianalgesic effects that result in restlessness and excitement when given to patients in pain. Thus although they can be used alone as sedative agents for noninvasive, nonpainful procedures, they are usually administered in combination with opiates when used in preparation for painful procedures [2,38].

Pentobarbital
Pentobarbital (Nembutal) and *secobarbital* (Seconal), which have a short to intermediate duration of action, and *thiopental* (Pentothal), with a short duration of action, are the agents most frequently used.

Complications
The barbiturates cause histamine release, which can prompt a fall in blood pressure in hypovolemic patients. Respiratory depression and arrest can occur when sedative doses are exceeded. Pentobarbital and secobarbital can have prolonged sedative effects lasting several hours in some patients. These agents can also produce a hangover consisting of mood alteration along with impaired judgment and fine motor skills that lasts for up to 24 to 48 hours [2,26,38].

Phenothiazines

Of the phenothiazines, *promethazine* (Phenergan) and *chlorpromazine* (Thorazine) have seen widest use because of their sedative properties and antiemetic effects, and because they were once thought to potentiate narcotic analgesia. More recent work has revealed that they actually have antianalgesic properties, and even their antiemetic effects when used for sedation have been called into question. Extrapyramidal reactions (although relatively infrequent) — dystonia and oculogyric crisis — and hypotension are the major adverse side effects of these agents [1,27,48–54].

Antihistamines

Hydroxyzine
Hydroxyzine (Vistaril) is the antihistamine used most often for sedation, typically in combination with a narcotic analgesic. In addition to its sedative properties, it has mild analgesic, anxiolytic, antipruritic, and antiemetic effects. It has been demonstrated to augment the analgesic effects of the opiates. Its major drawback is the fact that it can be administered only intramuscularly or orally [1,27,52,55–57].

Chloral Compounds

Chloral Hydrate
Chloral hydrate is commonly used as a central nervous system depressant and hypnotic agent because it has little effect on respiration and blood pressure in therapeutic doses. When administered orally, it must be diluted with a sweet-tasting liquid to reduce gastric irritation and disguise its unpleasant taste. It can, however, be given rectally. Having little analgesic effect, chloral hydrate does not reduce the pain of infiltration of local anesthetic; in fact, patients often awaken and become agitated or delirious when subjected to pain, thereafter proving difficult to console. Hence its major application as a sedative is for nonpainful procedures that require the child to remain quiet (e.g., computed tomography, magnetic resonance imaging, electroencephalography). Its use prior to plastic surgical repair should be discouraged. Other potential adverse effects include

lightheadedness, ataxia, dysphoria, nightmares, and subsequent hangover. Once administered, its effects are not reversible [2,38].

Ketamine

Ketamine is a derivative of phencyclidine that produces a trance-like or dissociative state characterized by pronounced sedation, excellent analgesia, and generally total amnesia. Its onset of action is rapid, and it does not depress cardiorespiratory function; rather, it increases heart rate, blood pressure, and pulmonary artery pressure. Purported not to interfere with protective airway reflexes, it induces marked hypersalivation and increased tracheobronchial secretions, which appear to have contributed to a number of cases of aspiration, even when administered in combination with atropine. It also has been reported to cause laryngospasm in a small proportion of pediatric patients. Ketamine causes increased muscle tone often accompanied by random movements, necessitating restraint [2,24,58–61].

Because ketamine causes cerebral vasodilation, its use is contraindicated in patients suspected of having increased intracranial pressure. Finally, recovery may be prolonged and can be accompanied by vomiting, nightmares, and periods of agitation unless audiovisual stimuli are strictly reduced (a feat often impossible in busy emergency departments). Ataxia and unsteadiness may persist for hours, and older patients have reported flashbacks, hallucinations, and bizarre dreams for weeks after the procedure. Concurrent administration of a benzodiazepine appears to reduce some of the unpleasant psychic emergence phenomena that otherwise can occur in up to 30 percent of patients [2,24,58–61].

Nitrous Oxide

Nitrous oxide, an inhalational agent, has strong sedative and anxiolytic effects and mild analgesic properties. It also has little effect on cardiorespiratory function. It must be administered mixed with oxygen to prevent hypoxia. Onset of action is noted within 3 to 5 minutes, and recovery is nearly as rapid once the source is removed. There is a fair degree of variability in response to the agent, with 10 percent or more of patients failing to derive benefit. Nitrous oxide requires special equipment for administration and special skill and training for the person delivering it (see Selection and Administration of Sedative Regimens below). Its disadvantages include nausea and vomiting (seen in 10–15 percent of patients), diffusional hypoxia, and expansion of gas-filled pockets, which contraindicates its use in patients with pulmonary disease, head injury, pneumothorax, possible intestinal obstruction, and even middle-ear effusions. Patients who have incurred significant facial injuries are likely to find the mask uncomfortable and may be at risk for expansion of intracranial air pockets. Use should also be avoided in patients with any depression of level of consciousness and in those known to have had or who are suspected of taking other depressant medications or alcoholic beverages. Younger pediatric patients may fear the mask or be unable to understand how to use the nosepiece [1,2,62–67].

SELECTION AND ADMINISTRATION OF SEDATIVE REGIMENS

Having discussed the salient properties of the more commonly used pharmacologic agents, we now address selection of regimen and describe techniques of administration. As noted earlier, the duration and complexity of the repair and the amount of pain likely to be incurred during infiltration of the local anesthetic must be considered when selecting a regimen. Associated or underlying conditions and prior ingestion or administration of medications may contraindicate use of some agents. The time and amount of last oral intake and the likelihood of vomiting also must be considered.

The facilities and personnel (and their availability, level of training, and expertise) in the emergency department are of prime importance in selecting a sedative regimen. All sedated patients require continuous monitoring with a cardiorespiratory monitor and must have a nurse or physician either in constant attendance or close by. Patients on regimens known to cause respiratory depression should also be monitored with continuous pulse oximetry and probably should be given low flow oxygen to reduce the risk of hypoxia [2,25]. Intravenous sedation necessitates the presence of a second physician or an anesthetist to titrate the medication and to monitor the level of sedation and effectiveness of respiration. Oxygen and a bag valve mask setup should be readily accessible in case respiration has to be supported, and personnel must be skilled in airway maintenance and respiratory support. Failure to heed these precautions can result in disaster.

When discussing regimens, it must be noted that although a large literature exists on the use of various methods of sedation in children, most of it is descriptive and anecdotal. There is little in the way of well controlled studies comparing safety and efficacy of regimens, and many dosage recommendations are empiric. Having made this point, we can now discuss individual regimens that we have categorized according to route of administration (Table 20-2).

Orally, Rectally, and Nasally Administered Agents

Although oral and rectal routes have the advantage of ease of administration and of being painless, as a rule agents given by these routes do not produce adequate sedation for surgical procedures. Hence their use should be limited to nonpainful, nonstimulating procedures; nevertheless, they can prove useful on occasion for older children with mild anxiety. Further disadvantages include the fact that pediatric patients may object to the taste of the medication and often find rectal administration unpleasant. There is also the problem of retention: Defecation can occur following rectal administration, and vomiting is always a possibility with use of oral agents. Onset of peak action is slower and less predictable than that of parenterally administered agents; and if the initial dose proves inadequate, significant delays can occur while personnel wait for a supplemental dose to take effect [2]. The intranasal route obviates problems of retention and shows significant promise for agents such as midazolam, which can be administered in small volumes and are rapidly absorbed through mucosal surfaces [42].

Table 20-2. Sedative regimens

Agent/regimen	Dose	Onset of peak effect (minutes)	Duration of action	Advantages	Disadvantages
Oral/rectal/nasal route					
Chloral hydrate	50–100 mg/kg (max. 1–3 g)	30–60	4–8 hr	Ease of administration; Little or no cardiorespiratory depression	No analgesic effect; Agitation when subjected to pain; GI irritant; Unpleasant taste
Diazepam	2–5 mg (max. 10 mg)	30–40 (unpredictable)	Unpredictable	Ease of administration; Anxiety reduction	No analgesic effect; Unpredictable onset and duration of action
Midazolam[a]	0.50–0.75 mg/kg PO	15–30	≈1 hr	Ease of administration; Anxiety reduction	No analgesic effect
	0.2–0.3 mg/kg IN	10–15	≈1 hr	Rapid onset; Brief duration	
Thiopental	25–45 mg/kg PR	10–15	30–45 min	Ease of administration; Rapid onset; Brief duration	No analgesic effect; Antianalgesic effect
Intramuscular route					
DPT	Meperidine 1–2 mg/kg (max. 50–75 mg); Promethazine 0.5–1.0 mg/kg (max. 25 mg); Chlorpromazine 0.5–1.0 mg/kg (max. 25 mg)	30–45	30 min–12 hr	Ease of administration; Strong sedative effect; Good analgesia	Respiratory depression; Histamine release; Potential for paradoxical agitation; Nausea and vomiting; Dystonic reactions; Frequent need for prolonged observation
Demerol/Vistaril	Meperidine 1.0–1.5 mg/kg (max. 50–75 mg)	30–40	1–2 hr (occasionally longer)	Ease of administration; Moderate sedative and analgesic effects	Often inadequate; Respiratory release; Histamine release
	Hydroxyzine 0.25–1.00 mg/kg (max. 50–75 mg)	10–20			
Midazolam[a]	0.1–0.2 mg/kg (max. 5 mg)	10–20	30–60 min	Ease of administration; Amnesia; Anxiety reduction	No analgesic effect; Relatively short-acting

	Dose	Onset (min)	Duration	Advantages	Disadvantages
Demerol/Versed[a]	Meperidine 1.5 mg/kg (max. 75 mg) Midazolam 0.1 mg/kg (max. 5 mg)	20	1–2 hr	Ease of administration Good analgesia Amnesia Anxiety reduction	Respiratory depression Histamine release
Ketamine	Ketamine 0.5–4.0 mg/kg with atropine 0.01 mg/kg	5–10	15–20 min of full sedation 1–6 hr for full recovery	Ease of administration Rapid onset Strong analgesia Amnesia Little or no cardiorespiratory depression	Hypersalivation and increased tracheobronchial secretions Aspiration Laryngospasm Random movements Agitation during recovery Nightmares, hallucinations
Inhalation Nitrous oxide	50:50 N_2O/O_2	3–5	10 min after source removed	Rapid onset Strong sedative Little or no cardiorespiratory depression Rapid recovery	Only mild analgesia Requires special equipment Special skill and training Nausea and vomiting Diffusional hypoxia Young children may have fear of mask, difficulty understanding use of nosepiece
Intravenous route Morphine	Titrated beginning with 0.1 mg/kg bolus, then add 0.05 mg/kg q 6 min as needed up to max. of 15–20 mg	~5–10	30 min–4 hr	Excellent analgesia	Only mildly sedating Respiratory depression Nausea and vomiting Histamine release
Fentanyl	Titrated beginning with 1 μg/kg bolus then add 1 μg/kg q 3 min as needed up to max. of 5 μg/kg	3 min	20–60 min	Excellent analgesia Rapid onset of action Short recovery period No histamine release Minimal cardiovascular effect	Only mildly sedating Respiratory depression Occasional paradoxical agitation Facial pruritus

Table 20-2. (continued)

Agent/Regimen	Dose	Onset of peak effect	Duration of Action	Advantages	Disadvantages
Diazepam	Titrated beginning with 1 mg/kg bolus, then add 1 mg/kg q 3–5 min as needed up to max. of 5 mg/kg	3–5	30–90	Anxiety reduction Amnesia	No analgesic effect Respiratory depression
Midazolam[b]	Titrated beginning with 0.1 mg/kg bolus, then add 0.1 mg/kg q 5 min as needed up to max. of 3 mg/kg or 5 mg total	5	15–60 min	Rapid onset of action Anxiety reduction Amnesia Rapid recovery	No analgesic effect
Morphine/diazepam	Morphine titrate 0.1–0.3 mg/kg, then diazepam titrate 1–5 mg/kg	10–20	1–3 hr	Good sedation Good analgesia Anxiety reduction Amnesia	Respiratory depression Histamine release
Fentanyl/diazepam	Fentanyl titrate 1–5 μg/kg, then diazepam titrate 1–5 mg/kg	10–20	20–60 min	Rapid onset Good sedation Good analgesia Anxiety reduction Amnesia Brief recovery	Respiratory depression Facial pruritus
Fentanyl/midazolam[b]	Fentanyl titrate 1–5 μg/kg, then midazolam titrate 0.1–0.3 mg/kg	5–15	20–60 min	Same	Same

[a]Optimal dosage and safety still under investigation.
[b]Optimal dosage, safety, and time interval between doses still under investigation.

Chloral Hydrate
As noted earlier, chloral hydrate is a hypnotic agent that produces only light sedation. Having little analgesic efficacy, it has the distinct disadvantage of producing agitation when children sedated with it are subject to the pain of infiltration of a local anesthetic. Thus although potentially useful for radiographic procedures required for planning definitive repair, its use in preparation for the actual surgical procedure should be discouraged. Although dosage recommendations range from 25 to 100 mg per kilogram to a maximum of 1 to 3 grams, in practice, doses toward the upper end of this spectrum are required to achieve sedation, whether administered orally or rectally. Onset of sedation usually occurs within 30 to 60 minutes. If no effect is seen within that time, an additional 25 to 50 mg per kilogram may be given. Duration of action ranges from 4 to 8 hours [2,26,38].

Benzodiazepines
When given orally or rectally, diazepam is rapidly absorbed and has mild sedative and anxiolytic effects. The suggested dose is 2 to 5 mg. Onset of action is not predictable, although some effect is usually seen within 30 to 40 minutes. Duration of action is also unpredictable; some residual sedative effect can be seen for 24 hours or longer. Administration by these routes in the emergency setting is perhaps best reserved for the anxious older child or adolescent with a relatively small, nonpainful wound who requires a relatively brief injection of local anesthesia or for whom TAC is applicable [1,2,26,38,39]. Midazolam, which can be given orally or nasally, is a promising new agent currently under study. With rapid onset of action (10–15 minutes following intranasal use) and short duration of effect (1 hour), it has the potential for being a useful pediatric sedative agent for the future. *Note:* It must be emphasized that at this time the optimal dosage of midazolam has not been clearly established, although in studies on preoperative patients oral doses of 0.50 to 0.75 mg per kilogram have been found to produce sedation within 15 to 30 minutes [68,69] and intranasal doses of 0.2 to 0.3 mg per kilogram in 10 to 15 minutes [42].

Barbiturates
Although oral administration of barbiturates is probably impractical in the emergency department setting (because of delay in onset and prolonged duration of action), success has been reported with use of rectal thiopental as a preoperative medication and as a sedative prior to nonpainful procedures. Hence it may prove useful for selected children in whom anxiety reduction (rather than analgesia) is the major need. When given rectally, absorption is slowed and duration of sedation prolonged in contrast to its ultrashort-acting effects when given intravenously. Dosage is 25 to 45 mg per kilogram. Onset of peak effect occurs within 10 to 15 minutes, and duration is in the range of 30 to 45 minutes. Respiratory depression is a possibility at higher doses [70,71].

Intramuscularly Administered Regimens

The intramuscular route has the advantage of taking little time for administration and of not requiring intravenous access (unless there is a complication). The injection is painful and typically upsetting to the patient for however brief a period. More importantly, absorption is variable, and there is usually some delay in onset of maximal sedative effect. Furthermore, as dose requirements of individual patients vary widely for many of the agents, especially the narcotics, the standard dose, although effective in most patients, proves inadequate for some and excessive for others.

Demerol/Phenergan/Thorazine
The combination of meperidine, promethazine, and chlorpromazine (DPT; also termed the "lytic cocktail") was initially formulated for sedating children who were to undergo cardiac catheterization and has since been widely used for a variety of procedures for many years [1,2,26,72,73]. Promethazine and chlorpromazine were thought to potentiate the analgesic and sedative effects of the meperidine, and both had the added advantage of having antiemetic properties. Whereas the sedative effect of meperidine is greatly intensified by the phenothiazines, there is now evidence that the assumption regarding analgesic potentiation was wrong [49–54]. Furthermore, phenothiazines increase the degree and duration of respiratory depression produced by meperidine and augment its hypotensive effects as well. Respiratory depression is a particular risk in patients with altered mental status and in those with chronic neurologic disorders [72]. Hence concern has arisen that use of this combination increases risk to the patient and subjects him or her to the possibility of all the other side effects of phenothiazines, including dystonic reactions. Nevertheless, the potent sedative properties of DPT, its ease of administration, and familiarity continue to perpetuate its use [1,2,26,72,73].

The recommended dosage range of meperidine is 1 to 2 mg per kilogram, and of promethazine and chlorpromazine 0.5 to 1.0 mg per kilogram each, up to a maximum of 75, 25, and 25 mg, respectively. In our experience, the higher end of the dosage range is required for plastic surgical procedures. Otherwise, up to 30 percent of patients prove to be inadequately sedated, requiring a supplemental injection and further delay. Onset of peak effect occurs within 30 to 45 minutes, and duration of sedation ranges from 15 minutes to 12 hours. The potential for prolonged duration of action can necessitate a lengthy period of monitoring and observation well beyond that required for the procedure [2,26,72,73].

Given the potential for depression of respirations and protective reflexes and for causing hypotension, continuous cardiorespiratory monitoring and pulse oximetry are mandatory. Naloxone and equipment for oxygen delivery, establishing a secure airway, and assisting ventilation must be set up and immediately available if needed (a likelihood in about 1–3 percent of cases). Because of likely impairment of protective airway reflexes combined with some increased risk of vomiting due to delayed gastric emptying, this regimen should be avoided in patients who have recently eaten. Personnel must also be prepared to contend with a disturbing paradoxical reaction consisting of restlessness, delirium, agitation, and screaming, seen in 3 percent or more of patients. This situation often prevents performance of the procedure and can persist for hours. Only a quiet environment with minimal stimulation appears to help ameliorate this reaction.

Despite the ease and inexpensiveness of its use, the unpredictable variation in onset, duration, and depth of sedation and its numerous potential complications increasingly seem to outweigh its benefits. As research and experience increase, it is likely to be replaced by newer regimens.

Meperidine and Hydroxyzine
The combination of meperidine (Demerol) with hydroxyzine (Vistaril) has the advantage of some potentiation of analgesic and sedative effects. Furthermore, hydroxyzine has anxiolytic, anti-emetic, and antipruritic actions that can potentially counteract adverse side effects of meperidine. The intramuscular route is necessary because intravenous administration of hydroxyzine is fraught with complications. The meperidine dose is 1 to 2 mg per kilogram (maximum 50–100 mg) and of hydroxyzine 0.25 to 1.00 mg per kilogram (maximum 50–75 mg). Peak sedation occurs within 30 to 40 minutes and lasts 1 to 2 hours. This combination provides improved pain relief and sedation over use of meperidine alone and is somewhat less likely to produce respiratory depression and hypotension than DPT; however, oversedation occurs on occasion. More commonly in our experience, sedation is inadequate (especially with lower doses), unless the period of pain and duration of the procedure are relatively brief. Furthermore, because of the potential side effects of meperidine, monitoring is required as for DPT, though generally for a much briefer period of time [1,27, 52,55–57,74–76].

Narcotic/Barbiturate Combinations
Morphine and pentobarbital have been used to provide analgesia and sedation for somewhat prolonged painful procedures that require a still patient. The dosage of morphine is 0.1 mg per kilogram (maximum 10 mg) and that of pentobarbital is 4 mg per kilogram (maximum 120 mg). The combination is given in a single intramuscular injection. Onset of sedation occurs within 20 to 45 minutes. If sedation is not adequate, an additional 0.05 mg of supplemental morphine per kilogram can be given. On average, sedation persists for 1 to 2 hours, although in some cases the duration may be prolonged. Analgesia is good with this regimen, and respiratory depressant effects are partially reversible with naloxone. This com-

bination requires the same type of monitoring as does DPT administration and shares the potential for prolonged recovery. Hangover from the barbiturate may actually be longer [2,77].

Midazolam or Midazolam and Meperidine

Midazolam (Versed) can be administered intramuscularly, either alone or in combination with a narcotic agent. Although optimal dosage is still being investigated, after intramuscular injection at a dose of 0.1 to 0.2 mg per kilogram onset of sedation has been reported to begin within minutes and appears to peak within 10 to 20 minutes, with a recovery period of 30 to 60 minutes [68]. Given its lack of analgesic effect, its use alone is best limited to procedures in which duration of pain is brief and relief of anxiety the major goal.

The combination of midazolam (0.1 mg per kilogram to a maximum of 5 mg) and meperidine (1.5 mg per kilogram to a maximum of 75 mg) given intramuscularly has an onset of effect in approximately 20 minutes and peak action at 30 to 60 minutes. Most patients can be discharged within an hour after the procedure [78]. The combination of midazolam with an opiate, however, carries with it a much greater risk of respiratory depression than when either agent is used alone. *Note:* the safety of this regimen is not clearly established at this time. Further study is required to determine if this combination is a safe and effect alternative to DPT [2,25, 79,80].

Ketamine

Intramuscular administration of ketamine has been used successfully in the emergency department setting for wound closure in children. Dosage recommendations range from 0.5 to 1.0 mg per kilogram [24] to as high as 4 mg per kilogram [61], which is given in combination with atropine 0.01 mg per kilogram to counteract hypersalivation and increased bronchial secretions. Onset of the full sedative effect typically occurs within 5 to 10 minutes in more than 80 percent of patients, at which point the patient manifests a wide-eyed stare, vertical nystagmus, a decreased or absent response to pinprick, and increased muscle tone. Some develop random, purposeless movements of the extremities that necessitate restraint. If full sedation is not achieved within 10 minutes, one-half to the full dose may be repeated. The duration of maximal sedation is 15 to 20 minutes, although full recovery may take 1 to 6 hours.

Small wounds can be closed under ketamine sedation without local anesthesia, but when the procedure is likely to exceed 15 to 20 minutes local anesthesia is necessary. Ketamine also can be given intravenously, in which case the onset of action occurs within approximately 1 minute, and titration is possible. However, its rapid onset of action when given intramuscularly and the convenience of intramuscular administration appear to have created a preference for this route [2,24,58–61].

Whereas ketamine has its advocates for use in the emergency department setting, it also has its detractors. Its use requires special training and skill on the part of the person administering it and a quiet environment, especially during recovery. Furthermore, there is concern that the margin between dissociative sedation and general anesthesia may be too narrow [26].

Inhalational Sedation

Nitrous oxide is the only inhalational agent that has found application in the emergency department setting. Its use requires a skilled operator and special equipment that must be meticulously maintained. Perhaps the safest means of administration is via a demand valve mask attached to a single tank containing a 50:50 mixture of nitrous oxide/oxygen. Some masks have a button the patient must press to release the mixture; others require the application of negative pressure on inhalation through the mask to initiate flow (Fig. 20-9A). The exhalation port in the mask is attached to a scavenging device to minimize release into the room. Errors in mixing are avoided with this system, and if the patient begins to become oversedated he either lets up on the button or becomes unable to exert sufficient negative pressure to release more of the anesthetic.

Alternately, a stand with separate tanks and a mixing valve may be used. This apparatus may be attached to a mask or a nosepiece (Fig. 20-9B). It allows the operator to regulate the ratio of gases but carries a greater risk of mixing errors. To prevent administration of a hypoxic mixture, the system must have a fail-safe device that shuts off the flow of nitrous oxide if the flow of oxygen is inadequate. The operator must monitor the patient carefully, stopping the flow of nitrous oxide if the patient becomes unresponsive to commands or difficult to arouse, shows changes in vital signs, or begins to gag or vomit. With both devices, the patient must be instructed not to breathe deeply or rapidly but, rather, to breathe normally so as not to undergo too rapid induction. Continuous pulse oximetry is also advisable. Nitrous oxide does have the advantage of onset of sedative effect within 3 to 5 minutes, followed by total recovery within 10 minutes of cessation of administration. Once administration of the nitrous oxide/oxygen mixture is discontinued, patients must be given low-flow oxygen for an additional 10 minutes to prevent diffusion hypoxia [1,67]. Considerable experience with its use has demonstrated efficacy, particularly when the time required for administration of local anesthetic is brief [1,2,62–66].

Special considerations are important when introducing nitrous oxide to children. Young patients may fear the mask or have difficulty understanding how to use the nosepiece; however, careful preparation enables many to use the agent successfully. The mask can be likened to that of a jet pilot or a spaceman, and the gas is termed "happy gas" for young patients who are then given the opportunity to practice. Children also should be forewarned to expect sensations such as tingling and floating.

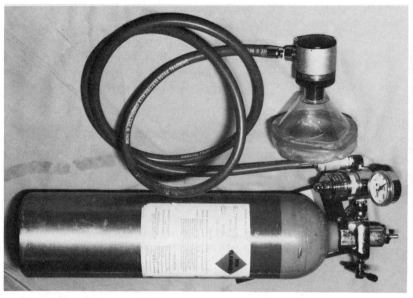

A

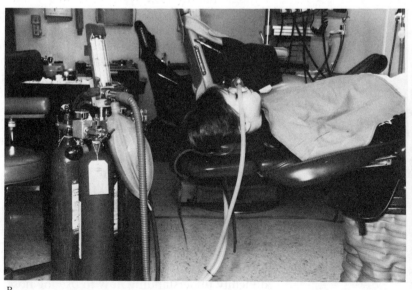

B

Fig. 20-9. Apparatus for administering nitrous oxide. *A.* Single tank containing a 50:50 mixture of nitrous oxide/oxygen attached to a demand valve mask. *B.* Separate tanks with a mixing valve attached to the nosepiece.

Intravenous Sedation

By definition, the intravenous route of sedative administration necessitates vascular access. Insertion of an intravenous line is painful and can prove difficult with pudgy toddlers in emergency departments where personnel have little experience starting intravenous lines in the very young. If multiple attempts have to be made to achieve access, the whole purpose of reducing the trauma of the procedure is defeated. However, in institutions where personnel are adept and well practiced at intravenous insertion, this route has numerous advantages. *Onset of sedation is generally rapid, and doses of agents given can be titrated to individual patient requirements, reducing the risk of complications* (although this point in no way obviates the need for careful monitoring). Furthermore, intravenous regimens typically result in shorter recovery periods, reducing the time required for observation after the procedure. Finally, if complications do arise, intravenous access is readily available for administration of naloxone and any other agents needed for resuscitative measures. Delays in starting the procedure can occur in patients with high dosage requirements, when titration can take some time [2,27,34].

Of the number of regimens available, three are discussed here: narcotics alone, benzodiazepines alone, and narcotic-benzodiazepine combinations.

Intravenous Narcotics

When pain control is the primary goal rather than sedation, intravenous narcotic analgesics may be used alone. This situation is more typical of older children in whom anxiety is not prominent and in whom the pain of injection of local anesthesia is likely to be the major problem, or when the wound to be repaired or other injuries are themselves painful. Morphine and fentanyl are perhaps the best agents for this purpose. The former is used when the wound is fairly large and the procedure is likely to be a lengthy one, whereas fentanyl's short duration of action makes it better suited to procedures of briefer duration, although supplemental doses may be given. Fentanyl is also safer when there is any concern about volume losses following trauma. Morphine is titrated beginning with an initial bolus of 0.1 mg per kilogram followed by incremental doses of 0.05 mg per kilogram, which can be given every 6 minutes (the approximate time of peak effect) up to a maximum of 15 to 20 mg. The initial fentanyl dose is 1 μg per kilogram, following which increments of 1 μg per kilogram can be added at 3-minute intervals up to a maximum of 5 μg per kilogram.

The goal is to produce a state in which the child is comfortable (with only mild pain or slight response to pinprick), calm, and a bit sleepy but readily arousable. If pain is totally ablated, the dose is too high. Both agents should be injected slowly to reduce the risk of respiratory depression, and should be followed by a slow flush of saline [1,2,26, 27,36].

Intravenous Benzodiazepines

The intravenous benzodiazepines can be used when the pain of the procedure is not likely to be severe or of long duration, and when patient anxiety is a major concern and amnesia a major goal. This situation, however, is rather uncommon in cases necessitating emergency plastic repair. Diazepam is the member of this group most commonly used for this purpose. The initial dose of diazepam is 0.1 mg per kilogram pushed slowly and followed by a saline flush. This dose can be repeated at 3- to 5-minute intervals until speech is mildly slurred and the patient highly relaxed (up to a maximum of 5 mg per kilogram). It is important to remember that some young children find intravenous diazepam painful and may become agitated during and after its administration [1,2,26,34,38].

Use of intravenous midazolam is currently being investigated in the pediatric population. Dosage recommendations and optimal intervals are not yet clearly established, although doses of 0.1 to 0.3 mg per kilogram are being used with some success, given in 0.05 mg per kilogram increments at approximately 5-minute intervals. Preliminary findings suggest that 0.1 mg per kilogram is adequate for school-age and adolescent patients and 0.2 mg per kilogram for younger children [78].

Narcotic/Benzodiazepine Combinations

As noted earlier, these combinations have the benefit of providing effective analgesia, good sedation, reduced anxiety, and some degree of amnesia. However, *they carry a substantially increased risk of cardiorespiratory depression over single-agent regimens* and take more time to administer. Regardless of the combination selected, each incremental dose must be administered slowly and the effect assessed at the expected time of peak action before titrating further. This point is particularly important with midazolam. We recommend administering the narcotic first to achieve mild sleepiness and decreased pain response (pain is not totally ablated), followed by titration of the benzodiazepine until speech is slurred. Combinations include fentanyl and diazepam or fentanyl and midazolam for brief procedures and morphine and diazepam or morphine and midazolam for longer procedures. Doses and onset of peak action are detailed in Table 20-2 [25,78–80].

We cannot overemphasize the importance of having experienced personnel who are familiar with these regimens. Without such personnel, intravenous sedation is best avoided.

PRACTICAL POINTS ON SELECTION OF REGIMEN

The "ideal" regimen for conscious sedation has been described as that which relieves pain and anxiety for the period required to perform the reparative procedure, after which its effects dissipate rapidly, enabling prompt discharge of the patient. It is easy and not painful to administer, has no significant side effects, and does not require sophisticated equipment for monitoring [26]. Clearly, no such ideal regimen exists, and therefore physicians must try to select the best, most practical regimen for the individual patient and the given emergency department. When making this decision, one must consider the following: (1) age of the patient, level of anxiety, presence of associated injuries, current medications, underlying medical problems; (2) degree of pain, duration of the procedure, amount of movement acceptable; (3) time required to achieve and duration of peak action of sedative regimen, time of anticipated availability of the plastic surgeon; and (4) personnel available and their level of skill, equipment, and monitoring capabilities. If results of sedation are to be optimal and complications minimized, medical and nursing personnel in a given emergency department must be familiar with and experienced in the administration of the specific sedative regimens used. Realistically, only some of the regimens are available in any given institution. Optimally, there would be regimens that produce sedation for differing periods of time and of differing depths.

Even in a fully equipped, well staffed emergency department, constraints may occur, especially during peak periods when activity in the department may make it impossible for senior level emergency physicians to expend the time (up to an hour) required for titration of intravenous regimens and for subsequent monitoring throughout the period of peak sedation. In such instances, an anesthesiologist may need to be consulted or an alternative, less labor-intensive regimen selected.

For practical purposes of selection, regimens can be grouped according to the degree of anxiety reduction and pain control needed and the duration of the procedure and degree of immobility required.

Anxiety reduction or sleepiness required
Oral or rectal chloral hydrate
Oral benzodiazepine
Rectal thiopental
Pain reduction in patient with minimal anxiety
Intravenous morphine
Intravenous meperidine
Intravenous fentanyl (brief duration)
Pain and anxiety reduction for brief period
Nitrous oxide
Intramuscular meperidine/hydroxyzine
Intramuscular ketamine
Intravenous fentanyl/diazepam
Intravenous fentanyl/midazolam
Anxiety reduction and amnesia for brief period
Intravenous diazepam
Intranasal, intramuscular, or intravenous midazolam

Pain and anxiety reduction for a moderately long procedure requiring immobility

Intramuscular DPT
Intramuscular morphine/barbiturate
Intravenous morphine/diazepam

Acknowledgments. We acknowledge the tireless efforts of Mr. David Kazimer in the preparation of the many drafts of this manuscript; the valuable assistance of Dr. William Magee of Pharmacology and of Mrs. Nancy Dunn and Mrs. Dolores Blumstein of the Children's Hospital Medical Library; and the helpful advice of Drs. Susan Asch, Laura Fitzmaurice, and Dee Hodge III.

REFERENCES

1. Thompson, A. E., and Frader, J. E. Pain management in children. In P. M. Paris and R. D. Stewart (eds.), *Pain Management in Emergency Medicine.* Norwalk, CT: Appleton & Lange, 1988. Pp. 401–417.
2. Zeltzer, L. K., Jay, S. M., and Fisher, D. M. The management of pain associated with pediatric procedures. *Pediatr. Clin. North Am.* 36:941, 1989.
3. Stewart, R. D. Local anesthesia. In P. M. Paris and R. D. Stewart (eds.), *Pain Management in Emergency Medicine.* Norwalk, CT: Appleton & Lange, 1988. Pp. 33–124.
4. Covino, B. G., and Vassalo, H. G. *Local Anesthetics: Mechanisms of Action and Clinical Use.* New York: Grune & Stratton, 1976.
5. Christoph, R. A., et al. Pain reduction in local anesthetic administration through pH buffering. *Ann. Emerg. Med.* 17:117, 1988.
6. DiFazio, C. A., et al. Comparison of pH-adjusted lidocaine solutions for epidural anesthesia. *Anesth. Analg.* 65:760, 1986.
7. Cousins, M. J., and Mather, L. E. Clinical pharmacology of local anesthetics. *Anaesth. Intens. Care* 8:257, 1980.
8. Braid, D. P., and Scott, D. B. The systemic absorption of local analgesic drugs. *Br. J. Anaesth.* 37:394, 1965.
9. Albert, J., and Lofstrom, B. Effects of epinephrine in solutions of local anesthetic agents. *Acta Anaesth. Scand. [Suppl.]* 16:71, 1965.
10. Stevenson, T. R., et al. Damage to tissue defenses by vasoconstrictors. *J. Am. Coll. Emerg. Physicians* 4:532, 1975.
11. Rothstein, P., Dornbusch, J., and Shaywitz, B. A. Prolonged seizures associated with the use of viscous lidocaine. *J. Pediatr.* 101:461, 1982.
12. Mofenson, H. C., et al. Lidocaine toxicity from topical Mucosal application. *Clin. Pediatr.* 22:190, 1983.
13. Wehner, D., and Hamilton, G. C. Seizures following topical application of local anesthetics to burn patients. *Ann. Emerg. Med.* 13:456, 1984.
14. Pryor, G. K., Kilpatrick, W. R., and Opp, D. R. Local anesthesia in minor lacerations: topical TAC vs lidocaine. *Ann. Emerg. Med.* 9:568, 1980.
15. Lyman, J. L., and McCabe, J. B. Improving the effectiveness of TAC application. *Ann. Emerg. Med.* 13:642, 1984.
16. Barker, W., et al. Damage to tissue defenses by a topical anesthetic agent. *Ann. Emerg. Med.* 11:307, 1982.
17. Dronen, S. C. Complications of TAC (letter). *Ann. Emerg. Med.* 12:333, 1983.

18. Dailey, R. H. Fatality secondary to misuse of TAC solution. *Ann. Emerg. Med.* 17:159, 1988.

19. Simon, R., and Brenner, B. E. Anesthesia and regional blocks. In R. Simon and B. E. Brenner (eds.), *Procedures and Techniques in Emergency Medicine.* Baltimore: Williams & Wilkins, 1982. Pp. 81–117.

20. Poulton, T. J., and Mims, G. R. Peripheral nerve blocks. *Am. Fam. Physician* 16:100, 1977.

21. Cousins, M. J., and Bridenbaugh, P. O. (eds.), *Neural Blockade in Clinical Anesthesia and Management of Pain.* Philadelphia: Lippincott, 1980.

22. Stoddard, F. J. Coping with pain: a developmental approach to the treatment of burned children. *Am. J. Psychiatry* 139:736, 1982.

23. American Academy of Pediatrics Committee on Drugs: Guidelines for the use of conscious sedation, deep sedation, and general anesthesia in pediatric patients. *Pediatrics* 76:317, 1985.

24. Bennett, C. R., and Stewart, R. D. Ketamine. In P. M. Paris and R. D. Stewart (eds.), *Pain Management in Emergency Medicine.* Norwalk, CT: Appleton & Lange, 1988. Pp. 295–310.

25. Gross, J. B., and Long, W. B. Nasal O_2 reduces risk of hypoxia during midazolam-meperidine sedation (abstract). *Anesthesiology* 71:A1182, 1989.

26. Cohen, D. E., and Broennle, A. M. Emergency department anesthetic management. In G. R. Fleisher and S. Ludwig (eds.), *Textbook of Pediatric Emergency Medicine,* 2nd ed. Baltimore: Williams & Wilkins, 1988. Pp. 53–65.

27. Paris, P. M., and Weiss, L. D. Narcotic analgesics: the pure agonists. In P. M. Paris and R. D. Stewart (eds.), *Pain Management in Emergency Medicine.* Norwalk, CT: Appleton & Lange, 1988. Pp. 125–156.

28. Jaffe, J. M., and Martin, W. R. Opioid analgesics and antagonists. In A. G. Gilman et al. (eds.), *The Pharmacological Basis of Therapeutics,* 7th ed. New York: Macmillan, 1985. Pp. 491–531.

29. Halpern, L. M., and Bonica, J. J. Analgesics. In W. Modell (ed.), *Drugs of Choice.* St. Louis: Mosby, 1982–1983. Pp. 194–235.

30. Tamsen, A., et al. Patient-controlled analgesic therapy in the early post-operative period. *Acta Anaesth. Scand.* 23:462, 1979.

31. Tamsen, A., et al. Patient-controlled analgesia therapy. II. Individual analgesic demand and analgesic plasma concentrations of pethidine in post-operative pain. *Clin. Pharmacokinet.* 7:164, 1982.

32. Dahlstrom, B., et al. Patient controlled-analgesia therapy. IV. Pharmacokinetics and analgesic plasma concentrations of morphine. *Clin. Pharmacokinet.* 7:266, 1982.

33. Austin, K. L., Stapleton, J. V., and Mather, L. E. Relationships between blood meperidine concentrations and analgesic response: a preliminary report. *Anesthesiology* 53:460, 1980.

34. Paris, P. M. Pain management in the child. *Emerg. Med. Clin. North Am.* 5:699, 1987.

35. Selbst, S. M., and Henretig, F. M. The treatment of pain in the emergency department. *Pediatr. Clin. North Am.* 36:965, 1989.

36. Billmire, D. A., Neale, H. W., and Gregory, R. O. Use of IV fentanyl in the outpatient treatment of pediatric facial trauma. *J. Trauma* 25:1079, 1985.

37. Adams, A. P., and Pybus, D. A. Delayed respiratory depression after use of fentanyl during anesthesia. *Br. Med. J.* 1:278, 1979.

38. Harvey, S. Hypnotics and sedatives. In A. G. Gilman et al. (eds.), *The Pharmacological Basis of Therapeutics,* 7th ed. New York: Macmillan, 1985. Pp. 339–371.
39. Geiderman, J. Benzodiazepines. In P. M. Paris and R. D. Stewart (eds.), *Pain Management in Emergency Medicine.* Norwalk, CT: Appleton & Lange, 1988. Pp. 239–270.
40. Reeves, J. G., et al. Midazolam: pharmacology and uses. *Anesthesiology* 62:310, 1985.
41. Rita, L., et al. Intramuscular midazolam for pediatric preanesthetic sedation: a double-blind controlled study with morphine. *Anesthesiology* 63:528, 1985.
42. Wilton, N. C. T., et al. Intranasal premedication (abstract). *Anesth. Analg.* 67:S260, 1988.
43. Walbergh, E. J., and Eckert, J. Pharmacokinetics of intravenous and intranasal midazolam in children (abstract). *Anesthesiology* 71:A1065, 1989.
44. Buhrer, M., et al. Comparative pharmacodynamics of midazolam and diazepam (abstract). *Anesthesiology* 69:A642, 1988.
45. Diamant, M. J., and Stanley, P. The use of midazolam for sedation of infants and children. *A.J.R.* 150:377, 1988.
46. Lichtor, J. L., et al. Increased anxiety after intravenous midazolam (abstract). *Anesthesiology* 69:A910, 1988.
47. Catoire, P., Hort-Legrand, C., and Vignoli, T. Reversal of midazolam by flumazenil: objective evaluation using evoked potentials (abstract). *Anesthesiology* 71:A116, 1989.
48. Baldassarini, R. S. Drugs in the treatment of psychiatric disorders. In A. G. Gilman et al. (eds.), *The Pharmacological Basis of Therapeutics,* 7th ed. New York: Macmillan, 1985. Pp. 387–445.
49. Dundee, J. W., and Moore, J. The myth of phenothiazine potentiation. *Anaesthesia* 16:95, 1961.
50. Moore, J., and Dunde, J. W. Alterations in response to somatic pain associated with anaesthesia. *Br. J. Anaesth.* 33:3, 1961.
51. Dundee, J. W., Love, W. J., and Moore, J. Alterations in response to somatic pain associated with anaesthesia. XV. Further studies with phenothiazine derivatives and similar drugs. *Br. J. Anaesth.* 35:597, 1963.
52. McGee, J. L., and Alexander, M. R. Phenothiazine analgesia — fact or fantasy? *Am. J. Hosp. Pharm.* 36:633, 1979.
53. Minuck, R. Postoperative analgesia — comparison of methotrimeprazine and meperidine as postoperative agents. *Can. Anaesth. Soc. J.* 19:87, 1972.
54. Beaver, W. T., et al. A comparison of the analgesic effects of methotrimeprazine and morphine in patients with cancer. *Clin. Pharmacol. Ther.* 7:446, 1966.
55. Beaver, W. T., and Feise, G. Comparison of the analgesic effects of morphine, hydroxyzine, and their combination in patients with postoperative pain. In J. J. Bonica and D. Albe-Fessard (eds.), *Advances in Pain Research and Therapy,* Vol. 1. New York: Raven Press, 1976. Pp. 553–557.
56. Hupert, C., Yacomb, M., and Turgeon, L. R. Effect of hydroxyzine on morphine analgesia for the treatment of postoperative pain. *Anesth. Analg.* 59:690, 1980.

57. Momsoe, T. Potentiation of postoperative analgesic agents by hydroxyzine. *Anesth. Analg.* 59:22, 1980.

58. Caro, B. Trial of ketamine in an accident and emergency department. *Anaesthesia* 29:227, 1974.

59. Dailey, R. H., Stone, R., and Repert, W. Ketamine dissociative anesthesia — emergency room department use in children. *J. Am. Coll. Emerg. Physicians* 8:501, 1979.

60. Vinnik, C. A. An intravenous dissociation technique for outpatient plastic surgery: tranquility in the office surgical facility. *Plast. Reconstr. Surg.* 67:799, 1981.

61. Green, S. M., Johnson, N. E., and Nakamura, R. Ketamine sedation protocol for emergency pediatric procedures (abstract). *Ann. Emerg. Med.* 18:442, 1989.

62. Stewart, R. D. Nitrous oxide. In P. M. Paris and R. D. Stewart (eds.), *Pain Management in Emergency Medicine.* Norwalk, CT: Appleton & Lange, 1988. Pp. 221–239.

63. Thal, E. R., et al. Self-administered analgesia with nitrous oxide, adjunctive aid for emergency medical care systems. *J.A.M.A.* 242:2418, 1979.

64. Griffin, G. C., Campbell, V. R., and Jones, R. Nitrous oxide-oxygen sedation for minor surgery, experience in a pediatric setting. *J.A.M.A.* 245:2411, 1981.

65. Stewart, R. D. Nitrous oxide sedation/analgesia in emergency medicine. *Ann. Emerg. Med.* 14:139, 1985.

66. Gamis, A., Knapp, J., and Glenski, J. A. Nitrous oxide analgesia in a pediatric emergency department. *Ann. Emerg. Med.* 18:177, 1989.

67. Fink, B. R. Diffusion anoxia. *Anesthesiology* 16:511, 1955.

68. Feld, L. H., et al. Premedication in children: oral versus intramuscular midazolam (abstract). *Anesthesiology* 69:A745, 1988.

69. Feld, L. H., Negus, J. B., and White, P. F. Oral midazolam: optimal dose for pediatric premedication (abstract). *Anesthesiology* 71:A1053, 1989.

70. White, T. J., III, et al. Rectal thiopental for sedation of children for computed tomography. *J. Comput. Assist. Tomogr.* 3:268, 1979.

71. Burckhart, G. J., et al. Rectal thiopental versus an intramuscular cocktail for sedating children before computerized tomography. *Am. J. Hosp. Pharm.* 37:222, 1980.

72. Terndrup, T. E., Cantor, R. M., and Madden, C. M. Intramuscular meperidine, promethazine, and chlorpromazine: analysis of use and complications in 487 pediatric emergency department patients. *Ann. Emerg. Med.* 18:528, 1989.

73. Nahata, M. C., Clotz, M. A., and Krogg, E. A. Adverse effects of meperidine, promethazine, and chlorpromazine for sedation in pediatric patients. *Clin. Pediatr.* 24:558, 1985.

74. Asch, S. Children's Hospital, St. Paul, MN (personal communication).

75. McEvoy, G. K. (ed.), *AHFS Drug Information.* American Society of Hospital Pharmacists, 1989. Pp. 1035–1036, 1231–1232.

76. Nathan, J. E., and West, M. S. Comparison of chloral hydrate-hydroxyzine with and without meperidine for management of the difficult pediatric patient. *ASDC J. Dent. Child.* 54:437, 1987.

77. Hodge, D. University of Southern California Medical Center, Los Angeles (personal communication).

78. Fitzmaurice, L. Children's Mercy Hospital, Kansas City, MO (personal communication).

79. Bailey, P. L., et al. Respiratory effects of midazolam and fentanyl: potent interaction producing hypoxemia and apnea (abstract). *Anesthesiology* 69:A813, 1988.

80. Versed: another dangerous drug slips through the FDA's sieve. *Public Citizen Health Research Group Health Letter* 4:1, 1988.

21 HEMOSTASIS DURING PLASTIC SURGERY

Krishna Narayanan
Marc D. Liang
Jeanine M. Walenga

Adequate hemostasis is an important concern in emergency room treatment of wounds. Hematomas often lead to disruption or infection of surgical and traumatic wounds. Lack of mechanical control of bleeding vessels is the most common cause of poor wound hemostasis. However, rarely there is an intrinsic clotting disorder in the patient. This chapter focuses on the basic biologic defects of hemostasis and their acute management.

Hemostasis is the culmination of a complex interaction between the vessel wall, platelets, and proteins involved in coagulation (Fig. 21-1). A primary hemostatic plug is usually formed within 4 to 7 minutes of the acute injury, diffusion of fibrin around the plug represents the secondary stage of hemostasis, and clot retraction constitutes the final stage. Abnormalities in any of the mentioned pathways can result in continued bleeding (Fig. 21-2).

EVALUATION

A careful history is of paramount importance in the detection of pathologic bleeding disorders. A personal or family history of bleeding disorders or a history of previous episodes of bruising, prolonged bleeding, hematuria, or joint swelling provides useful information regarding the possible existence of a congenital bleeding disorder. Screening for the use of aspirin or other anticoagulation agents is necessary, and a history of smoking or oral contraceptive use may be significant.

Routine clotting studies include platelet count, partial thromboplastin time to evaluate the intrinsic coagulation system, prothrombin time to evaluate the extrinsic coagulation system, and bleeding time for an overall assessment of hemostasis. Normal values for these studies are found in Table 21-1. Additional assays that can provide further information during a bleeding episode are fibrinogen measurements and the thrombin time assay (checking for lysis after 5 minutes).

Adequate fibrinogen is necessary to form a hemostatic plug. Levels over 100 mg per deciliter are required during major surgical procedures. The thrombin clotting time not only provides an indication of

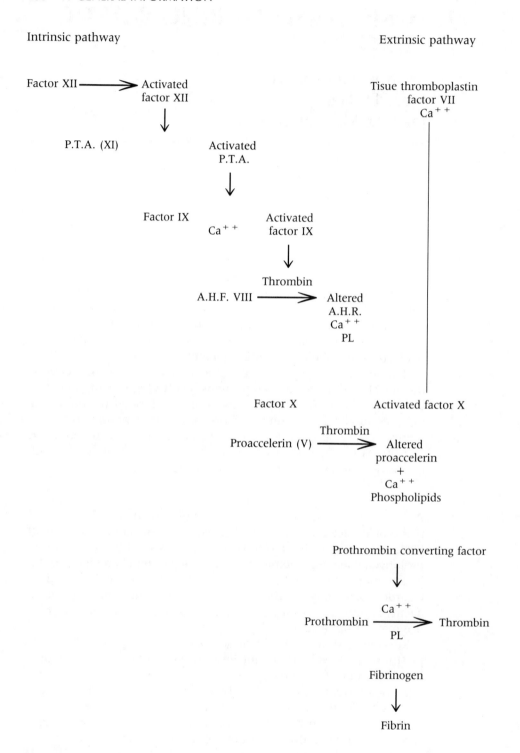

Fig. 21-1. Two major pathways of thrombin formation.

I. Disorders of the vessel wall
   Vasculitis
   Capillary fragility
   Von Willebrand's Disease

II. Platelet abnormalities
   Decreased or ineffective production
      Congenital
      Acquired
   Increased metabolization
      Immune (collagen disorders)
      Nonimmune
      Ristocetin Tx
      Heparin Tx
      Hypersplenism

III. Coagulation protein deficiencies
   Hemophilia
   Christmas disease

Fig. 21-2. Causes of abnormal hemostasis.

Table 21-1. Correlation between laboratory assay values and clinical and surgical bleeding

Test	Normal value	Minor bleeding[a]	Major bleeding[b]	Spontaneous bleeding
Bleeding time (min)	<6	<6	<8	>15
Platelet count (/mm^3)	>200,000	>100,000	>50,000	<10,000
Prothrombin time (sec)	11.5 (100%)	14 (>50%)	16 (>40%)	36 (<10%)
Partial thrombo-plastin time (sec)	30	<35	<45	>60
Thrombin time (sec)	8	<11	<16	>60
Heparin (unit/ml)	—	0.05	0.2	0.5
Euglobulin lysis time (whole blood) (min)	>90	>90	>60	<30
Fibrinogen (mg/dl)	200–400	150	100	30

[a]Adequate hemostasis for major surgery.
[b]Adequate hemostasis for minor surgery.
Source: Adapted from *Blood Coagulation Clinical and Laboratory Aspects*. Michigan State University, East Lansing, MI: The Kellogg Center for Continuing Education 1983. With permission.

fibrinogen activity, it is affected by excessive levels of fibrin(ogen) split products, which can act as anticoagulants, and heparin. Another clotting assay, the Reptilase time, which is not affected by heparin, can be used to differentiate the cause of the prolonged clotting time.

Consultation with a hematologist should be considered for patients with newly diagnosed or long-term bleeding disorders.

BLEEDING DISORDERS

Von Willebrand Disease

Von Willebrand disease is the most common inherited bleeding disorder and is caused by a deficiency of Von Willebrand factor (vWF), a protein associated with the factor VIII macromolecule. The function of vWF is to bind platelets to the endothelial surface. Some patients have a concomitant decrease in factor VIII:c levels as well. Varying degrees of bleeding tendency are associated with this disorder. The diagnosis can be made by the presence of a prolonged bleeding time, which is the hallmark of the disorder. The prothrombin time and partial thromboplastin time are often normal in these patients.

Other tests are more complex but are useful in the diagnosis and management of the disease. They include the vWF assay and the ristocetin-induced platelet aggregation test to determine the functionality of vWF.

With acute trauma, after mechanical control is obtained active surface bleeding is controlled by normalizing the bleeding time and factor VIII:c activity with fresh frozen plasma, cryoprecipitate, and in difficult cases platelet concentrates. The use of desmopressin (DDAVP), with the guidance of a hematologist, can successfully prevent hemorrhagic complications following surgery.

Aspirin must be avoided in these patients. Fibrinolytic inhibitors may be useful for management of bleeding of the head and neck regions of these patients because of the high fibrinolytic activity here. Again, these agents should be used under the guidance of a hematologist.

Hemophilia

Hemophilia A is a deficiency of factor VIII and is the more common type of hemophilia. Hemophilia B is a deficiency of factor IX and is less common. These disorders are clinically indistinguishable. The degree of disorder depends on the relative deficiency of the factor in the patient.

The acute management includes normalizing the levels of these factors: for factor VIII to a level of 50 units per deciliter; and for factor IX to 30 to 40 units per deciliter. However, it must be remembered that bleeding from cuts and bruises (as with minor trauma) often responds to firm pressure or topical application of thrombin. One unit of fresh frozen plasma contains 0.7 to 0.9 units of factors VIII and IX per milliliter.

Cryoprecipitate is a concentrate of factors VIII and IX and contains 80 to 100 units when obtained from 200 ml of plasma. However, it may also contain cold insoluble globulins, which can cause allergic reactions.

Human factor VIII concentrates are made from pooled plasma and form the mainstay of treatment for hemophilia A. Prothrombin complex concentrates and lyophilized plasma, prepared from large plasma pools, are the primary treatment for hemophilia B.

Other Causes of Bleeding

Many drugs and diseases can cause bleeding by disrupting the balance of hemostasis. The use of anticoagulants, antiplatelet agents, and fibrinolytic agents is rapidly growing. These drugs should be discontinued before surgery if possible. If not possible, the surgeon must take their antihemostatic properties into account. Furthermore, studies have shown that antibodies, alcohol, and various cardiac, antiinflammatory, and antihypertensive drugs alter platelet function. Presurgical histories and laboratory screening of patients has become an important part of proper patient care.

Liver diseases, disseminated intravascular coagulation, and vitamin K malabsorption manifest with bleeding complications during surgery and can usually be treated with fresh frozen plasma. Specific platelet disorders such as thrombocytopenia, including immune thrombocytopenia purpura and thrombotic thrombocytopenia purpura, or thrombocytopathies in which platelet function is defective can lead to severe side effects after trauma. Platelet concentrates can reverse bleeding due to platelet defects.

The often overlooked fibrinolytic system — that part of hemostasis responsible for breaking down the clot when it is no longer needed — may also be responsible for bleeding. If inhibitors are abnormally low or if activators are present in excess, fibrinolytic activity may be higher than normal, which would lead to an enhanced rate of clot lysis. If this problem is specifically diagnosed, the fibrinolytic activation can be reversed with epsilon aminocaproic acid.

EXPANDING HEMATOMA OR UNCONTROLLED BLEEDING

Uncontrolled bleeding is an emergency. Almost uniformly it is caused by an uncontrolled injured vessel. These patients are best served by control in the operating room where the surgeon has adequate lighting, instruments, and methods of hemostatic control. It is often necessary to extend the injury or incision to provide adequate exposure of the bleeding source. One should design these extensions in such a way that they do not cross flexion creases and remain as aesthetic as possible. Simple suture ligation or electrohemostatic control are obtained.

It must be mentioned that clamping of vessels in the emergency room often is associated with inadequate visualization of the vessel and sometimes leads to injury of associated neurologic structures. This practice is to be avoided at all costs.

MINOR WOUNDS   Bleeding from minor wounds can often be controlled by 5 minutes of pressure and elevation. Injections with local anesthetics containing epinephrine are useful for local hemostatic control. They should not be used in patients with severe hypertension or ischemic heart disease or in areas with end-vessel blood supply (fingers, penis, and toes).

SUMMARY   Bleeding in the surgical patient is a serious and potentially life-threatening complication. Thus diagnosing the cause of the bleeding and applying the proper treatment is critically important. Efforts should be made to diagnose and correct any deficiency prior to surgery in order to avoid intra- and postoperative complications. If intraoperative problems arise, it is important to obtain laboratory evaluations prior to treatment. Clearly hemostatic disorders are many and varied, and in order to avoid inappropriate or unnecessary treatment a proper laboratory diagnosis is essential.

The use of transfused blood or blood components should be minimal but sufficient to maintain adequate hemostasis and to avoid the risks associated with excessive or inappropriate transfusion. Hemostasis is a fine balance between two evils — bleeding and thrombosis. We know now that hemostasis is a complex process involving coagulation, fibrinolysis, platelets, endothelium, leukocytes, other cellular elements, and blood flow properties. The stresses of surgery, anesthesia, wound trauma, foreign bodies, drugs, fluids, and so on have become a major component in the hemostatic balance. Acute awareness of changes in hemostasis — presaging a bleeding or a thrombotic complication — is necessary for comprehensive patient care.

INDEX

INDEX

The abbreviations *f* and *t* stand for figure and table, respectively.